FIRST STEPS *on the* PATH *of* YOGA

Nicki Doane and Eddie Modestini

Published by Maya Yoga Press
Huelo, Hawaii

Copyright © 2020 by Kaitlin Childers, Edward Modestini and Nicole Doane.

All rights reserved. No portion of this book may be reproduced, stored in a retrieval system or transmitted in any form or by any means without the written permission of the authors.

Front and back cover photographs by Jerad Hobaugh /Picaflor Films. Cover design by Nicole Racquel Ryan and Kaitlin Childers. Book Design by Nicole Racquel Ryan. Photography by Pasha Rose / Pasha X-Pose-U & Jerad Hobaugh /Picaflor Films.

Printed and designed in the USA.

ISBN 978-0-578-87741-9

"Anyone who wants to learn yoga and go deeper into the practice and philosophy will love this book. I highly recommend First Steps for any student or teacher of yoga. Beginner or advanced yogis will find so much wisdom to help guide their practice. So grateful for these teachers and their teachings."

—RYAN LEIER, *Founder of One Yoga & Lululemon Athletica Global Ambassador*

"Nicki and Eddie taught me the roots of my practice starting with detailed attention to the breath, hands and feet. I wasn't sure why at the time, but today I credit them for helping me have 19 years of being on the mat without ever having a yoga related injury. Their practice is about the process of healing, the body, heart and soul - not just making pretty poses for Instagram. Whether you're new on the mat or have been going deep for decades they will inspire you with the subtleties of yoga, the storytelling and meaning behind each posture and their never-ending sense of humor. Oh and if you DO wanna make beautiful poses for Instagram, they'll teach you how to get there safely!"

—MICHAEL FRANTI, *Musician, Activist, Yogi*

"With their new book, master teachers Nicki Doane and Eddie Modestini have created an essential foundation for the practice of yoga. They respectfully honor the lineage of their teachers and the natural evolution of their own practice in a way that is informed, balanced, sustainable and encourages listening. First Steps on the Path of Yoga is an invaluable resource for students and teachers alike … whether just beginning on the path or enhancing a lifelong journey."

—DAPHNE LARKIN, *Owner, Sanctuary for Yoga*

"Opening First Steps on the Path to Yoga is like stepping into the wisdom, power and vibrancy of the Maya Yoga studio on Maui. Now that incredible energy, community and deep integral practice is available to the wider public in this amazing book. With clear photos and detailed instructions, students at every level will find it will deepen and enhance their practice. I am so incredibly grateful to have studied with both of these amazing teachers throughout the years. With this book I can now continue this work as I strive to develop my personal practice through the ancient and individualized sequences provided."

—SARAH NELSON, *Maya Yoga practitioner and lifelong friend*

The world's largest living organism is a strand of aspen trees in central Utah, nicknamed the Pando clone. These trees appear to stand alone but each individual tree is united to the whole by a shared root system. They are bound together in their creation, their survival, and their demise.

These trees are a perfect metaphor for yoga. We are all connected, and to evolve as a whole we must first address the environment we live in and experience. Your personal path toward healing and connectivity will absolutely benefit those around you and in doing so will contribute to the evolution of our species and the preservation of our delicate planet. As you put your feet together in *samastiti* you stand in the same spot every yogi has stood: Pattabhi Jois, BKS Iyengar, T Krishnamacharya, and all the great teachers. We are all within each other. We're just like the aspen trees; a living organism united by our shared roots and collective responsibility.

With this book we hope to add our voices to the chorus of dedicated teachers and practitioners seeking to reestablish faith in yoga so it may continue to heal our planet. Thank you for taking the time to do this practice. Yoga is a culmination of all its students, and in practicing yoga you are adding your energy to the spiritual regeneration of the planet.

FOREWORD

With the madness in the world continuing to rise, there is no better time for Eddie and Nicki to share their wisdom through this book.

We were fortunate to move to Maui in 1998, the same year as Eddie and Nicki, but we planted roots on the opposite side of the island almost a two-hour drive to their studio. On more than one occasion, we would drive out the night before, sneak into the studio to sleep and wake to Nicki sweeping the room for the 7:30am class. We would roll up our blankets, roll out our mats, and these were usually the only times we were on time for class.

We participated in their very first teacher training on Maui in 2003, and have attended week-long retreats and workshops both on island and abroad when our schedules line up. Our friendship has grown over the years, inside and outside their studio. In 2006, they brought their 2 young children to a tiny village nestled in the hills of the Amalfi Coast to help welcome the birth of our third daughter. They continue to be a strong support for our family.

Various forms of yoga have been part of our lives since the early 1990s, but what Eddie and Nicki offer is a sense of safety, individualized attention and the importance of true foundation. In one of our first classes we spent over 45 minutes setting up for and moving into downward dog, so we knew we were going deep into study. The level of integrity and compassion they bring to their teaching is admirable. Their passion and understanding of various systems of yoga that they continue to study, play with and make their own proves their commitment to teaching.

What they have to offer is more than yoga… they inspire and spark a desire to be a better human. One of their beliefs that they often share in class is, "We are all beginners," inviting us to listen and learn and not get stuck in our heads about what we are supposed to accomplish or be, but rather put the focus on the process of becoming.

To this day, we learn something new and deepen our understanding of the poses when we "take it to the mat," another one of their wisdoms that translates to everyday life. As we settle into savasana, Nicki reads passages from Rumi, Hafiz or her other favorite writers and poets adding another layer of mental yoga to the experience. We walk out of class feeling better physically and mentally, which carries us through our day more centered and capable to deal with what life throws our way. We miss them when we are not together and rejoice when we can spend time in the same place. They have and continue to be great spiritual teachers, committed cosmic cowboys searching for greater truths and epic friends.

—WOODY AND LAURA HARRELSON

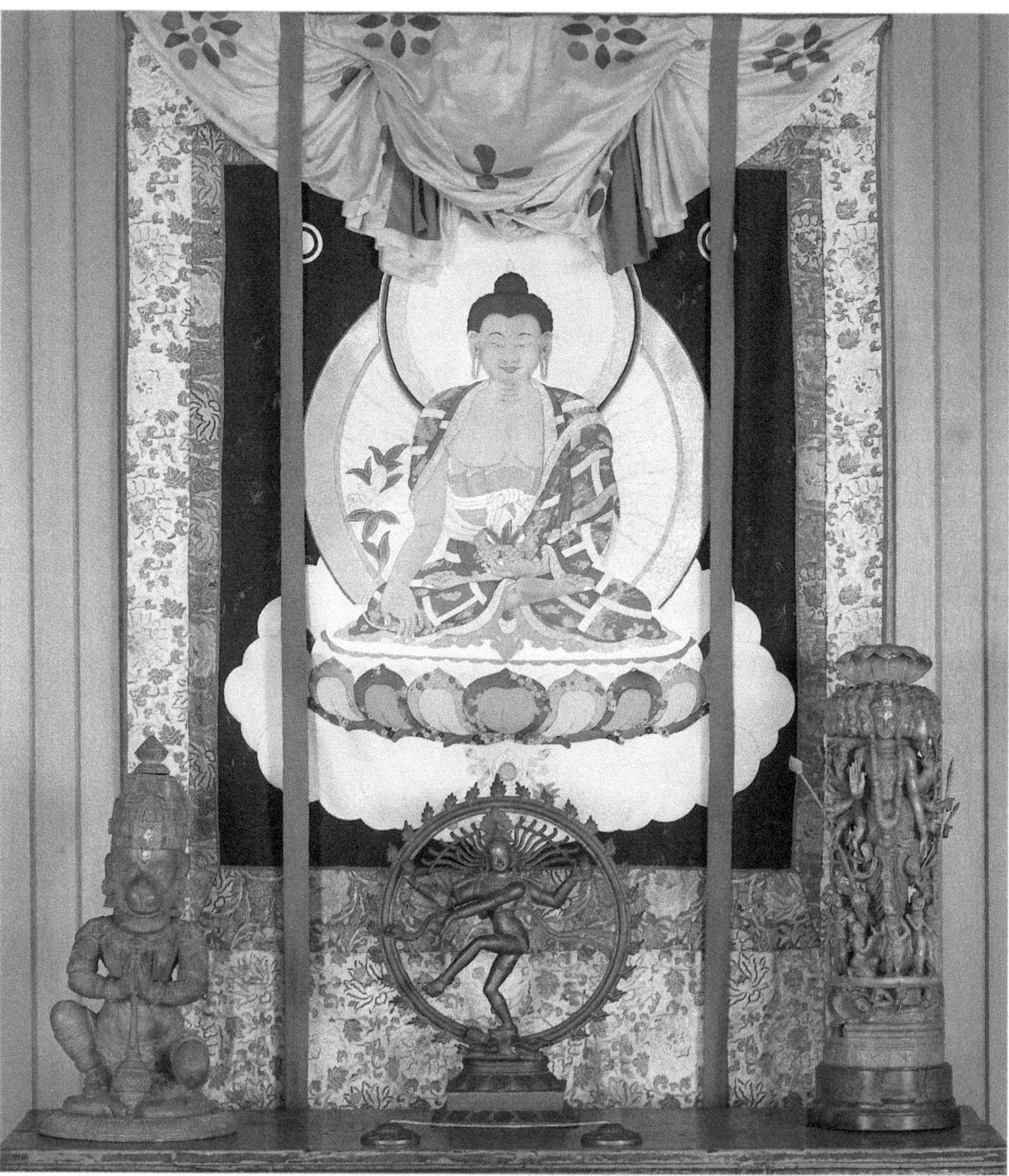

I would like to say a few words. Nowadays, the attitudes of people in our society are changing. They look at all their affairs as business ventures and think only in terms of making a profit or loss. This outlook is on the increase. This attitude is becoming an obstacle to our spiritual progress. It is pathetic and sad that this instant gross business-oriented attitude meant to be applied during transactions with a road-side vendor has been applied to even matters involving spiritual truths.

One cannot have such a trivial attitude as expecting immediate benefits in auspicious matters like [yoga] as though one were a laborer who does one hour of work and expects immediate payment. They should not lament that they have not received even one [cent] for all the time spent on this. When this pattern of thinking begins, we enter a phase of deterioration day by day.

—SRI T. KRISHNAMACHARYA, *Yoga Makaranda (The Essence of Yoga),* 1934
Translation by Sri C.M.V. Krishnamacharya

TABLE OF CONTENTS

1	**Aloha**	**1**
	Product vs. Process	2
	How to Use This Book	3
2	**How We Found Yoga**	**4**
	Nicki Doane	4
	Eddie Modestini	19
3	**Foundations**	**26**
	Breath	26
	Bandha	29
	Props	35
	Pain	37
	Hyperextension	42
	Recruiting	44
	Check, Check, and Check Again	45
	Hands and Feet	46
	Thresholds	50
	Personal Practice	53
4	**Warm Up Poses**	**56**
5	**Surya Namaskar A**	**96**
6	**Lunges**	**110**
7	**Surya Namaskar B**	**124**
8	**Standing Poses**	**134**
	Straight Leg Standing Poses	134
	Bent Knee Standing Poses	157
	Balancing Poses	165

9	**Backbends**	**172**
10	**Twists**	**183**
11	**Inversions**	**190**
12	**Seated Hip Openers**	**206**
13	**Pranayama**	**238**
	Preparatory Asana	239
	Surya and Chandra Bhedana	244
	Viloma	247
14	**8 Limbs of Ashtanga Yoga**	**252**
15	**The Yoga Sutras of Patanjali**	**260**
	Nicki's 10 Foundational Sutras	265
16	**Functional Anatomy**	**278**
	Bones	278
	Spinal Anatomy	279
	Segments of the Spine	289
	Pelvic Anatomy	300
	Hip Anatomy	303
	Knee Anatomy	306
	Shoulder Anatomy	308
	Connective Tissue	310
	General Contraindications	319
17	**Practice Sequences**	**326**
	List of Asana	349

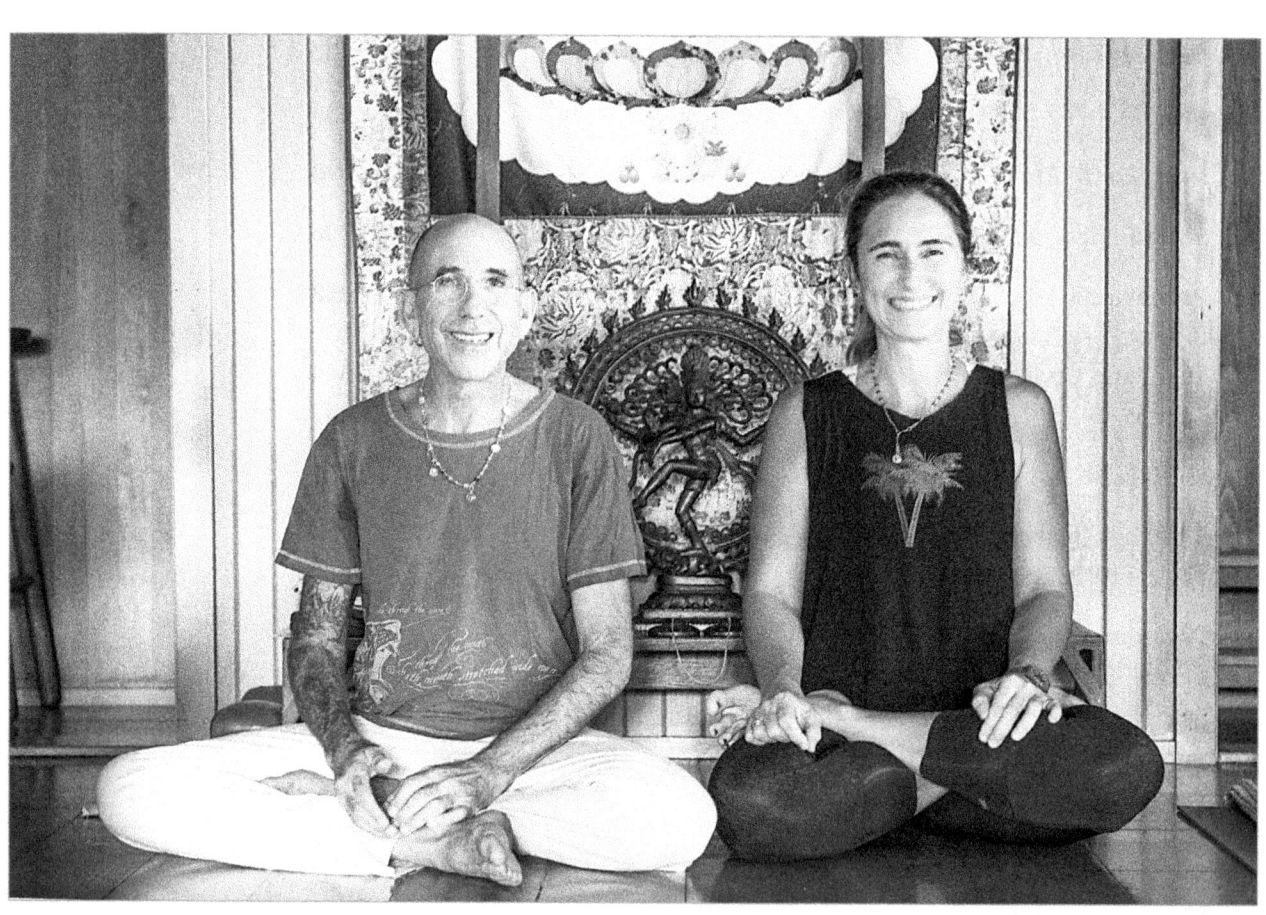

ALOHA

PRODUCT VS. PROCESS

Hello. You are holding a book that has two authors: Nicki Doane and Eddie Modestini. This book represents our 30+ years of experience practicing, studying and teaching yoga. We believe that yoga is the most effective healing modality on the planet. The pages of this book will take you through its introductory poses and practices to begin a lifetime of self-reliant health.

With this book we add our voices to the chorus of dedicated practitioners seeking to reestablish faith in yoga. Much of modern yoga is more about products and playlists than practice and process. It has become the yoga of attainment; once you attain the pose, you attain yoga, regardless of the process that brought you there. This product-oriented mentality is pushing people into difficult poses without proper instruction, and people are getting hurt. It's difficult for us to watch because the yoga we know doesn't cause pain. Our yoga is about healing and ultimately about love.

We are interested in yoga as a *process*, not a product. The poses are just anatomical geometry. The process is much more interesting and it lives in you. Yoga as a process is harder to understand, practice and teach, but it is also much more interesting. It is a process of creating positive change in your body to stimulate positive change in your mind. Every *asana* (pose) is a tool in this process, and to use a tool effectively you must understand the action by which it works. Replicating the final form of a pose without understanding its anatomical actions can be both ineffective and injurious.

This book will teach you to understand *asana* in a process-oriented way. It will demonstrate how each pose works in your body and detail the steps that will bring you toward it. Whether or not you "complete" the pose, or achieve its final form, is irrelevant; it is the process that will change you.

And yes, understanding yoga as a process will require more attention to detail. But in today's increasingly disconnected world, the time you spend connecting with yourself on a cellular level is invaluable. We believe you have the mental and physical bandwidth to do this work. You are completely worth it.

HOW TO USE THIS BOOK

Aloha

EDDIE:
You have to be open to what yoga is telling you because it may be different from what you're telling yourself. It may even be different from what we are telling you. That's the beauty of personal practice; it makes yoga the teacher. Make space for external guidance but maintain freedom in your mind. Be receptive to your process.

We believe each individual person is more important than any yoga system, rule, or pose. Yoga is not defined by us and our ideas, nor the ideas and objectives of any other system because yoga is about **you**—your healing and personal evolution—and you are completely unique. So how can we create your specific system and a system for all our other readers in a single book? Well, we can't. But we can provide you with knowledge to begin looking at yourself in the context of structural alignment, and from there you can determine the instructions that best serve you.

Start with our Foundations section to explore yoga's underlying anatomical principles, and then move on to The Practice. Read our directions and try the practice sequences, paying close attention to yourself in all the poses. Find the ways your unique anatomical shapes diverge from the principles of alignment and use our instruction to navigate the props and poses that will bring you closer to the lines of yoga. If something about this practice causes you pain, please listen to that pain. Find a way to navigate your discomfort while moving in the direction of yoga; that is, toward the fundamental structural alignment of the pose, which will point you in the direction of your true Self.

The Practice section is not intended to be an exhaustive list of poses. Our practice section focuses on the handful of poses that have proved invaluable in our 30+ years of experience with yoga; the ones we consider to be foundational to all yoga practitioners, regardless of their circumstance or experience.

We hope this work will encourage you to develop a personal practice. Going to a yoga class is not the same as having a personal practice. Classes are a fantastic way to learn from your teachers and develop your *sanga*, or community, but the real work is done at home. Developing a personal practice means doing the poses you need, not just the ones you like. Your personal practice is the list of poses that will most accurately attune your body to the lines of yoga, and it's difficult to find that in a yoga class. Yoga is a **self**-reliant healing system.

We invite you to read and practice, practice and read, and use our sequences as a guide. Give yourself freedom to explore. Let your personal practice be your primary teacher. We are presenting this information to help you explore yoga, but when it comes to your personal practice, you're in charge. Be patient with yourself and your ability. Yoga takes time. Do not break your body to fit these poses. Stay connected to the process, not the product.

HOW WE FOUND YOGA

Maya Yoga is our unique style of Hatha yoga. It developed organically through years of experience with both Ashtanga and Iyengar yoga, coupled with decades of personal practice and an unwavering faith in yoga. The story of Maya Yoga is really our stories: how we found yoga and fell in love with it and how it brought us together to teach.

Nicki Doane

I was born in Nicosia, Cyprus. My dad was a diplomat in the Foreign Service and we moved to a new country every two years. When I was in high school my mom took us back to the States to prepare me for college, and at the time, it felt like a prison sentence. I had spent most of my life moving seamlessly among international cultures and the mainland seemed endlessly boring. I was in for a big surprise.

We settled outside of Washington, DC and I finally received a real education, although not in the subjects my mom intended. I learned about the Grateful Dead, vegetarianism, and alternative living—the whole hippie scene. It was an eye-opening experience of peace, love, live music and flowing skirts. Yoga was certainly a part of the culture, but for me, it was peripheral. I saw people doing yoga at Dead shows and heard people talking about it but never tried it myself. I was mostly into the live music and all the other stuff that came with it.

I took my first yoga class at the University of Massachusetts at Amherst when I was 18. At that point I was a real hippie; I followed the Grateful Dead religiously and sustained myself on brown rice and tofu. The food at the university cafeteria was awful—in fact, it turned me into a lifelong vegetarian—and my rebellion against hotdogs and meatloaf introduced me to a large community of like-minded people. The alternative living community was inclusive, supportive, and overwhelmingly hip, and as a State Department kid, I had never really had that before. I soaked it up like a sponge. A friend recommended I take a yoga class, which sounded cool, and then I discovered I could use yoga as a gym credit, which was perfect. I needed three gym credits to graduate and was ready for something new.

The school offered three kinds of yoga: Hatha yoga, Iyengar yoga, and Kundalini yoga. Hatha was the easiest to pronounce so I signed up. I got my schedule

How We Found Yoga

and was bummed to see that Hatha yoga was on Tuesday and Thursday mornings at 8:00 am. I was not a morning person. It was January in Western Massachusetts, and instead of snuggling up and sleeping in I had to get up at 7:30 am for yoga. I dragged myself out of bed and trudged across the frozen campus, thinking that yoga had better be really, really good.

Yoga was better than good, it was life-changing. I absolutely loved it. I couldn't believe how much I loved it. It was like I had found a comfortable old pair of shoes that fit me perfectly. I left class and started banging on my friends' doors, totally excited to tell them about this awesome yoga class. They were all asleep, of course, but I stayed excited. I didn't miss a single class the entire semester—well, I may have missed a few during the Dead's spring tour—and I fell in love with how yoga made me feel. There was a sense of ease I had never felt in anything else. I was hooked.

The next semester I tried Kundalini yoga but didn't have the same "wow" experience. The instructors were beautiful and brilliant people but sitting and chanting just didn't resonate with me at the time. I was 19 and probably a bit too distracted. I needed something more physical.

The last class on the list was Iyengar yoga. I had decided to take it after Kundalini but all my friends warned me not to. They said the instructor was terrible. He had a horrible reputation; students said he kicked, slapped, and yelled at them. It didn't sound like the kind of yoga I wanted, so I skipped it. Little did I know, the dreaded Iyengar teacher was actually Eddie Modestini—the co-author of this book.

I skipped yoga that semester but kept it in my life, casually practicing the few poses I had learned from the Hatha yoga class. In my senior year I lived with some girlfriends in a house off campus and one of them was taking Eddie's Iyengar yoga class. One day she taught us *surya namaskar A* and it was WOW all over again. *Surya namaskar* was totally different from what I had experienced in previous yoga classes and I absolutely loved it. It felt like I had discovered some long-forgotten secret. I was hooked all over again.

The class was still called Iyengar yoga but Eddie had been introduced to Ashtanga yoga by Tim Miller. He was teaching Primary Series in his Iyengar class. Every week my friend came back from his class with a little bit more of the Ashtanga system and I just couldn't get enough. I decided to take the Iyengar class for my final semester, despite Eddie's bad reputation. Anyone teaching this amazing stuff couldn't be that bad.

I was late to my first day of class. I ran into the room and frantically removed layer upon layer of clothing—it was January, so there were a lot of them. I finally tossed it all off and turned around and Eddie was sitting at the front of the room, looking right at me. Locking eyes with him sent this crazy electrical jolt through my body. I knew I would have some kind of connection with him. I never dreamed it would become what it did but I immediately knew there was something there. Intuition is a powerful thing.

Eddie was teaching the Primary Series of Ashtanga yoga and I loved it. I had enjoyed the other types of yoga but Ashtanga really resonated with me. It was fun, challenging, and I could DO it; I was naturally flexible and athletic, and at the time I thought yoga was all about flexibility.

I went to every single class that semester and started going to Eddie's classes outside of the university as well. I just couldn't get enough of the yoga, and I definitely had a crush on Eddie. He didn't really notice me at first (although he now claims he did) but he did tell me about his teacher, Tim Miller. Tim was coming to Amherst for a weeklong *asana* intensive so my friends and I decided to stick around after graduation to take it.

The intensive was amazing; I was totally lit up and asked Tim how I could get more Ashtanga yoga. Tim lived in Encinitas, California, and gave me an open invitation to visit. My friends and I were already planning a cross-country road trip but didn't really know where we were going. Encinitas was a long shot, but I took his information anyway.

Before we left for the road trip I asked Eddie if there were any books I could use to study Ashtanga yoga on my own. There weren't any Ashtanga books available at the time but he told me to get BKS Iyengar's *Light on Yoga*. He also showed me a list of the poses in Primary Series. I didn't have any paper on hand so I tore open a brown paper grocery bag and wrote down the name of each pose with a little stick-figure diagram to illustrate it. For the next few months that little piece of paper bag was either in my pocket or unfolded next to my mat, everywhere I went, all over the country. It became my lifeline. It was my humble connection to the art of yoga, a connection that has shaped my life ever since. I still have that little piece of paper bag today.

My friends and I eventually made it to Encinitas and I showed up at Tim Miller's studio hoping to take a few classes. The woman behind the desk told me I had just missed him; he was teaching a workshop on Maui. We chatted for a bit and she told me that Tim's friend from the East Coast was visiting him at

How We Found Yoga

How We Found Yoga

the studio. It was Eddie, but of course, he had also gone to Maui. We got back on the road and ended up in Santa Cruz, which is where all the hippies were, so I decided to stay. I had been on this road trip for several months with my best friend and her boyfriend, and we were all pretty sick of each other.

I found a place to stay in Santa Cruz and decided to call my mom. I had not spoken to her in over a month; there were no cell phones or email back then. She was happy to hear from me but couldn't believe I was calling at that exact moment because some guy claiming to be my yoga instructor had just called the house. It was Eddie! I was blown away, partially by the incredible timing of the call but mostly because I still had a bit of a yoga-teacher crush on him. She told me he was going to a Grateful Dead show in San Francisco that night and hoping to find me.

Hoping to find me? It was a Dead show in San Francisco, there were thousands of people there. I know it sounds crazy, but if I had been there he would have found me.

Everyone in Santa Cruz was at that show, except me. I was living in a house with a bunch of hippies and was pretty sick of them. I had decided to stay home and skip the show, which was totally weird for me. I was really, really into the Dead and going to shows. I could not believe my rotten luck.

I gave my mom the Santa Cruz phone number and told her to give it to him if he ever called back. Eddie called my mom the next morning, bummed he hadn't found me at the show, and got my number in Santa Cruz. We talked the next day. He knew I had been in Encinitas and wanted to study with Tim, and he was driving back down to Encinitas the next day. He offered to give me a ride and to set me up with a work trade position at the studio.

I was pretty free at the time, with just my bag and my yoga mat, so I decided to go. I left a note on the kitchen table with a couple bucks for rent and I was gone. Well, I might have left without a couple bucks for rent, but oh well. Sorry guys.

I stayed at Tim's house for about a month, doing yoga and working at the studio. I was having an absolutely amazing time but I still thought it was temporary. Yoga was just a hobby. I had a relatively conventional path ahead; I had studied Russian in college and fully expected to start a career as a translator. It was 1991, the Berlin wall was down and there was a lot of opportunity in that field. I had a couple of jobs lined up but wouldn't hear back from them until

November so I was content to hang out in Encinitas.

While I was at the studio, Tim, Eddie and a few other people went off to Mysore to study with Pattabhi Jois. Eddie was sick when he left, became sicker while he was there, and ended up coming back to California early. He stayed in Encinitas to get better and we started hanging out a lot. He told me he was going back to Mysore as soon as possible and I should go with him. I was hesitant, mainly because I was 22, totally broke, and not sure it was the "right" thing to do—I still thought I was going to get a "real" job relatively soon. I also didn't have a passport because my diplomatic passport had expired when I turned 21. Eddie wanted to leave in less than a week and not having a passport was a deal-breaker.

Luckily, one of my dad's friends was stationed at the US consulate in Tijuana, Mexico. I borrowed a car, crossed the border and got totally hooked up by the consulate staff. They had a new passport ready in just a few hours and even gave me a ride back to my car at the border. I was still broke, but Eddie loaned me the money for a ticket and we went to India on November 1st, 1991. That trip sealed the deal for Eddie and me, and for our life with yoga.

When we got to Mysore, Eddie sent me to Guruji's house to register and pay for classes. I really didn't know much about Pattabhi Jois, only what I had seen and heard in Encinitas. Tim's studio had the classic picture of a young Guruji in *samastiti* and he always seemed larger than life. He was tall, handsome, and seemed to possess a quiet, intimidating strength. I was expecting a pretty imposing figure, or at least a tall one, and was kind of nervous to meet him.

Guruji's studio was in the back room of his house but I went to the front door and knocked. There was a little sign that said "Ashtanga Yoga Research Institute, Pattabhi Jois," and the door opened to a small, robust old man. He was almost a head shorter than me and I'm not very tall. A little unsure, I asked if I could find Pattabhi Jois. He gave me a huge smile, exclaimed, "Yes!" and opened the door wider. I was totally blown away; here was my yoga luminary, the teacher of teachers, answering his own door to the humble home in which he lived and worked.

Guruji walked me through the house, where he had been doing his laundry, and took me up to the office to register. The registration process was totally old-school. He took out a little key from under the rug, unlocked his desk drawer and pulled out a small registration book. He carefully put on his glasses and asked a bunch of random questions, including my mother's maiden name and

How We Found Yoga

How We Found Yoga

my place of birth, and then I gave him cash to cover the classes. He told me to come back the next morning at 6:00 a.m. I was still not a morning person but he said, "Yes, six o'clock, you come." The other resident yogis told me I should be stoked because newbies usually started at four or five. I thought those people were nuts.

Before we went to Mysore, I still used my little paper bag list of postures every time I did yoga. Eddie told me, as we left California, that studying with Guruji meant showing up in the morning and doing Primary Series on your own. There was no general instruction and no cheat sheets. You did the series on your own and he stopped you wherever you need to be stopped. I knew I needed to memorize the series but, as usual, I waited until the absolute last minute; I memorized the entire sequence on the plane to India. My first day practicing in Guruji's studio was also my first day doing Primary Series without that security blanket, and it was intense.

The room was very small and there were eight people in it, plus Guruji. It was intimate, probably about six people too many for an American sense of space, but you get used to it. Newcomers waited on the stairs outside the room and when someone finished the series you would take their spot. I was extremely nervous. When a spot opened up, in the very front, I moved in and immediately started practicing.

Somewhere in the middle of the series, around *janu sirsasana*, I heard someone speaking in another language at the back of the room. Another person joined the conversation and they went back and forth for a while. It was Guruji and Sharath, his grandson, and I was getting really nervous but just kept going. Eventually I heard one of them snort, as if shrugging their shoulders, and they stopped talking. Miraculously, neither of them interrupted my practice. I did the entire Primary Series on the first day, which was very uncommon. Guruji or Sharath usually stopped and dismissed people when they felt the postures were too advanced for the student, and that happened to almost every newcomer.

The Primary Series ends with a sequence of radical backbends. You start with *urdhva dhanurasana* (upward-facing bow) and then walk in to grab your feet, and then maybe your ankles, calves, and up toward your thighs. On the very first day, Guruji had me grabbing my ankles. It progressed daily for the first few weeks and then he began to add Intermediate (Second) Series postures, moving me deeper and deeper into extreme backbends. I was still very much a beginner but I was doing really strong poses. These are poses I would never recommend to a beginner but I was able to do them because I am very flexible. I remember Guruji walking up to me in one of these backbends and smiling, saying, "Yes, very supple, very good."

I am a naturally flexible person and I had always thought being flexible was a huge advantage. It seemed like everyone was doing yoga to become flexible and I was already there. I had no idea there was any kind of mind-body connection because the physical practice had always been readily available. The postures had never challenged my body so they never got into my mind. It was easy. But after a few weeks in Mysore it was not so easy. Eventually my hands were above my knees in *urdhva dhanurasana*, walking toward my butt. That means I am standing with my head and torso bent backward to the point that my hands are on my thighs and I am staring at the back of my knees. It's an extreme backbend and I was doing it almost every day. My back started to hurt, just a little at first and then more and more. I was confused because I had never had back pain. I assumed it was a phase and would eventually go away; as Guruji often said, "One, two weeks and all better, no problem."

Our mornings in the studio with Guruji were relatively short—about two hours—but very intense. Time and space were major commodities because there were always too many people in the room and more people waiting to take their place. Most students rushed in and rushed out and then spent the rest of the day processing their experience. My first trip to Mysore was definitely the least rushed because there weren't many people trying to study with Guruji. But I was always a little bit different, even when the lines out the door became totally packed, because I took my time with the series. Tim had told me an ideal breath was a ten-second inhalation and a ten-second exhalation, which is massive. Every movement in Ashtanga yoga is connected to a single breath to create a *vinyasa*, and if you're spending ten seconds on each breath, those *vinyasa*s will last forever. I spent a lot of time working to develop that ten-second lung capacity and it made me slower than everyone else.

Guruji knew Eddie was an Iyengar yoga teacher and he really liked that. He loved that a certified Iyengar instructor had come to study his system, especially because the two systems had become so adversarial. It was like a check on his bucket list: one more student on my side. But he was also very respectful of Eddie's experience and taught him in a process-oriented way; he broke down each individual pose of the Ashtanga sequence and whispered their benefits into

Eddie's ear. He didn't do that for anyone else.

Eddie and I had gone to Mysore together so Guruji gave me a certain amount of leeway. We both practiced a little bit slower than the other students and he didn't seem to mind. But one morning, about two months into our stay, Guruji yelled from the back of the room, "Nicki! Why you going so slow? You Iyengar student!" It was like a slap in the face. That was the first time I had felt an emotional explosion from the practice and I was totally unprepared. I grabbed my mat in a huff and ran upstairs, into the room where everyone did the finishing poses. I flopped over into *paschimottanasana* and stayed there, crying at the top of my lungs.

There were no doors in that part of Guruji's house so I'm sure everyone downstairs could hear me. I carried on for a good ten minutes before Eddie came upstairs and said Guruji wanted to see me. I refused, with the usual sob story; he's mean, he hates me, there's no way I'm going to talk to him, blah blah blah. Eddie told me to take my time, calm down, and then go downstairs and talk to him.

I was still sniffling and my eyes were all puffy but I finally got up and walked downstairs. Guruji was standing in the hallway outside of the yoga room, and as I started down the stairs he asked, "Nicki, why crying?" I blubbered on for a minute about him being mean and yelling at me, and he finally said, "Nicki, you crying, I'm crying. You smiling, I'm smiling." I started crying even more. He said, "You come," and brought me back into the yoga room. He always kept a stool in the corner, where he often sat, and he motioned for me to sit on the floor next to it. He sat on the stool, put his hand on my head, and told everyone else to keep practicing.

Every day, for the next two months, I would go downstairs after finishing my practice and sit on the floor next to his stool, with his hand on my head. I fell in love all over again, with him and with yoga. He became more than just a teacher, he became my Guruji. With those very simple words, he had taught me yoga is all about love. The transmission was so clear; telling the story still makes me emotional. I get chicken skin every time.

Guruji was full of love and intelligence, but his method was fierce. The adjustments, even then, were very strong. People were definitely pushed. If you said no, he would ask, "Why fearing?" Whatever came as a result of being pushed into poses was "your karma," and he expected you to deal with it yourself. His answer was always, "Oh, one, two weeks and all better, no problem." That was obviously not always the case but I knew there was a deep compassion in him. He was an endlessly loving individual. Toward the end of his life his grandson, Sharath, took over much of the *asana* instruction and the intensity that came with it, and Guruji maintained a gentle, graceful presence. He was all about love.

Guruji was always joyful and he never turned people away. There was always room for one more person. People eventually started to complain because the room was way too small for the number of people practicing: it had gone from an intimate eight-person setup—four people on each side of the room, facing forward—to ten people and then twelve people, with two people in the middle of each row. Then there were people practicing on the steps outside the door, and everyone was getting kicked and knocked around from all the jumping back and through, but he would never turn people away. Yoga was for everyone. Guruji eventually built a yoga *shala* that holds 75 people (in 2003), and his inclusive spirit stayed with us. We never turn people away from our classes. I don't care how many times you have to move your mat to make space for another person, just do it and get on with your practice.

After four months in Mysore my back really hurt. The flexible veneer was wearing thin and I was starting to wonder what to do about it. The daily backbends definitely weren't helping, but I wasn't willing to stop practicing or to back down from the poses that brought such a joyful sense of accomplishment. I was too "advanced" to go backward. But our time in Mysore was almost up so it was time to go elsewhere.

Eddie's father was Italian and was living in Florence, Italy, so we decided to visit him on our way back from India. Eddie knew an Iyengar yoga instructor also living in Florence, a woman named Gabriella Giubilaro, and we decided to study with her for a few weeks. Gabriella is a student of Dona Holleman, one of BKS Iyengar's original senior students. She comes from that very rigorous and authentically Iyengar teaching style. Studying with her was very different, especially after coming from our sweet, smiling Guruji, but it was also very accurate and effective.

Gabriella kicked me on my very first day in her class. I was in *trikonasana* (triangle pose) and I remember thinking, *Who the hell are you, and why did you do that?* Guruji had adjusted me but no one had ever, ever kicked me in a yoga class. But in truth, she had kicked me in the exact place my tissue was sleepy. The method was abrasive but the instruction was totally on point. After class she showed me that I wasn't really working my legs and that my back was hurting

How We Found Yoga

NICKI:
It is important to give each teacher your full attention, but spending your life within a single system will put walls around your knowledge. It will limit your ability to help yourself and your students because every single person is different. There is always more than one way to follow the path of yoga.

because I was only bending in one place. It was eye-opening. Gabriella is a magnificent teacher and she was exactly what I needed at the time.

Gabriella really liked to work hard and we loved that. The "can-do" attitude is a big part of the Ashtanga system and we had just come from its Mecca. Gabriella's Italian Iyengar scene was a little different; they loved anything *supta* (reclined) and spent half the class talking about lunch. Eddie and I were all jazzed up about yoga and the three of us fed on each other's energy. She pointed out my weak spots and taught me how to address them using Iyengar's laser-sharp alignment principles. I was hinging in my lower back and didn't know how to share backbends with the rest of my spine, so she pushed me toward the foundational work of standing poses and hip openers. We spent six weeks with Gabriella, and by the time I left, my backbends were completely pain-free—and still are to this day.

Studying with Gabriella completely changed my perspective on yoga. I came to yoga at a time when Ashtanga and Iyengar were more like cats and dogs than yin and yang. Teachers and practitioners swore dogmatic allegiance to one or the other, and people who studied both were treated like outcasts. It had already happened to Eddie; the Iyengar institute had taken his certification away when he decided to study Ashtanga with Guruji. I didn't get it. I knew, in my mind and body, that the teachings of BKS Iyengar and Pattabhi Jois were complementary. My Ashtanga yoga practice was better than ever thanks to the teachings of Iyengar yoga. What was the big deal?

I later found out BKS Iyengar and Pattabhi Jois had the same teacher (T. Krishnamacharya), and that confused me even more. I heard Ashtanga practitioners bad-mouthing Iyengar yoga but knew they had never tried it. I heard Iyengar students dissing Ashtanga yoga and again, they had never tried it. It was so unnecessarily political.

The animosity really hurt me because I knew they were complementary systems. Ashtanga yoga was joyful and exciting but it didn't teach very much detail, and Iyengar yoga was precise and accurate but much less uplifting. Practicing both of them saved my life with yoga. If I had stayed only with Ashtanga yoga, I may have stopped doing it because of my back pain. If I had only been introduced to Iyengar yoga, I probably would have stopped doing it because I needed more movement and joy. I am absolutely certain I progressed as far as I did into the Ashtanga system, and remained injury-free, because of the teachings of Iyengar yoga.

The rift between the two systems has never made sense to me. We oscillated between them for our first ten years together and it made us the teachers we are today. It was a yearly pilgrimage: went to Italy for Iyengar yoga, to India for Ashtanga yoga, and then spent the rest of our time teaching. The Ashtanga yoga community had a pretty big network of teachers in the US, and there was always a studio that needed a sub because everyone visited Guruji at different three-month intervals. The Mysore-style Ashtanga series was consistent everywhere we went so subbing classes was easy. That was our life for many years.

One of our subbing locations was Nancy Gilgolff's Ashtanga studio on Maui. We loved being on Maui because of the big Ashtanga community and also because it's Maui. What's not to like?

We liked it so much that in 1995 we bought a piece of raw land on the north shore along the Hana Highway north of Paia. We continued to travel and teach but added Maui to our list of yearly destinations. We cleared the land and built a tiny cabin, about 12' x 12', running on solar power and water from a catchment system. We also began to build our own personal yoga studio, a beautiful hardwood structure overlooking the ocean. People visiting the property were always confused because the yoga studio was ten times larger than our house. Most people spend their time and money building a comfortable home but we lived in a tiny cabin and built a big, beautiful yoga studio. It had been Eddie's lifelong dream to build his own yoga shala and equip it with a full set of Iyengar props. There was no business plan; it was just a private space for us and our friends to practice yoga. We never dreamed it would become the thriving community it is today. It was just our little space in the jungle and we loved it.

In 1998 I became pregnant with our daughter Maya and we decided to make Maui our permanent home. Eddie and I were stoked to be around our beautiful studio full-time, and our friend Casey asked to come by and practice with us. We were working on Intermediate Series together, despite my growing belly, and it was a very strong practice. On our first day in the studio together, Casey's husband came with her and begged Eddie to teach him too. Stan was not a yogi but wanted to be. We see that a lot in yoga, the stiff guy following his flexible wife to class, and it's challenging because they need completely different poses.

Eddie consented, but only if the guy would come six days a week for a month. That was the Mysore commitment. Students couldn't just drop into regular classes with Guruji; they had to make a month-long commitment to the Ashtanga system, to Guruji's teaching, and to themselves. We still feel strongly about

How We Found Yoga

How We Found Yoga

commitment because it's a huge part of an effective practice. It's difficult to really learn something if you do it sporadically, and it's not fair to judge something unless you've given it your full attention.

We decided to split the room in half: Casey and I worked on advanced Ashtanga poses, and Eddie and Stan worked on basic Iyengar-style standing poses. The very next morning, there was someone waiting on the steps outside our studio. We politely asked what she was doing there because we're not exactly easy to find; we live down a long dirt road in the jungle so she probably wasn't just lost. She said she was there for yoga class. Rick Bickford, one of the carpenters who helped build the studio, had told her there was a studio out here. We invited her in, honoring Guruji's inclusive spirit, and that's how it all started. Every day there would be another person, sometimes two or three, who just showed up on our doorstep for class. We never advertised or put up fliers, it was all word of mouth and it grew quickly.

We still had the room split between the Ashtangis and the Iyengar-style beginner classes, but after a while it was too distracting to have two very different classes happening simultaneously. There were just too many people. We integrated the classes and started teaching basic Ashtanga yoga, Primary Series, to everyone who came. Eddie and I taught together, giving us the ability to address students on an individual level while keeping the flow of the series.

As the years went by we found ourselves teaching less and less of the Ashtanga set series. We wanted to serve all the individuals who showed up in our studio and it didn't feel right to force them into poses that were inappropriate for their anatomical reality. Instead, we began to focus on reoccurring anatomical themes: stiff hips, stiff shoulders, closed chests, and sluggish hands and feet. Almost all of the students who walked through the door needed help in one or all of these areas, and everyone benefited from practicing them, regardless of their previous experience.

We began to develop a blend of Ashtanga and Iyengar poses that safely addressed these anatomical sticky spots and it was a huge hit. We watched several of our close friends work through major, chronic pain, and finding relief from pain is like getting a whole new life. People even look different when they're released from pain; it's a total mind-body transformation. And it was completely self-sufficient. Yoga was the roadmap and we were the guides, but people were doing the work themselves. It was great. We taught this hybrid style in our studio, six days a week, for eight or nine years. Our classes were packed but it was still very laid back. The studio didn't even have a name. We finally decided to call it the Maya Yoga Studio after our daughter Maya. I love Sanskrit and Maya is a Sanskrit word meaning "illusion." The "illusion" reference has become more fitting than I could ever have imagined, as it later became the name for our entire teaching method: Maya Yoga. Maya Yoga is always changing to meet the needs of its students, and it's never quite what you think it's going to be. It's the perfect illusion.

Several years later, one of my regular students told me she was bringing a friend from the East Coast to class. He showed up looking like he had just walked off the beach and didn't seem to be much of a yogi. Eddie and I welcomed him and guided him through the practice anyway, and he turned out to be the director of the Omega Institute in Rhinebeck, New York. He invited us to teach at the institute and we happily obliged, and it became the first of many off-island teaching invitations.

For the next few years we taught all over the country and in Canada. My family still lives on the East Coast so every year we would drag the kids through an exhausting six-week tour of teaching gigs and family visits. Eventually I started teaching solo, leaving Eddie and the kids on Maui for a few days or weeks at a time. It was very hard to leave them but it's far better than taking the whole carnival on the road.

Our home studio continued to grow and our students started asking us to have a teacher training. We finally agreed but the registration was totally island-style: we had only three people signed up to take the training but on the first day there were 24 people in the room. Our studio has always been very "organic" like that. That first training was very strong because most of the students had been coming to our studio for years. We started out with 20-minute headstands and 40-minute shoulderstands, and it was incredible to have cultivated that kind of energy in our community.

Eddie and I started teaching at larger and larger conferences and we needed a name for our style of yoga. We thought about calling it Hatha yoga because it draws heavily on the traditional poses, but Hatha yoga has a very passive, gentle connotation. If you've practiced with us you know our teaching is not exactly passive. We finally decided to call it Maya Yoga, after our studio, and the "illusion" reference became more fitting as our practice evolved. Maya Yoga is an illusion of a system: it maintains the foundational elements of both Ashtanga and Iyengar yoga but is, at the same time, completely different from either one.

How We Found Yoga

How We Found Yoga

NICKI:
Eddie often says our students are like snowflakes: no two are exactly the same. There has never been another person like you on this planet and there never will be, and that is so incredibly cool. Your individuality is a good thing and it shouldn't be constricted by the rules and regulations of a single system. It is our responsibility as teachers to meet you at your level, instead of expecting you to be at the level we want to teach.

We have deep respect for both the Ashtanga and Iyengar systems and always acknowledge the parts of those lineages that have been incorporated into Maya Yoga. We give credit where credit is due. In fact, we teach both the Ashtanga and Iyengar rules as part of our teacher trainings because it is important to know the rules. As you become a more mature teacher, you learn when and how appropriate it is to break the rules. But you have to know them to break them.

Breaking rules is how we began to work with individuals. That's exactly what most people are: unique exceptions to the rule. Developing Maya Yoga was, in many ways, a process of breaking the rules of Ashtanga and Iyengar yoga to better to accommodate the individuals in our classes. But breaking the rules of those systems is very different from breaking yoga's universal principles of alignment, which we have always honored. We always follow the lines of yoga.

When students now ask me, "What do you teach?" I tell them, "People." Most teachers have a system—Iyengar, Ashtanga, vinyasa, whatever—but the underlying truth is we should be teaching people, not systems. Teaching people means you are focused on individual healing; teaching systems is more about tradition, memorization, and repetition. Systems can become stagnant, and yoga is as alive and dynamic as you are.

Yoga affects us in different ways. Some of us get very emotional right away and others are slower to find the mind-body connection. And by "emotional" I mean the whole spectrum of human experience—sadness, joy, frustration, jealousy—whatever yoga draws out of your psyche. I was definitely slow to make the mind-body connection because yoga postures were easy. They never made me deal with myself. That's what freaked me out so much in India; I had always been in control of my practice and suddenly I had this explosive emotional reaction. But that's when yoga really gets interesting. It's not just about your body; it's about using your body to get to your mind. When the emotions start to bubble, you know you're really penetrating. That's how you know your practice is truly effective.

If you are just doing the postures and nothing else in your life is changing, please question your practice. Just because you can put your foot behind your head does not mean you're an evolved being—there's more to it than that.

Trying to better understand the mind-body connection led me to the Yoga Sutras of Patanjali. The Yoga Sutras are a set of ancient aphorisms (small words with big meaning) that outline the psychology of yoga. But studying them was not easy because most of the available interpretations are long, academic, and dry. Even the thin ones can be daunting. I spent months falling asleep to various translations and finally put them aside, thinking I was just not ready.

Years later, with the help of Bhavani Maki, a friend and colleague, I discovered I was already teaching the yoga Sutras in my classes. She linked my teaching philosophy to the underlying meaning of the Sutras, and a light bulb went off in my head. I realized these teachings are already inside of us, and it is through our practice that the work is revealed. It is almost like the Sutras are written in code and you have to do yoga to decipher them. Yoga is your Rosetta Stone to the infinite wisdom that lives inside you.

How We Found Yoga

Eddie and I no longer teach together as much as we used to. Our practices and our lives have evolved in different directions but I am endlessly grateful to him for leading me toward yoga. Without him I would not have my children, my home, or my path through yoga, and I probably wouldn't be teaching. He truly pushed me through my hesitation and encouraged me to become a great practitioner and a great teacher. I also believe some of it was already in me because yoga felt familiar from the very beginning. On my first trip to India Pattabhi Jois said I had very good *samskara*s, which are your past life impressions. He told me I had been doing yoga for many lifetimes and I truly believe that; if you are doing yoga in this lifetime, you have done yoga before. We do not find yoga, yoga finds us.

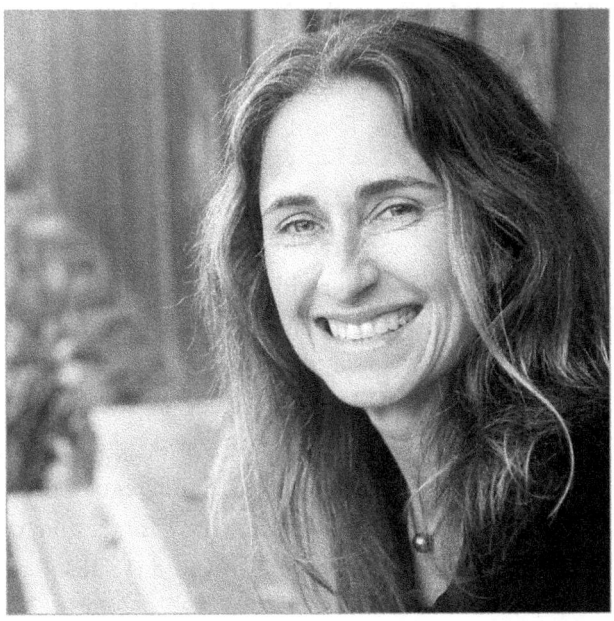

Eddie Modestini

I healed two slipped discs in my back through daily practice and faith in yoga. No doctors or surgeries, just me and my practice. It's a real story and a huge part of who I am and why I teach yoga.

I am a really stiff guy. I had my left kidney removed when I was 12 years old, and to get it out, the doctors cut a line from my belly button to my spine. They levered my hips away from my ribs and compressed all the discs in my lumbar spine (lower back). It hurt like hell and back pain became my life.

Pain can make you angry, pretty much all the time. You can never get away from it. It starts to cloud everything you do and it can eventually chase you out of your body. Your skeleton bends and shifts away from the pain without your knowledge, creating a new structure based on antalgia: the body's natural ability to compensate for pain through posture and motion. It crippled me.

I was stiff to begin with but pain made me even more twisted and congested. Americans don't usually look inward for healing so we project our pain, in the form of anger, onto everyone around us. I was definitely not the nicest person back then.

In 1982 I was really living with my back pain. I had bought a 30-acre farm in Colorado and was installing a 12-foot elk fence, driving massive posts into the rocky ground. It took me a couple years to complete, and by the time I finished, my back was done. I was hobbling around on a cane at 28 years old. The pain was completely debilitating.

I was diagnosed with two slipped discs in my lower back and the doctor recommended a double laminectomy. A laminectomy fuses two vertebrae together by removing their intervertebral discs, and a double laminectomy fuses three vertebrae by removing two discs. Intervertebral discs are the resilient cushions that sit between each vertebra, the bony segments of your spine. Removing these discs means a permanent loss of flexibility and shock-absorption. I didn't want to do it. I had no idea what I could do to escape my back pain but I knew I had to start looking.

I started by selling the farm; my back was so broken I couldn't do the work any longer. I moved to California looking for something to heal me and found the Optimum Health Institute in San Diego. I fasted for three weeks and learned the healing powers of nutrition, raw foods and wheat grass, and it helped my back a lot. I'm not strictly raw and I don't subsist on wheat grass, but at the time,

How We Found Yoga

EDDIE:
Yoga created the skeleton that walks inside my body. It changed my bones, and changing my bones changed my life.

those two things were revolutionary to me. Changing my diet dealt with the inflammation around my injury and gave me a starting point for really getting into my pain. After that I went to Heartwood Massage School in northern California and studied deep tissue massage and postural integration with Jim Spira. I figured that learning more about the body would help me fix my back, and I was on the right track.

Jim turned me on to Tai Chi and meditation. I was a dedicated student and meditated a lot but I mostly meditated on the pain in my back. I couldn't get past it, mentally or physically. At first I tried to suppress the pain and then I tried to transcend it, but neither worked. I was also extremely stiff, which didn't help. After six months of intense practice I asked Jim, "Hey man, how am I doing?" I was really struggling, sitting cross-legged with my knees way off the ground, shoulders hunched over, and chin jutting forward to keep my head up above my stiff neck. And Jim, being the honest, intelligent man that he is, said I was really, really stiff and needed something stronger. He said he would take me to a yoga class.

On July 1st, 1983, Jim took me to an Iyengar yoga class with Gayna Uransky. Gayna was several months pregnant and teaching *surya namaskar A* with a huge belly. I couldn't keep up with her! When we did standing poses, I fell out of triangle pose in the middle of the room. I was a complete mess: embarrassed, helplessly stiff, and completely outside of my body. But I immediately knew I had found my path. I knew yoga would fix my back. It was the first time since I hurt my back that I could say to myself, *Wow, this is really going to work*. I signed up immediately and did yoga at least three times a week for the next few months.

Finding yoga was like getting thrown a life preserver. I was still in the water and had a long way to go, but I finally knew I wasn't going down; the pain wasn't going to pull me under. I had been living in fear for so long, and yoga gave me hope. It also gave me a road map: it showed me the way to heal my pain long before I actually got rid of it. The journey from discovery to healing would span almost ten years but I always had faith in yoga, from the very first moment I found it.

My girlfriend was moving from California to Massachusetts and she invited me to come along. I told her I would love to come but I had to do yoga. I wasn't going to move until she assured me there was a good Iyengar yoga teacher in town. I'm not sure why she still wanted to date me after I told her yoga was more important, but she called me a week later and said she had found a junior-inter-

How We Found Yoga

mediate Iyengar instructor named Jyothi Hansa. I moved to Massachusetts and studied with Jyothi for about nine months. The girlfriend didn't last, but my life with yoga was on fire.

I started teaching yoga at the University of Massachusetts at Amherst on January 21st, 1984. I had only been doing yoga for several months but it's not like there were a lot of yoga teachers back then. I was working at a bakery, getting up at 3:00 am to make bagels and croissants for $7.00 an hour, and the university offered me $25.00 an hour to teach yoga. That was more money than I had ever been paid in my life. I taught three classes a week at the University and also started teaching in town. I kept the bakery job though, up until I went to study in India, and still love to make bread. I've always been drawn to things that require infinite patience and meticulous attention to detail like baking, jewelry making, and Iyengar yoga. Some people think it is tedious and frustrating work but I see the beauty. It's fine art.

I was ready to take the next step toward yoga so I spent two months at the Iyengar Yoga Institute in San Francisco, studying mostly with Manouso Manos. I attended the first Iyengar Yoga Convention in San Francisco in 1984 and took classes with all the senior teachers. These are great, great teachers: Victor Van Kooten, Angela Farmer, Kofi Busia, and all the Iyengar bigwigs. Many of them have since been de-certified by the Iyengar system, just like me, but that was much later.

I left the conference wanting more yoga and decided that becoming a certified Iyengar instructor was probably the best way to do it. Certification was way more intense than it is today. Doing *asana* was just one part of it; you also had to practice for five years, make at least one trip to India and study with a select group of senior teachers for a certain period of time. Then you were eligible to take the assessment, given by the Iyengar Yoga National Association United States (IYNAUS), and most people failed it multiple times.

I took the first Iyengar yoga certification assessment to be given on the East Coast of America. To pass, you had to be proficient in the poses and teach them correctly, including the fundamental structural alignment of every beginning posture, and also be able to adjust your students. The most difficult part of the exam was the dreaded hat; each student pulled three poses out of a hat and was given one minute to properly sequence them and then had to teach them in front of seven senior Iyengar teachers. You could have pulled anything—standing poses, inversions, backbends, forward bends, or twists, all written in their

Sanskrit names—and you'd have to figure it out in a split second with all the senior teachers watching. And the teachers were intimidating as hell; they were true Iyengar types, strict and unflinching. I passed the exam and received my Introductory Certificate to teach Iyengar yoga in 1988. Twenty-five people took the test and only three of us passed: Theresa Roland, Kevin Gardner, and me. It was intense.

At around the same time as the Iyengar certification, somewhere between '88 and '89, I received a BA in exercise physiology and physical rehabilitation from UMass at Amherst. I had been enrolled at Amherst while studying yoga and the more "conventional" path of study was incredibly helpful to my yoga experience. The university classes taught me anatomy, which was huge, and also gave me another frame of reference for studying the body in movement. A few years into my BA, I also stared teaching yoga and anatomy at Stillpoint Massage School and developed a yoga curriculum with Susan Little, Tias Little's mother. I was still teaching regular yoga classes at UMass, and by the time I received my Iyengar certification I was probably teaching about 14 yoga classes a week. All that teaching was a huge factor in my ability to pass the Iyengar certification. I was already an experienced teacher, even if I didn't have the credentials yet.

Also in that same time period, although it's hard to remember exactly when, I got a degree in developmental sequence movement and physical rehabilitation from the Institute of Educational Therapy. The institute focused on self-reliant healing, as opposed to the Western model of other-dependent healing, and it resonated strongly with my yoga experience. Most therapeutic techniques are other-dependent, meaning someone has to facilitate and execute your healing process (massage, acupuncture, medicine, etc.), but yoga teaches people to rely on themselves for healing.

Studying at the institute and teaching massive amounts of yoga played a major role in developing my ability to see and understand bodies. It allowed me to begin helping my yoga students on an individual level and to develop techniques suited to each student's needs.

I started doing Ashtanga yoga less than a year after getting my Iyengar certification. I guess I was the black sheep of my Iyengar certification group. I had read about Pattabhi Jois in *Yoga Journal* and tracked down Tim Miller in Encinitas. Tim taught me Ashtanga yoga for several months and then he and I went to Mysore to study with Pattabhi Jois.

How We Found Yoga

EDDIE:
Our teaching is based on the work of our teachers, our individual practice, and human physiology. It is a combination of art and science because yoga follows the lines of human anatomy.

How We Found Yoga

I immediately fell in love with the Ashtanga system. It thrived on flexibility and agility, two things I had gained through the practice of Iyengar yoga, but studying with Pattabhi Jois was completely different than working with BKS Iyengar. He was often just as intense, but he was also extremely kind and treated me like family. BKS Iyengar was a magnificent teacher, perhaps the best on the planet, but calling him a "loving" teacher is certainly a stretch. Pattabhi Jois taught with love and he became my Guruji.

I had to renew my Iyengar certification every year, and during the renewal process IYNAUS asked if I was studying any other kind of yoga. I was honest; I told them I had been studying Ashtanga yoga and they rescinded my certification. It was very frustrating. I had done the work for the certificate and was continuing to practice Ashtanga and Iyengar yoga, but in the end I was happy to let it go because I didn't want to be part of a system. I have deep respect for Iyengar yoga and still teach it to this day, but I was starting to see that yoga is bigger than the systems. I wanted to move in the direction of yoga, and at the time, moving toward yoga meant moving away from the system that had brought me to it.

I was authorized to teach Ashtanga yoga by Pattabhi Jois in 1993. The "authorization" was a verbal blessing and it allowed me to teach First and Second Series. At that point there were only a handful of people studying with him on a regular basis so it was very informal. You just asked Guruji if you could teach, and when you were ready he would give you his blessing. Eventually the system became more organized and began granting Ashtanga certifications but I did not pursue one. I chose, instead, to focus on using my combined experiences to heal my body and the bodies of my students.

I no longer consider myself an Ashtanga or an Iyengar practitioner but dedicating myself to those systems and exploring them to the extent that I did definitely made me the teacher I am today. I tried to fit into the system of Iyengar yoga and I succeeded, to some extent. Then I tried to fit into the system of Ashtanga yoga and again succeeded to some extent. But I never fully fit into either one. As I continued to teach, I began to see lots of other people who did not fit. I didn't think they needed to "fit in" to practice yoga because yoga is about healing, not rules. Healing is inclusive; rules will always exclude certain individuals. I began to customize my teaching to be personally significant to each person, rather than making them fit the criteria of any system. I discovered an avenue toward the individual rather than toward the system, essentially making the individual more important than the system. I didn't really realize it at the time, but this work was creating a radically inclusive style of yoga.

My current teaching evolved from that approach: putting individuals above the system. I do not fit people into a system; I teach each individual a system that will work for them. And I use the word "system" because yoga is systematic: it starts with the foundations and builds in a very precise and methodical way. We believe that this system—the method and hierarchy of poses—must be tailored to the individual because no two people need exactly the same thing.

How We Found Yoga

Nicki and I taught this style of yoga together for many years. We no longer teach together but our path has always been toward yoga. Over the years we have helped each other maintain integrity in our teaching and a strong faith in yoga. We also work to ensure that yoga is always bigger than our personalities because yoga has a fundamental structural alignment that is not based on personality. Part of being a good teacher is bringing your students to yoga without putting yourself in the way. Yoga is rich and engaging, it does not need to be embellished with an extra song and dance. It is so much bigger than either of us.

I owe everything to yoga; it gave me my heath, my children, and my livelihood. Thank you for taking the time to do this practice. Yoga is a culmination of all its students, and in practicing yoga you are adding your energy to the spiritual regeneration of the planet.

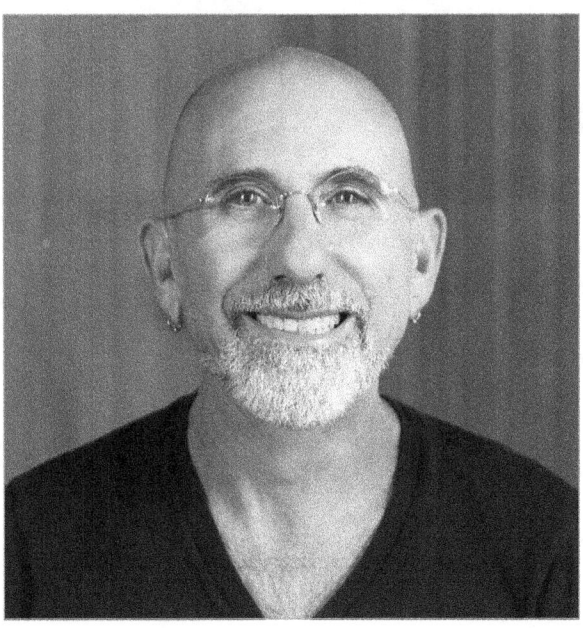

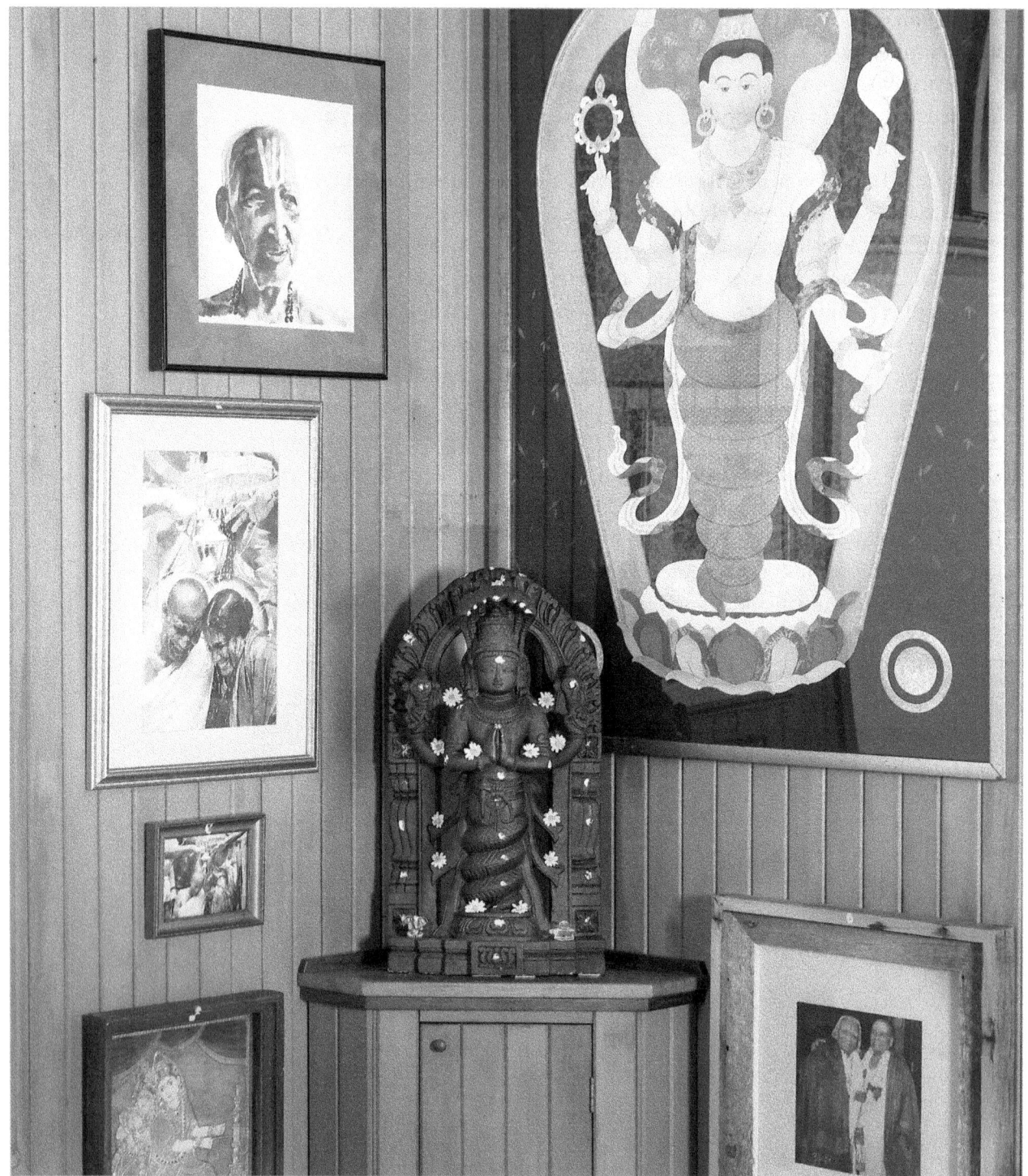

FOUNDATIONS

BREATH

Imagine you are on a beach. The waves are rough. A glass bottle is being tossed and turned near the shore, filled with a murky mix of water and sand. Pick it up and place it gently upright, away from the churning waves. The water and sand will continue to swirl inside the bottle, governed by a kinetic memory of the ocean's pull, but after a few moments of stillness the contents begin to settle. The sand becomes heavy and the water less opaque. After several minutes away from the churning sea, all the sand has settled to the bottom. The water is clear, calm, and completely transparent. The bottle and its contents become individuated, and in their clear individuation they become a single equanimous being.

Yup, you guessed it: you are the glass bottle. Your mind and body are subject to the push and pull of everyday life, compounded by the action and reaction of your own subconscious tendencies. Your psyche becomes cloudy, agitated, and deluged by chatter. Yoga is an opportunity to pluck yourself from this tidal wave of distraction. It allows you to sit quietly and settle so that you may see yourself more clearly and in that clarity develop the tools for a happier, healthier life. It is a journey toward stillness and ultimately toward unification of body, mind, heart, and soul. The most fundamental tool in this journey is your breath.

Breath as a Mirror

Your breath is a powerful tool of self-observation. It holds a wealth of information about the state of your mind and perfectly reflects the energetic currents flowing through your body. When you're angry or nervous, your breath is short, fast and shallow. When you're relaxed or sleepy, it is long, steady, and slow. Your breath also reflects emotions held in the subtle body, the quiet, vibrational being that operates below your conscious realm. Learning to observe your breath will help decipher the deep-seated patterns living in your subtle tissue and allow you to release them to better suit your mental and emotional evolution.

Breath is your strongest connection to the present moment. Our lives are full of thoughts, things, and technologies that distract us from the present moment, especially when we are challenged in yoga. When the *asana* gets tough, most people space out. They stop thinking about the pose and start thinking about lunch, work, kids—anything but the present moment. It's okay, we've all done it. We are inclined toward mental escapism because our minds can be anywhere at any time. But your breath doesn't have that option. It can only exist in the present moment. It cannot be in the past or in the future; it can only be right here, right now. It never leaves. It is the source of your energy and your life, and *ujayii pranayama* will keep your attention firmly rooted in its meditative rhythm.

Foundations

Ujayii Pranayama
ooh·**jai**·ee praw·nuh·yaa·muh | *victorious breath*

> **NICKI:** Becoming fully present in each and every breath will literally lengthen your life. The more conscious you are of your breath the more life you have to live.

Ujayii pranayama is the heartbeat of *asana*. *Ujayii* means victorious and *pranayama* is a method of assimilating *prana* into the body. *Pranayama* usually translates to a "study of breath" but *prana* is more than just the air you breathe. *Prana* is the universal life force. It exists beyond us and within us, saturating the air we breathe, and is the single most important factor in our longevity. *Ayama* means to extend or lengthen so *pranayama* is truly an extension of your life force.

Yogis believe that we are born with a predetermined number of breaths, set in a finite cycle of inhales and exhales. The best way to influence your destiny is to exert measured control over each breath through the practice of *pranayama*. Lengthening your breath will lengthen your life.

> Sit in a comfortable upright position and close your eyes. Use your tongue to wet your lips. Close your mouth and place your lips lightly together. Release any tension in your tongue, jaw, throat, and face. Breathe through your nose.

In the beginning your breath may scrape through your outer nasal cavity, a quick, shallow, and noisy cycle that originates more in your nose than in your body. *Ujayii* is an internal practice. Soften your nostrils and allow your breath to pass through lightly and silently, as though your nostrils are straws sipping breath deep into your body.

> Continue to breathe through your nose. Attach every ounce of consciousness to observing the sound and texture of your breath. Determine its origin within your body and slowly bring it deeper inside.

Ujayii pranayama originates at the base of your throat and creates a soft rushing sound, similar to a light breeze moving through the forest (or air being let out of a tire, for the less poetically inclined). Use the sound of *ujayii* to cultivate symmetry between your inhale and exhale, with a slight natural pause in the middle. Think of your breath as a long piece of silk moving through the eye of a needle and use your awareness to smooth out any wrinkles in the fabric.

> Keep breathing. If you feel tension gathering in your body or mind, simply relax the intensity of your effort. Soften everywhere and breathe freely. When the tension has dissolved, resume *ujayii pranayama* and try to remain soft.

Softness is more receptive than strength, and *pranayama* is subtle-body work. It's about connecting with the quiet Self hidden underneath your personality, and it requires time and space. It cannot be forced. If it takes too much effort to think about the slight natural pauses, or about where your breath is coming from, then don't think about it. Just keep breathing, and with time and practice all those elements will fall into place.

Ujayii Pranayama in Asana

Pattabhi Jois taught "free breathing" during *asana*. His very delicate grasp of the English language made him speak in little Sutra-like aphorisms that left little room for interpretation, but that was part of the charm. We finally got him to clarify that "free breathing" just meant **keep breathing**. Don't stop. Avoid holding, grasping, or gripping your breath. Let your breath be fluid, graceful, and most importantly, constant.

Always begin *asana* by observing your breath. Establish *ujayii pranayama* in a simple, still position so it can follow you into more vigorous *asanas*. Vigorous *asanas* may make your physical tissue hot but *ujayii* will keep your nervous system cool, calm, and receptive.

Use *ujayii* to match the energy of each physical action: inhale for expansive actions (lifting, reaching, extending) and exhale for contractive actions (folding and emptying). Every movement should be fully encapsulated in breath: begin your inhale before you begin the movement and finish the movement before you finish your exhale. Movement is initiated by breath and breath extends through movement. That is the nature of *vinyasa*: breath and movement are co-dependent partners. One should only go as far as the other will allow.

Ujayii pranayama should be audible to you, and perhaps the people right next to you, but not everyone else in the room. It shouldn't sound like Darth Vader or scuba gear, and it certainly shouldn't be aggressive or forceful. Your breath mirrors your energy and personality. If your breath is aggressive your practice may reflect those aggressive tendencies. If your breath is soft and shallow, you're just skimming the surface. The goal of this practice is to refine your breath-body connection in a way that integrates the subtle layers of your being. It is not intended to reinforce your current patterns. Use *ujayii* to cultivate balance in your breath and your practice. Balance facilitates sustainability.

Ujayii pranayama is a perfect barometer for your *asana* practice. It measures your connection to your physical experience and tells you when you have surpassed your thresholds. When that happens—your breath becomes lost in heat, tension or effort—take the time to rest. Your breath is always more important than the pose because *ujayii pranayama* is what separates simple heart-pumping calisthenics from the precise, deliberate, and spiritual practice of yoga. When you lose your breath you lose your connection to your Self, and thus your connection to yoga.

Ujayii pranayama is your mantra, your mandala, the thing that keeps you tethered to your experience. Take the time to cultivate its natural meditative rhythm: a delicate but deliberate channeling of your life force and a subtle yet highly conscious connection between your awareness and your physical experience.

BANDHA
baun·dah | *lock*

*Bandha*s are physical and energetic seals that keep energy properly placed within your body. They work together to support the length of your spine and maintain energetic relationships appropriate for each area: strength in the pelvis and lower back and softness in the neck and jaw. The four main *bandha*s cultivated in *asana* are *mula bandha, uddiyana bandha, jalandara bandha,* and *jiva bandha.*

The *bandhas* involve a very subtle physical engagement that creates an extremely powerful energetic response. *Mula bandha* prevents your bodily energy (*prana*) from leaking out at the base of your spine. *Uddiyana bandha* moves this energy toward the sacrum (base of your spine) to support your pelvis. *Jiva bandha* uses your tongue to prevent the effort of *asana* from gathering tension in your face and jaw. *Jalandara bandha* is the most advanced of the *bandhas* and prevents the pressure of *pranayama* from spreading to your head.

Mula and Uddiyana Bandha
moo·lah & ooh·dee·ya·nuh baun·dah | *root & upward-flying-belly lock*

Mula and *uddiyana bandha* are the cornerstones of a healthy *asana* practice. They are acknowledged by most yoga systems but are widely misunderstood and rarely taught in all their explicit detail. Their application in modern yoga has become synonymous with "core work" and "tightening," indicating grunting abdominal exercises that are better suited to the gym than the yoga studio. In reality, *mula* and *uddiyana bandha* have nothing to do with forming a six-pack. Conventional core work creates short, inflexible abdominal muscles that can make backbends difficult and painful. The *bandha*s are designed to strengthen your practice, not create more restrictions within your body. There is more strength in length than in bulk, so let's take a closer look.

Mula and *uddiyana bandha* are the true foundations of "core" strength, but your core is not your abdomen. Your core is your spine. *Mula* and *uddiyana bandha* work together to support the base of your spine, and their points of action are deep below the superficial tissues of your belly and butt. Teaching the real work of *mula* and *uddiyana bandha* requires some PG-13 vocabulary, namely the words "anus" and "genitals," which rarely make their way into a yoga studio. Very few yoga teachers are stoked to talk about genitals in a room of strangers wearing form-fitting clothing, and that's completely understandable. But we owe it to our students and to the lineage of yoga to explore this practice with precision, leaving nothing to the imagination.

Mula means root. *Mula bandha* is appropriately located at the base of your spine, where you contain your bodily energy. The physical point of action is a small muscle called the perineum, located between your sit bones, anus and genitals. The muscle fiber of the perineum runs from front to back. The anus is a sphincter, with muscle fiber that forms a circle. We're not trying to be unnecessarily graphic here; it may be helpful to visualize these muscular directions when you begin exploring *mula* and *uddiyana bandha*.

Uddiyana means flying upward. The physical point of action for *uddiyana bandha* is in your lower abdomen, between your pubic bone and your navel. It does not include your navel or the tissue of your upper abdomen; both of these areas should remain soft when *uddiyana bandha* is contracted.

Mula bandha and *uddiyana bandha* are practically impossible to separate. They contract and release in unison. *Mula bandha* pulls bodily energy upward

Foundations

NICKI:
My favorite illustration of *uddiyana bandha* is the statue of Ganesha in our studio. Ganesha is the beloved elephant-headed Hindu deity, and he has a round, jolly, protruding belly—one that looks like it shakes when he laughs. But if you look closely, the skin just underneath his belly is pulled tightly toward the top of his pelvis in the action of *uddiyana bandha*. The size of his belly is irrelevant because *uddiyana bandha* is not about your navel; it's about your lower abdomen.

from the connection of the perineum to the anus and *uddiyana bandha* pulls it straight back toward your spine. These two energetic actions meet at the top of your sacrum, where the base of your spine meets the bowl of your pelvis, to create a strong muscular-energetic seal. On a skeletal level, *mula bandha* stabilizes the three fused bones of the coccyx (tailbone) and *uddiyana bandha* solidifies the five fused bones of the sacrum (the bottom of your spine). The resulting energetic seal creates a container for the bottom of your subtle body, like a cinch at the bottom of a bag.

Mula and *uddiyana bandha* are best explored by sitting on a block in *virasana*, also known as "hero's pose." We will give a quick description here but full instructions (and contraindications!) for the pose are included in the Seated Hip Openers section.

Foundations

NICKI:
The purpose of the *bandhas* is to awaken and control the subtle pranic energy present in our bodies.

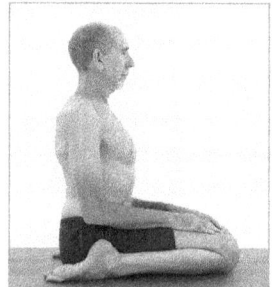
Virasana

Start on your hands and knees. Look between your legs and set your feet slightly wider than your hips, with the tops of your feet on the floor and your toes pointed straight back. Place a block between your feet and sit on it with your thighs parallel in front of you and your feet on either side of your hips. Walk your torso back until your head and shoulders are directly over your hips. Rest your hands on your thighs. The front edge of the block should be just in front of your sit bones to keep them fully supported.

Lift the flesh of your buttocks up and back to bring your sit bones in contact with the block. Use your hands to find your frontal hip bones and bring your pelvis to neutral: visualize your pelvis as a bowl of water filled to the brim and try not to spill a single drop. Align your sternum directly over your pubic bone and rest your hands on your thighs. Close your eyes and lower your head. Keep your chest lifted and your spine tall. Your shoulders should be directly over your hips with your sit bones heavy on the block.

Imagine that your perineum—that little muscle between your genitals and anus—is a rainbow. The rainbow is currently lying flat on the block between your sit bones. The action of *mula bandha* will lift the rainbow to create an arc that reaches up toward *uddiyana bandha* in your lower abdomen. *Uddiyana bandha* will meet *mula bandha* in the center of your pelvis to pull the rainbow back toward your sacrum, and from there, the energy will move upward from the base of your spine.

Bring your awareness to these physical landmarks. Inhale fully, soften everywhere, and exhale completely. At the bottom of your exhale, when you are completely empty, lift the tissue between your genitals and anus. Pick up the rainbow. Pull the lowest part of your abdomen toward the base of your spine. Inhale and feel the energy of *mula* and *uddiyana bandha* travel upward from the base of your spine, as though the rainbow was reaching up your spine toward your chest. Pause at the top of your inhale and then exhale completely. At the bottom of your exhale, lift the rainbow again. Use your breath to explore these corresponding actions.

Uddiyana bandha is a spontaneous reaction of *mula bandha*. You can't do one without the other. Always initiate them at the bottom of your exhale, just before you begin your next inhale.

Pinpointing the *bandha*s in your subtle body without engaging superficial tissues may seem difficult but it is certainly possible with practice. Refining your *bandha*s will teach you to gather strength where strength is needed and cultivate softness everywhere else. Softness is the best way to uproot the stress, tension, and congestion that govern our lives. But remember: practice implies repetition. Once is never enough.

Jiva Bandha
gee·vuh baun·dah | *soul lock*

Jiva means soul. *Jiva bandha* is created from the action of your tongue, which is the gateway to your subtle body. Engaging *jiva bandha* relaxes your face, unclenches your teeth and prevents your jaw from locking. There is a visible softening of the cheeks, lips, and throat. It is especially helpful when you are being challenged, and easily translates from your *asana* practice into everyday life.

Your jaw is intimately connected to your mental and emotional state. It softens when you laugh and smile and tightens when you are challenged, frustrated, or in pain. These are lightning-fast, unconscious reactions traveling along well-established neurological passageways between your brain and face. Using yoga to connect with tissue further away from your brain—such as lifting your quadriceps in a standing pose—challenges your nervous system and sends messages along these well-established pathways. Your brain is trying to talk to your quadriceps but your face, tongue, and jaw are more neurologically connected. They're the path of least resistance. You tighten your jaw, furrow your brow, and clench your teeth; a series of subconscious neurological reactions to the physical and mental challenge of *asana*.

Unfortunately, you cannot do an *asana* with your face. If your neurological intelligence stops at your face, you'll never get to your quadriceps. You need to extend your neurological communication beyond these readily-accessible tissues and *jiva bandha* will help you bridge this formidable gap. It allows you to relax the intensity of your effort and use the clarity of cool, unpressurized awareness to develop new patterns in your neuromuscular communication.

> Separate your lips and wet them with your tongue. Put your tongue back in your mouth and set your lips lightly together. Make the tip of your tongue very pointy inside your mouth. Gently place this point onto your upper palate, right above your two front teeth. The point of contact is where the ridges of your hard palate begin; most people have a vertical ridge in this exact spot. Your tongue should not touch the soft palate at the roof of your mouth or the enamel of your two front teeth. The pressure between your tongue and upper palate should be light, like a butterfly landing on a flower.

The energy of *jiva bandha* lives right in the tip of your tongue, at the point of connection. Allow the rest of your face and throat to soften completely. Always initiate *jiva bandha* at the top of your inhale when you are completely full of breath. Use it to soften your body and mind around the fullness of your breath and to dissolve any tension you have gathered in your pose, your practice, and your life.

On a vibrational level, *jiva bandha* connects a large energetic circuit in your subtle body. This circuit goes over the crown of your head, down your spine, across *mula* and *uddiyana bandha*, and up your solar plexus. It reconnects through *jiva bandha* when the tip of your tongue touches your upper palate. It's huge. Your body is comprised of these large connecting circles, and using the *bandha*s to link them together creates a subtle vibrational unity in your body.

Jalandara Bandha
jah·lawn·daur·rah baun·dah | *throat lock*

Jalandara bandha is primarily used in the practice of *pranayama*. *Pranayama* generates a significant amount of energy in your nervous system and *jalandara bandha* keeps this pressure from affecting your head. *Jala* means "net" or "web." *Jalandara bandha* is like a spider web at the bottom of your throat that seals the space between your chest and head. Guriji called it "throat lock," but it is not really a constriction or closure of the throat. *Jalandara bandha* is created from the precise placement of the head and chest, and it requires openness in your chest, neck, and shoulders.

> Explore *jalandara bandha* in a comfortable seated position, such as *virasana*. Sit up straight and tall with your sit bones evenly weighted on the block. Inhale and lift your chest toward your chin. Exhale and maintain the lift of your chest but soften your throat and shoulders. Inhale to lift your chest even more, and as you exhale reach your chin forward and release it to your chest. Extend your chin forward as it lowers. Do not force your chin down to your chest; instead, lift your chest to meet your chin. In the full pose, your chin rests just on top of the clavicular heads—those two bony knobs at the base of your throat that mark the top of your sternum.

Jalandara bandha should not cause pressure or pain in the back of your neck. If the back of your neck is uncomfortable your chest may not be lifted high enough to create the seal. This is an advanced *bandha* so please don't force it. Take the time to open your chest, shoulders, and neck, and allow *jalandara bandha* to naturally evolve into your practice.

Bandhas in Asana

Mula, uddiyana, and *jiva bandha* are perfect energetic companions to the rhythm of *ujayii pranayama*. Eddie often calls it "starting your engine" for *asana* practice.

Begin by establishing *ujayii pranayama*. At the very bottom of your exhale, when you are completely empty, engage *mula* and *uddiyana bandha*. Inhale fully, and at the top of your inhale find *jiva bandha*. Allow *jiva bandha* to soften the tissue of your face, throat, and jaw, including the space between your ears, and then exhale completely. Begin the cycle again and keep it with you for the duration of your practice.

This may sound like a simple task but developing subtle breath-*bandha* relationships is a lifelong practice. Be patient and remember that refining your breath requires mental, emotional, and physical receptivity. Cultivate strength in the specific places where it's necessary and cultivate softness everywhere else, because softness is more receptive than strength.

PROPS

Foundations

Krishnamacharya—the father of modern yoga—said there are as many *asana*s as there are living creatures on the planet. His statement reinforces our belief that anyone can do yoga, regardless of their current shape or size. There is an *asana*, or a way of approaching an *asana*, that is available to every person on the planet. Our goal is to safely guide your unique shape toward these *asana*s and toward the lines of yoga they illustrate.

EDDIE:
I have a very strong seated practice. I spent years developing openness in my hips and legs and cultivated long timings in poses like *virasana, baddha konasana,* and *padmasana*. But in 2012 I broke my ankle skiing and it forced me to rewind some of that work. I had to bring back props I hadn't used in years. It was disheartening but so necessary. If I had pushed forward and held stubbornly to my yogic achievements, I would never have reintegrated my ankle back into my leg. I used props to maintain my practice while giving my body the time to heal, and now my seated practice is prop-free and deeper than ever.

Building your anatomy in the direction of yoga may require the use of props. Props create the action of the *asana* in your body while protecting your joints, ligaments, and any other anatomically vulnerable areas specific to your unique shape. They move your body in the direction of yoga, and with enough practice, you will achieve proper alignment without their assistance. A gradual transition away from props indicates that your body has changed to reflect the lines of yoga; if your props do not facilitate change you must reevaluate both the prop and your method of using it. If you're using the same prop ten years from now you may not be using it effectively; you might be using it as a crutch.

Props should not be used to alter the lines of yoga or to permanently change the *asana* to better fit your shape. *You* are supposed to change, not the pose. The word "prop" is actually a less than perfect fit for these fantastic tools: a "prop" is something you lean on but **yoga props** push you deeper into your experience. They will not necessarily make the pose easier, oftentimes they make it more challenging, but when used correctly they greatly increase the efficiency of your effort. And that's what this is all about: creating an effective, integrated, sustainable practice to support your life.

If your path through yoga requires props they must be constantly evaluated and adjusted to reflect your personal evolution. You are not the same person every single day, and you certainly will not be the same person 10 years from now. The ever-changing patterns of your life create new anatomical realities on a daily basis and your use of props must honor that natural progression. Do not become attached to your props, or to the poses that "need" them, because yoga is about change. Be willing to let them go when they are no longer necessary and to let them in when they're needed, even if you didn't need them in the past.

Yoga has several highly effective props that can be found in almost any studio: blocks, belts, blankets, and bolsters. There are also several less recognizable but equally effective ones, including wedge boards, benches, chairs, ropes, swings, and the "horse." There are thousands of ways to use each of these props and hundreds of everyday items that can be used in their stead. Yoga's methods are as rich and varied as the individuals who seek to employ them.

We will mention specific props in relation to specific *asana*s but we cannot, within the confines of this book, explain the innumerable ways props can support your individual yoga practice. What we can do is provide a few general guidelines. When deciding whether you need a prop for a particular pose, consider the following things:

1. What are the principles of alignment in the pose; i.e. what is the posture trying to address or activate in your body today?

2. What action is created in the pose to achieve those principles?

3. What part of your anatomy needs additional guidance or protection to achieve this action?

4. What prop and method of use will most effectively achieve that result?

Let's use this reasoning for a very common posture: *uttanasana* (standing forward bend).

1. *Uttanasana* opens the legs and hips by stacking the bones of the leg in a straight line and rotating the pelvis around them.

2. The primary actions are: arrange your foot, ankle, lower leg and upper leg in a straight line; engage your quadriceps; internally rotate both legs; fold forward from your hips; rest your hands on the floor; soften your spine and look at your knees.

3. The most common anatomical impediment is tight hamstrings; they keep your pelvis stuck in place, and when you fold forward, the action pulls on your lower back instead of stretching your legs.

Foundations

EDDIE:
Props helped me develop enough clarity in my skeleton to practice without their assistance, and I did so for many years. Now, with a very mature practice, I am again learning to embrace props as a way to deepen my practice. Props give me the ability to have effort without tension. They allow me to evolve toward the intelligence of the pose, to start receiving its wisdom. It is deep work that will shape my practice for decades to come. Yoga is boundless, it just keeps on giving.

Pulling on your lower back in a forward bend can destabilize your lumbar intervertebral discs and contribute to chronic back pain.

4. Moving deeper into the forward bend pulls on your back instead of your legs, so to put the stretch back into your legs you need to back off of the forward bend. Eddie calls this "rewinding" the pose. To rewind *uttanasana* you must create a platform for your hands that is higher than the floor. A block is the simplest prop; place your hands on a block to decrease the bend in your back and simultaneously work the action of your legs and the rotation of your pelvis. Straighten and engage your legs, lift your sit bones and soften your spine. If the block is not high enough to relieve your back, go higher; use the seat of a chair or put your hands against a wall.

The action of the pose belongs in your pelvis and legs; use as many props as it takes to facilitate that work. Once you find the most effective prop, use it intelligently. Incorrect use of a prop can hold you back but correct use will propel you forward.

PAIN

Pain is an essential feedback mechanism that operates between your body, your nervous system, and your brain. It is your strongest indicator of danger and an important part of your ability to avoid injury. In that light, dealing with pain in yoga seems pretty straightforward: if something hurts, don't do it because you're going to cause an injury. But pain is closely intertwined with anger, fear, and anxiety; and these tangled emotions create a confusing gray area. Most people choose to avoid it completely and that's a personal choice. But your pain is part of you, and if you ignore it, it will become an even bigger part. Exploring and understanding your pain is at the heart of yoga and is perhaps the most important undertaking of your life. So let's take a closer look.

Pain is often at the root of human actions but it's not always the bone breaking, joint-wearing pain you would expect. Our lives are often driven by pain's sneaky counterparts: anger, fear, anxiety, frustration, and the whole spectrum of defensive emotions. These emotions may have originally stemmed from pain—mental, physical, or emotional—but they hang around long after the pain itself has subsided, a stubborn scab of suffering layered over past wounds. These emotional scars work deep below the surface of your rational decision-making process, and when you encounter them the immediate instinctive reaction is to retreat.

In reality, physical pain is the sole indicator of actual threats to your body. Anger, fear, anxiety, and all those defensive emotions represent perceived, imagined, and self-perpetuated threats, but they elicit the same response as actual pain: immediate and nonnegotiable retreat from the source. This retreat is a learned, conditioned response based on past experiences, not an actual red flag from your nervous system. And in the presence of actual pain, that host of defensive reactions can amplify the pain itself—the "mountain out of a molehill" effect—creating ever-stronger feedback loops between anxiety and the perception of pain. They throw a protective shroud over the roots of your pain, and in that darkness, the pain expands like a boogeyman in the closet. This inability to distinguish actual pain from perceived pain may control a lot of your actions and in doing so, dictate your life and its outcomes.

Bridging the gap between perception and reality requires that you explore everything about your pain, including your reaction to it. Your yoga practice can be a personalized laboratory for understanding your pain; each *asana* is a research project to help locate it, and once found, to develop a better dialogue with it and its root causes. The end result is an increased sensitivity to pain, in terms of prevention, understanding, and awareness, but a decreased reactivity to pain. There will be more intelligence and less knee-jerk reaction. It's an extremely important personal process because the way you react to pain on the mat is probably the same way you react to pain in the rest of your life. Gaining a better understanding of your pain will give you better control of yourself and your actions. It puts you back into the driver's seat of your own life.

Just to be clear, we're not saying pain is all in your head. Physical pain is very real and can be very debilitating—trust us, we've been there. But pain does not have to be a dead end. Physical pain can evolve and in many cases it can be alleviated. But to embark on that process you have to look the tiger in the eye; you must be willing to face your pain and determined to understand it. You have to hunt it down, find its anatomical root causes and chase it out of your body. It rarely leaves of its own volition, and in our experience it rarely resolves in response to other-dependent healing modalities. And pain, much like tension and congestion, can be very sneaky. It moves from one place to the next and getting it to truly leave your body requires intelligence, sensitivity, determination, and faith in yoga.

Foundations

NICKI:
We have the unfortunate tendency to layer suffering on top of our pain. If we do not release it, the suffering can become larger than the pain itself. And suffering is a choice. You can be in pain without suffering, and you can suffer without being in pain.

Pain and Yoga

BKS Iyengar said pain in the body is disease that has not yet manifested. That is an extremely profound statement. Yoga has the power to evict pain before it threatens your life. It gives you the ability to change your life, as it has changed ours. This sentiment is captured in one of Nicki's favorite Sutras, *heyam dukham anagatam*; your present practice can alleviate your future suffering.

That brings us to the most important point about pain in yoga: yoga does not create pain, the pain is already there. It exists in your muscles, tissues and bones, and yoga simply reveals its presence.

Some of us have more pain than others but all of us have it, and an effective yoga practice will definitely bring it to the surface. Pattabhi Jois called it karma. That pain in your hamstrings when you do *uttanasana*? That's your karma—maybe you didn't do enough yoga in your past life. But that pain is not coming from *uttanasana*, it's coming from your tight hamstrings. You may not have known it was there but that's why you're doing yoga. These postures reveal the secret hiding spots of pain and congestion in your body so you can banish them before pain and all its debilitating defensive emotions consume your life.

So where does this pain come from? The roots of pain are diverse and personal. Sometimes pain comes from quiet, lifelong imbalances that have slowly shifted your skeleton off course, and other times it comes from jarring, traumatic experiences. But the roots are ultimately irrelevant because determining what "caused" your pain isn't necessarily going to help you remove it; in fact, those emotions can become a barrier to your progress. They create a defensive emotional excuse to continue running from the pain, and oftentimes, that emotional defense imbeds itself deep into your personality. You have to let go of the anger, fear, confusion, and memories surrounding your pain and use yoga to address the pain itself.

So if yoga does not cause pain, why are so many people getting hurt in yoga today? It may be hard to digest, especially because Western society is more litigious than reflective, but these are largely self-inflicted injuries. They come from pushing too far, too fast, and ignoring early indications of pain. We know because we've done it. Both of us have really hurt ourselves in yoga but our injuries were not the inevitable result of a difficult pose. They were the result of our desire to "get" the pose before our bodies were ready. There was usually some amount of ego involved, a mind-over-matter mentality, but yoga always put us

Foundations

EDDIE:
Our primary responsibility is keeping our students safe. We don't teach things that jeopardize an individual's safety but that doesn't mean we simply ignore certain poses. It means we don't teach every pose to every person. We look at each individual and teach them what's right for their reality at this moment and give them the tools they need to evolve.

back in our place. There is a Sutra for this, one of our favorites: *te prati prasavah heya sukshmaha*. It means the moment you think you "know it all" is the most dangerous moment of all.

That brings us to another ugly truth about pain in modern yoga: many injuries arise from careless teaching. There is growing pressure for teachers to differentiate themselves by teaching more and more advanced postures, often at the expense of necessary foundational work. This is an extremely dangerous trend, and in our minds, it is also highly unethical.

We feel it is essential to teach to the anatomical and personal reality of the people in front of us. We don't teach the poses we like to do or the poses our students want to do; we teach them what they need, right now, and focus on postures that will help them the most. These are usually not the most "fun" or "advanced" poses but yoga is not just about a sense of accomplishment. Yoga is about healing, integration, and sustainability. That is our job as yoga teachers, handed down to us from Pattabhi Jois and BKS Iyengar: to guide students safely along the path of yoga, and unfortunately, there aren't very many shortcuts.

Finally, pain can also come from misalignment and repetition in that misalignment—such as doing a hundred rounds of *surya namaskar A* (sun salutation A) with your hands and feet in the wrong place. That's why we're such sticklers for proper alignment.

In the end, addressing pain in yoga brings us back to one of yoga's core principles: personal responsibility. When undertaking this work, you are responsible for taking care of yourself. That includes taking responsibility for your pain and your role in addressing it because only you know what you're really feeling. It also includes studying with teachers you trust and focusing on poses that are safe for your anatomical reality. No yoga teacher can force you to do anything you don't want to do. If you feel pressured into a particular pose, don't go back to that class. You are more important than any teacher, pose, or system of yoga.

Pain and Your Practice

We firmly believe there is some pain on the path to freedom—after all, we come with pain and yoga reveals it—but yoga should decrease the amount of pain in your life. If yoga does not decrease your pain it's time to question your practice. Eddie sums it up nicely: if there is pain and intensity in your *asana* but no pain in your life, then your yoga practice is effective. If there is no pain in your *asana* but lots of pain in your life, then your yoga practice is ineffective.

Foundations

EDDIE:
Sitting on a couch doesn't hurt but sitting on the floor in a yoga pose might. Does that mean the yoga pose caused your pain? No, the pose simply revealed it. The couch is a band-aid, a way of pushing pain down the road. Yoga will bring that pain into focus and provide tools to remove it from your body, but it's important to remember that yoga is the messenger not the culprit.

Foundations

Developing an internal dialogue with your pain is essential to a sustainable yoga practice but it's difficult to make a discussion of pain relevant to everyone. Pain thresholds vary widely from one person to the next and only you know what you really feel. We can, however, establish certain guidelines in relationship to pain. First and foremost, always move away from pain in your joints, especially white, sharp, hot pain. The ligaments that connect bone to bone in your joints are not vascularized, meaning there is no blood flowing through them. Stretching them usually results in pain that feels white. Ligaments can't bounce back like muscles; instead of stretching and contracting they may loosen or tear.

All of your joints are crisscrossed with ligaments so don't overlook even the slightest discomfort in your knees, shoulders, ankles, etc. The tiniest twinge, while easily ignored, can be the beginning of a much larger problem. Taking care of your body means listening very carefully to what it is telling you.

Pain in your muscles is generally safer unless it's located very close to where the muscle meets a joint. Muscles become narrow as they insert into the connective sheath that attaches them to your bones, and that's where they are most vulnerable to rips and tears. You definitely want to avoid pain in those areas, such as the top of your hamstrings where they attach to your sit bones. Always try to move the stretch (and the sensation it brings) into the middle of the muscle, where it is broadest, strongest, and most resilient. And that pain, the pain of urging sleepy tissues into action and imploring your stiff, congested areas to open up, is exactly the pain we expect to find on the path to freedom. Guruji called it "sweet pain."

If you are following the lines of yoga and still encountering pain, don't give up. Yoga is boundless and there are many tools available to you. The first is to simplify: deconstruct the main elements of the pose and approach each action individually. Box on the wall is a great example: if *adho mukha svanasana* (downward facing dog) hurts your wrists, do box on the wall instead. It teaches the same work as *adho mukha svanasana*, primarily the strengthening of the inner triad of your hands, but creates less pressure in your wrists and lower back. After a few days or weeks of box on the wall try *adho mukha svanasana* again, and see if you have developed enough strength in your arms and legs to do the pose safely and effectively.

You can also use another pose, or series of poses, to teach your body the necessary actions. Backbends are a great example: if backbends hurt your lower back it may mean your quadriceps and psoas are tight. Spend a few weeks or months opening those areas with our lunges and a great pose we call King Arthur, and then slowly incorporate backbends back into your practice.

There are many overlapping anatomical actions in yoga, and that overlap reinforces the importance of understanding the principles of posturally integrated alignment. You need to understand what each *asana* is trying to DO in your body. Once you do, you'll find there are many other *asana*s utilizing the same action but approaching it from a different direction. This will help you identify a more accessible version of the pose while continuing to develop your anatomy in the direction of yoga.

The End of Pain

Personal yoga practice is always about you: your healing and personal evolution. If something about your practice causes pain, listen to it. There is no sense in becoming a martyr to your yoga practice.

Taking personal responsibility for your pain means understanding that not every *asana* is perfect for you. Some poses, regardless of how easy or attractive they may seem, might not be appropriate for you right now. Other poses might never be appropriate, and that's totally fine. There are many, many other *asana*s—as many *asana*s as there are living beings on this planet.

Yoga has a lot more to offer than the pursuit of a single pose or of a single sequence. It's not really about poses; it's about changing your body. The poses are just tools. If one of them is painful or ineffective, try another one. BKS Iyengar said your body is a temple and *asana*s are your prayers. There are thousands of prayers, and no one can say one prayer is more important than another. The gods will listen to them all.

HYPEREXTENSION

Joints are areas of the body where bones come together to facilitate movement in the skeleton; i.e. your knees, elbows and neck. A joint's natural range of motion is defined by: 1) bony restrictions and 2) the presence of ligaments, which are inflexible white tissue. Hyperextension is the extension of a joint beyond its natural range of motion via an extension of the joint's ligaments. Ligaments, unlike elastic muscle tissue, will not return to their former shape or length once they have been extended beyond it. Extending a ligament breaks down the architecture of the joint and in doing so renders it 1) susceptible to long-term

Foundations

NICKI:
It's okay to have poses you don't like but you have to think about why you don't like them. Is it because they're hard or because they're painful? I had to work really hard to get *pincha mayurasana* (forearm balance) out of my lower back. My shoulders were stiff and it was so hard to press my hands down and stretch my legs up to get the pressure out of my lower back. But I had faith in yoga. I knew I could get rid of the pain if I did the work, and I did. But it's a fine line. If the pain is hot and sharp, like a knife, don't force it. But if the pain is in the middle of a muscle, don't worry about it too much. Sometimes we need to push ourselves past our limitations to find relief.

damage and 2) less capable of performing its intended function, such as keeping your knees in place.

Hyperextension is detrimental for another reason, one closely connected to the subject of flexibility. If you're recruiting the flexibility to do a specific pose by hyperextending your ligaments, you're not actually penetrating the muscles or set of muscles the pose is designed to affect. And if you're not creating the intended action of the pose, you're not moving your anatomy in the direction of yoga. Correcting hyperextension puts the work of *asana* back into your muscles, thereby protecting your joints and ligaments and moving your body toward posturally integrated alignment.

Foundations

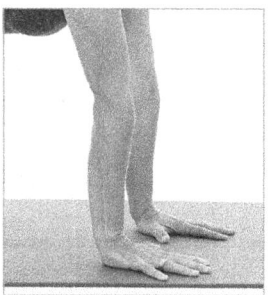

Hyperextended arms

Avoiding hyperextension seems like it should be easy; just back away from any "stretching" feeling in the white tissue of your joints: the front of the knee, back of the knee, front of the shoulder, inner and outer elbows, etc. But the tricky thing about hyperextension is it usually doesn't hurt. People who are prone to hyperextension in their joints don't feel like they're hyperextended; their hyperextension feels totally normal and straight. Furthermore, hyperextension can be very difficult to observe in your own body. You may be able to see it in a pose like downward dog but detecting hyperextension in *uttanasana* is nearly impossible.

We'll explain various ways to look for hyperextension in specific postures but the general rule is this: draw a line between three connecting joints, and if the middle joint is 1) outside of that line and 2) moving counter to the joint's normal range of motion, it is hyperextended. In your arm, the three joints are the wrist, elbow and shoulder; in your leg they're the ankle, knee and hip. Pay close attention to your arms and legs to figure out if they're straight, and if they're not (i.e. they're hyperextended) micro-bend them until the hyperextended joint is back in line with its neighboring joints. Most people need only the tiniest adjustment, hence the "micro" bend; bending the line in the opposite direction is equally ineffective. Straight is straight and bent is bent, and you must learn to see the difference.

Hyperextension is not limited to the movement of your knees, elbows and wrists; it can also apply to extremely important structural components like the sacroiliac joint, the 12th thoracic vertebrae, and the occipital condyles at the base of your skull (where your head attaches to your neck). Hyperextension and hypermobility in these areas usually go unnoticed until there's an injury, which underlines the importance of working with experienced instructors who understand the lines of yoga.

RECRUITING

Recruiting is similar to hyperextension: it involves a lack of structural integrity that obstructs the intended action of the *asana*, thus rendering your effort ineffective. The root cause of recruiting is very simple. Your tissue is always looking for the path of least resistance, and when it encounters stiffness in a particular area it avoids the stiffness by recruiting flexibility from somewhere else.

You can recruit flexibility in any *asana* but lunges are particularly susceptible. The lunges open your hips by moving your legs around your pelvis and spine, but your spine is inherently more flexible than your hips; it is a chain of small, connected joints working together to provide a range of movement far surpassing that of your gargantuan hip socket. When you confront your stiff hips in a lunge they may simply pull on your spine instead of doing the work themselves. It may feel like you're doing the pose, but in reality you're recruiting flexibility from your back instead of developing it in your hips and legs.

To illustrate, try this simple experiment. It works best when standing in front of a full-length mirror. Stand with your feet together and your hands on your hips. Bend your right knee and lift it to the height of your hips, keeping your left leg as straight as possible. If you are having trouble with balance, put one of your hands on a wall to stabilize yourself. Now use your hand(s) (or the mirror) to check out your hips. The action of lifting your leg probably shifted your hips to the right, lifted your right hip higher than your left, and made the right side of your waist shorter than the left.

Why did lifting half of your leg affect the rest of your body? Because the leg bone is connected to the hip bone, and the hip bone is connected to the back bone, and the back bone is connected to the…Well, you get the point. That ripple effect is the result of recruiting. Lifting your leg would not affect your back if your hips and legs were open; your femur would slide smoothly in your hip socket, your pelvis would remain neutral, and your spine would stay equally extended. But most of us do not have perfectly open hips and legs so the action comes from your spine instead.

If your hips didn't move at all in that exercise, they may be relatively open. Flexibility is a good thing, right? Unfortunately, the more flexible you are the more careful you have to be about recruiting. Try straightening your right leg and lifting it higher. See how far you can go before your hips start to pull on your spine (or your left leg, which may start to bend). Watch your feet, ankles, legs,

Foundations

Foundations

pelvis and spine; once your hips run into stiffness, they'll borrow flexibility from anywhere they can get it. And if you're naturally flexible you will have a lot of places to get it from.

Recruiting is bad for two reasons. First, it prohibits you from getting into those really stiff, congested areas, such as your hips. They'll keep hiding behind the veil of your more flexible joints: lower back, knees, ankles, etc. Second, recruiting creates dangerous patterns that contribute to long-term destabilization of those "flexible" joints. Sure, they're more flexible than your other joints, but they are simply not designed to get dragged around all the time. Recruiting can wreak havoc on wrists, ankles and knees and contribute to serious injuries such as slipped discs; when legs and hips are stiff, your lower back may do all the bending intended for your pelvis. Remember: you're doing yoga and yoga demands personal responsibility.

Yoga is not about finding the easiest way to do each pose it's about finding the most effective way to do each pose. When you're doing a particular *asana* keep the action of the pose focused on the area that needs its attention. This is especially relevant for flexible people. Being flexible gives you the capacity to recruit both flexibility and strength from the wrong places. Recruiting in this way may prohibit you from uncovering hidden stiff spots and may also keep you from gaining structural balance in your muscles and bones.

CHECK, CHECK, AND CHECK AGAIN

Yoga is a sequential process; you have to accomplish the first anatomical action before you can proceed to the next one. But it's not a simple single-directional task. Each additional principle of alignment builds on the previous action and each new action can affect the previously established foundations. As you progress through a pose you have to 1) check and maintain your foundations and 2) review the previous anatomical actions in sequential order. You have to check, check, and check again. If you cannot maintain one action of the pose don't move on to a more complicated one.

Yoga will challenge your internal somatic perception. Your mind is full of misleading notions about where and how you hold your body, what muscles you use, and the areas of your anatomy under your control. Yoga is the process of moving from who you think you are to recognizing who you really are, and it requires that you undergo personal scrutiny. There's a Sutra for it: *te prati prasavah heya sukshmaha*. The moment you think you know everything is the most dangerous moment of all. Those moments require you to be hyper-vigilant; to check, check, and check again.

This approach might seem nit-picky and tedious but it's important because it's YOU. This is your body, not someone else's, and taking the time to look at yourself is the first step toward self-realization. Every little anatomical refinement is another opportunity to explore your body, your vessel, your temple, the glorious creation that is you. How much time do you have in your busy life to truly look at YOU? Probably not very much, so appreciate each moment. You have an amazing body and yoga is an invitation to do the best you can with it. Hopefully this process will teach you to accept yourself and love yourself completely because you are absolutely deserving of love.

Yoga is a metamorphosis; you start as a caterpillar and end up as a butterfly. Your skeleton should change, and when it changes to reflect the lines of yoga, you've tapped into the deep undercurrent of collective human consciousness. That's why we're such sticklers for proper alignment; doing yoga is like using your bones to tune your mind to the frequency of the universe.

HANDS AND FEET

Yoga is meticulous about foundations. The foundations of *asana* are almost always your hands and feet, and we teach very specific alignment principles for each one. They are called the alignment of the foot and the inner triad of the hand. Both principles are designed to extend the inner line of your arms and legs because most of us are longer on the outside of our limbs than on the inside. This imbalance comes from stiffness in your hips and shoulders; they pull on the inseam of your arms and legs like a big congestion magnet. You can see it in a beginner's seated forward bend: the big toe bone is sucked backward and the pinkie toe falls forward. In a beginner's downward dog, the knuckle of the index finger is pulled away from the mat and weight falls into the outer wrist.

The alignment of the foot and the inner triad of the hand assert the inseam of each appendage because these areas have the greatest ability to penetrate the large joints above them. The inner heel and big toe bone connect to the pubic bone, thus organizing the bones of the pelvis, and the inner triad of the hand connects to the center of the shoulder. Building clarity in your hands and feet will develop clarity in your joints, which will ultimately clarify your spine. It all eventually goes back to the spine; we're talking about organizing your hands and feet but those appendages are really just a gateway to your central axis. That's

EDDIE:
I had an opportunity to teach in front of BKS Iyengar and several of his most advanced students in Massachusetts when I had only been studying yoga for a few years. I was supposed to get the students warmed up before he arrived but I ended up teaching the entire class. I was terrified. After the class I had the nerve to ask him how I did, and he said, "You talk, and your students don't move." It was so profound. I knew all the directions and was moving through the poses on auto-pilot, despite the fact that most of the students weren't getting past the first instruction.

Those words completely changed the way I teach and the way I practice. You have to complete every action before you move to the next one, and if the action is difficult to complete, you have to stay there and figure it out. Luckily for us, there is always another way to explore the anatomical action; if you can't do downward dog, do box on the wall instead. Yoga is boundless like that—the ceiling is very high. But there are no shortcuts. You cannot develop a sustainable practice if you skip the foundations.

yoga's amazing progression. It starts on the outside with simple appendages but eventually moves inside to support your spine, brain and major organs. This physiological journey mirrors the metaphysical journey from your gross body, the *shtula sharira*, to your subtle energetic body, the *sukshma sharira*.

Alignment of the Foot

Foundations

Your feet are almost always connected to the ground. They're the first point of contact in your lifelong communication with the earth, and yoga is like a game of telephone: if your feet don't get the message, your hips are never going to get it. Exploring the alignment of the foot can be done in many poses but we'll use a simple standing posture.

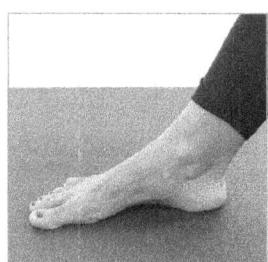
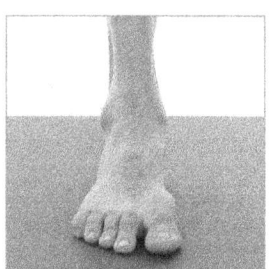
Alignment of the foot

1. Stand with your hands on your hips and step your right foot forward two to three feet in front of your left, enough to see it clearly.

2. Shift your heel slightly to the right to make the outer edge of your foot roughly parallel to the long side of your mat. Notice we said *roughly* parallel; the back of your foot is narrower than the front of your foot so it's not going to make a perfectly straight line. The goal is to put the center of your heel directly between your big toe and pinkie toe to create an even-sided triangle. Use your judgment.

3. Lift all five toes. Spread the big toe and pinkie toe away from each other, and then spread your second toe away from the third and the third away from the fourth.

4. Lift your right inner arch. If you can keep your arch lifted without lifting your toes, place your toes back down on the mat. If they start to become tense or grip the mat, lift them up again. Keep the weight of your foot squarely in the body of the foot itself, not in your toes.

5. Press firmly into your big toe bone. The "big toe bone" is not the big toe itself; it's the knuckle below the big toe and the corresponding "ball" underneath. Press firmly enough to create a depression in the skin between your big toe bone and your second toe bone. Root that area to the mat.

6. Lift your inner ankle bone to put your ankle directly over the center of your heel without disturbing the placement of your heel itself. Use the knobby bones on either side of your ankle as guides; make them level, without distorting your inner arch or making your big toe bone light. Press evenly between the knuckles of your foot and the center of your heel to spread the energy of your foot forward and down, like a root.

Once you've made it to the end of the list return to the very first direction. Watch how each step affects the next and figure out which actions are the most difficult to maintain. Repeat those actions, over and over again and in different poses, until your foot gets the message.

We call this work "organizing" the foot. It will develop a cellular memory of structural alignment in your feet and ankles. You'll have many opportunities to practice it in the upcoming section and it will eventually become second nature. But for now, remember to check, check, and check again. The alignment of the foot is especially important in the lunges and standing poses because feet and ankles are typically more flexible than hips. They're often the first thing to get pulled when you encounter stiffness, and if you recruit flexibility from your feet and ankles it will be difficult to develop flexibility in your hips.

Yoga is about developing connective passageways between your brain and your tissues, allowing you to fully occupy your own body. We want you to saturate your body with your awareness. The longest gap in this process exists between your brain and your foot: they're further apart than anything else. Extending your consciousness all the way to your big toe establishes the longest passageway.

The Inner Triad

The inner triad of the hand consists of the index finger knuckle, the base of the thumb, and the base of the inner wrist. These three points create a triangle and this triangle should carry the majority of weight in all poses that use the hands as a foundation. Pressurizing the inner triad protects the pisiform bone, a tiny bone in your outer wrist that is the smallest bone in the appendicular skeleton. Allowing weight to fall to the sides of your hands in a pose like downward dog forces the pisiform to bear the brunt of the pose—and that's not sustainable.

Foundations

EDDIE:
This work should carry through your entire practice. When we say to "organize" your foot and ankle in a specific pose, we want you to do everything on this list. Learn it well and it will become second nature.

Using the inner triad to organize the weight in your hands also balances the muscles of your lower and upper arm. It develops a straight line through the wrist, elbow, and shoulder of each arm. This straight line translates the energy of the pose from your hands to your shoulders and from your shoulders to your spine.

1. Start on hands and knees with your wrists directly underneath your shoulders.

2. Look at your wrist creases—the horizontal line where your hand meets your wrist—and make them parallel to the front of your mat.

3. Lift the middle finger of each hand to expose the bone that runs from the knuckle of your middle finger to the center of your wrist. Make those bones perpendicular to your wrist creases and then put your middle fingers back on the mat.

4. Point your middle fingers straight forward and spread the rest of your fingers evenly. Keep your pinkie and thumb as evenly spaced as the rest of your fingers. Let your thumb follow the natural line of your palm; overstretching your pinkie and thumb will narrow the carpal tunnel at the base of your wrist.

5. Bring your awareness to the inner triad: the base of the index finger knuckle, the base of the thumb knuckle, and the base of the inner wrist. These three points should form a relatively even triangle.

6. Connect your mind to the points of this triangle and press it firmly into the mat. Check to see if that action disturbed the alignment in your wrists or fingers. Adjust as necessary, reapply the action of the inner triad, and then check again. The knuckle of the index finger should be the center of the action, moving energy forward and down. This action decreases pressure in the outer wrist and translates the action of the pose from hands to shoulders.

Holding weight in the inner triad must be practiced diligently until the shape of yoga is written into your hands and clearly visible in every weight-bearing pose. *Adho mukha svanasana* is the easiest pose to examine and solidify this relation-

Foundations

EDDIE:
Press the knuckle of your index finger into the mat so firmly I wouldn't be able to peel it off. Press it down and keep it down. Don't let it get light at any point because if it's light, it's ineffective.

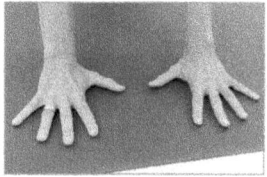
Inner Triad - proper placement

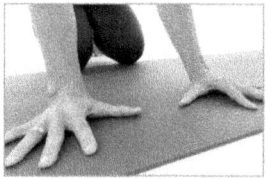
Improper placement - index finger knuckle is lifted off the mat

ship so try to make it a daily practice. Put every ounce of your consciousness into refining the structure of your hands before moving on to more difficult arm-balancing *asanas*. This concept of building sequentially and intelligently is at the core of yoga.

THRESHOLDS

Thresholds represent your personal edge. They are the line between what you currently know and what you are capable of learning. Navigating your threshold is like being on a cliff; you have to walk to the edge to see the incredible view, but if you get too close you'll fall off. Likewise, you learn the most when you explore the edge of your practice. It gives you a glimpse of what's beyond without actually taking you there, which is why Prashant Iyengar says the pose always "begins" when you want to come out. That's when you've found your edge. The things that speak loudest to you in that moment are the elements that require the most attention. They illustrate your individual road map to anatomical freedom. Going beyond your threshold is the anatomical equivalent to falling off the cliff: it removes your ability to interpret your body's feedback.

There are three indicators of being at (or beyond) your threshold. The first is breath. *Ujayii pranayama* measures your connectivity to your physical experience. If you are gasping for air, breathing out of your mouth or holding your breath, you should retreat from the edge. Find a more restful pose, like *balasana* (child's pose), return to steady *ujayii pranayama* and then resume your practice.

The second indicator is the shaking of the limbs, known in Sanskrit as *anga-medjayatva* (awn-guh-me-jai-uht-vah). Doing something new with your body—like lifting your kneecaps—requires a reprogramming in the neurology of the muscles. You are developing new passageways between mental synapse and muscular response. Shaking is indicative of this process and it is totally normal. You're approaching the load capacity for your internal circuitry so things are bound to get a little shaky. The fact that this shaking has a Sanskrit name means people have been dealing with it for thousands of years. You are not alone in your experience. But if you can't control the shaking with your mind or your breath, you must come out of the pose before you blow a fuse.

The third indicator of being at or beyond your threshold is when the pose has plateaued and your actions are no longer ascending. It's when you've lost the thread that connects you to the lines of yoga; when you feel totally defeated in your body and mind. When that happens do not stay in the pose by willpower alone. When you're done, you're done. And while retreating from the edge may feel like a crisis or a lack of determination you must learn to see it as an opportunity. Exploring those moments and the feedback they create is crucial to understanding and unraveling your limitations. They sit at the apex of who you are and who you are able to become.

Front Door vs. Back Door

Foundations

Most students have different thresholds for different poses; maybe you happily spend ten minutes in *balasana* (child's pose) but race through *chataranga dandasana* (four-limbed staff pose) like you're being chased. It's okay; we all have poses we like and poses we dislike. The poses you like tend to be the ones that are easy for you to do. Most students gravitate toward these poses, especially in the beginning, because ease and accomplishment are appealing emotions. We call these "front door" poses because you can breeze right through them. There's nothing particularly wrong with the front door but yoga is a practice of finding balance. If you spend all your time at the front door you'll lose the key to the back door.

NICKI: You have to be willing to dig underneath your aversion to those poses and to dig underneath your aversion to other things in your life because aversions will really limit you. Be open.

Your "back door" is made up of all the poses you dislike. It's the poses you skip through as fast as possible, the ones that reveal your weaknesses and restrictions. Start paying attention to those poses. Study their principles of alignment to identify the parts of your body that deviate from the lines of yoga, and use that information as a blueprint for your personal practice. Start knocking on the back door. Unlocking it will let the light into your practice and your life.

Kiki

Yoga reveals what is already inside your body and mind. The poses do not create pain or frustration; they do not clench your teeth or leave you in despair, nor do they contain any of the negative energy you may ascribe to them. Those elements are already inside of you, the poses simply reveal their presence. It is a difficult concept to process because our culture does not encourage personal responsibility. We are socialized to project frustration and negativity onto everything and everyone around us. Sometimes that means blaming yoga for your back pain, which is only detrimental to you and your relationship with yoga, but it more often entails projection onto your most personal relationships—partners, children, and friends—and those projections almost always bring us pain.

Personal responsibility is at the core of yoga. Pay attention to the poses you don't like because they hold the greatest opportunity for change. These poses represent both a crisis and an opportunity, a concept neatly enshrined in the Japanese word "kiki." The poses you do not like are the kikis of life. In the beginning they are a crisis. They push you around and uncover your stiffness, and your first reaction is to retreat. *I don't like that pose. I don't want to do it.* Underneath this defensive reaction lies your greatest teacher, the catalyst of personal evolution. If you let down your walls and turn the projections inward these poses can set you on the path to personal awareness. Changing your relationship to these poses is equivalent to changing your relationship with yourself. It's personal evolution, and collectively, it has the power to create a profound spiritual revolution.

PERSONAL PRACTICE

Yoga is a self-reliant healing system. It teaches you to look inward for answers because you possess the ability to help yourself. You can be the solution to your mental, physical, and emotional problems of the past, present, and future. But you have to work for it. Healing yourself through yoga is an independent task. The *asana*s are your roadmap and we can be your guides but the work is entirely your own. It's just like Rumi said: "How can you get the pay if you haven't done the work?"

You are completely unique and your personal practice should reflect that. It should be comprised of the *asana*s that most effectively integrate your unique body with the lines of yoga. Your personal practice is not something you can find in a regular yoga class because you do not require the same work as the person next to you. Modern yoga generally puts the flow of the class above the needs of the individual but yoga should be an involution; it should focus on your personal needs and experience. Classes are a great way to check in with your teachers and with the *sanga*, or community, but the real work is personal. You owe it to yourself to develop a personal practice that contains enough mental and physical space to connect with you.

When it comes to developing your personal practice dedication is more important than duration. Your practice doesn't have to be several hours long and it doesn't have to follow the format of a modern yoga class. It should be a regular practice (at least three to five days of the week) and that means it has to fit into your daily life. You're a busy person so start small and simple. Pick three

Foundations

NICKI:
On my first trip to Mysore, Guruji told me the two highest forms of yoga are being in a relationship and having a child. In my first few years of Ashtanga yoga, my practice dictated my life. Having children finally taught me *vairagyabyam*, which is non-attachment. I had to let go of some of the physical aspects of the practice to make room for my children. My early years with yoga were very self-indulgent but that's not what yoga is about; it's not about isolating yourself to polish your spiritual mirror. It's about relationships: relationships with yourself and with the people around you. It is a life support system. Some days I only get to do a 15 minute practice and I am grateful for that because it means my life is full of other meaningful relationships.

postures that are personally significant to you and do them as often as you can manage. Don't pick three postures you're really good at, pick three postures that challenge you. Apply yourself to those three poses, even if it's just for ten minutes every day, and we guarantee you they will change. And if the poses are changing, you are changing too.

Those small changes develop *shraddha*: faith in yoga. You have to see and feel the changes in yourself, big or small, to develop the faith to move forward.

We want you to develop a long-term relationship with yoga. Hopefully the positive effects of a small, simple personal practice will inspire a more substantial practice, but it's okay if it doesn't. Doing a little bit of yoga on a regular basis is much more effective than doing massive amounts of yoga sporadically. But remember, yoga can only give as much as it receives.

Guiding Your Personal Practice

Working with an experienced yoga teacher (or teachers) is essential to developing and guiding your personal practice. Your body may require very specific instructions and you cannot get that kind of personalized attention from a book—nor from a mediocre yoga class. It is important to check in with your teachers frequently because your specific instructions will change as your body moves toward the lines of yoga. Directions that are appropriate for you now may not be appropriate a few months from now. Any anatomical direction can be overdone, sometimes to the point of injury, and a good teacher will help you safely navigate this personal evolution.

Choose your teachers carefully. There are many brilliant teachers out there who are deserving of your time and respect and this book will never be able to take their place. Selecting your yoga teacher should be just as important as selecting a physician, and deciding which yoga classes to attend should be just as important as deciding to pursue a particular medical treatment.

Finally, don't stop going to yoga classes. We have been practicing yoga for decades and we still make time to study with our teachers because there is always more to learn. We hope you will be more discerning about the teachers and classes you choose but your personal practice cannot replace your *sanga*, or community. Guruji was always very clear about that: as students it was our responsibility to return to our community and cultivate yoga. Many of his Western students would want to stay in India forever but he would push them away because they were not from India. They needed to go home, to their families and

---

Foundations

NICKI:
The teacher breathes life into the teachings. This practice is about connections: connections between you and your teacher, between you and yoga, and between you and your Self.

NICKI:
It is important to explore different teachings but you can't just dabble. Different systems emphasize different things and if you flutter between them none of it will penetrate. Find a teacher or a system you like and give them at least a year of your attention and practice. Once you have truly learned their work you can decide if it is right for you.

communities, and share this work. Yoga has a profound vibrational effect that must be shared to be realized.

Lighten Up

The concepts in this section probably make yoga seem pretty heavy but it doesn't have to be serious all the time. It doesn't even have to be spiritual; doing yoga to gain flexibility and physical fitness is perfectly valid. You don't have to be looking for personal evolution every time you get on your mat and you don't always have to chase your pain. You are absolutely welcome to practice for the sake of practicing. Use the postures to work up a sweat, connect to your breath, and quiet your mind. Sometimes the best way to get rid of your stress and anxiety is to stop giving them your attention.

Yoga is all about balance. If your practice is getting you down, stop overanalyzing it. It shouldn't be a form of self-flagellation. Try to move a little bit more; use a dynamic sequence to lighten your being and cultivate joy. If your practice is not affecting your consciousness at all, start analyzing it. Try staying in the poses long enough to let them reveal your patterns and use that feedback to discover yourself. Whatever your practice may be, make sure it truly serves you.

Your life does not need to revolve around your yoga practice. Your yoga practice should support your life, whatever it is you choose to do. It should integrate your life, not disintegrate it. Sometimes your practice will fall apart but it will always be there for you, waiting patiently, until you are ready to put it back together. And sometimes your life will fall apart and yoga will be right there, patiently waiting to remind you that you are completely deserving of your own love and attention.

Let your practice be something that makes you happy. An *asana* is a posture of the mind and heart, just as much as a posture of the body. All of these *asana*s are tools and when you use them effectively they will begin to open the windows of your body and soul—whether or not you're looking for it. Eddie calls it using your bones to tune your mind to the frequency of the universe. Every pose turns the dial and eventually you'll stumble upon the right channel. In other words, if you're doing the poses accurately spiritual evolution will find you.

Foundations

EDDIE:
Stay simple. You can't remodel the whole temple of your being in a single day because you have to keep living there. Don't break down all the walls of your anatomy at once. Move slowly, sustainably, and be compassionate. We want you to be happy.

NICKI:
I still practice the Primary Series of Ashtanga yoga on a regular basis because it's fun. It's familiar, it's joyful, and it lightens my being—and sometimes I need that. I also do poses that challenge me but yoga isn't always about digging into the darkest parts of your psyche. It is also about love, compassion, and joy. Please don't get too serious about this stuff. It's hard enough as it is.

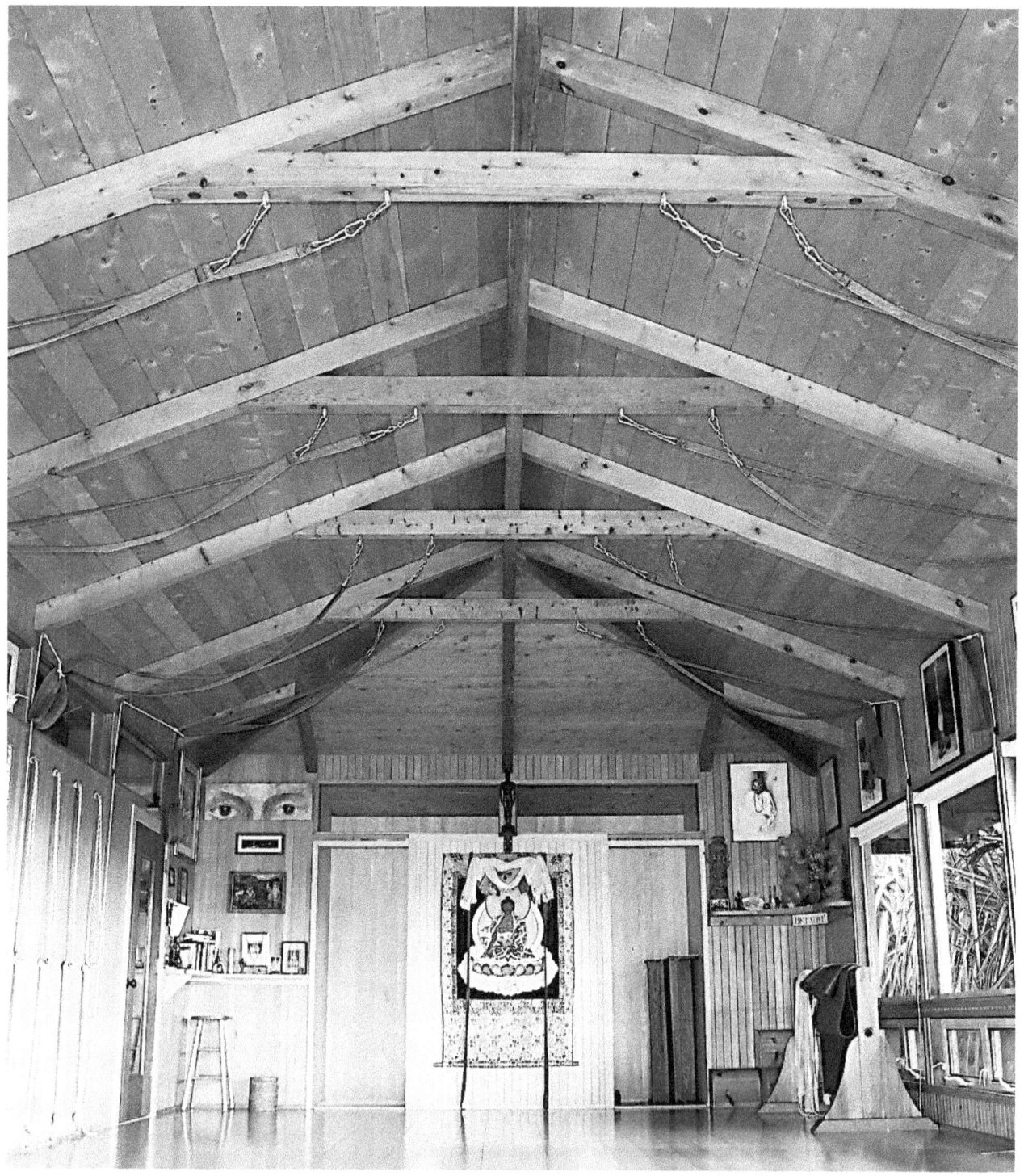

WARM UP POSES

Yoga is 99% practice and 1% theory.
—PATTABHI JOIS

The following chapters describe fundamental *asanas* (poses) in the order we introduce them to beginning practitioners. You can use them as a manual for your entire practice or as a reference for specific *asanas*. The book concludes with several introductory sequences, all of which draw on the poses described within. Poses are presented in the following format:

Pose Name
Sanskrit pronunciation | Sanskrit translation

Pose introduction (when necessary).

1. Numbered instructions

STEP 1: Expanded instructions for specific steps, including energetic action and the anatomical rationale behind individual movements.

SHANTI PATH MANTRA

The Student-Teacher Agreement

Our Sutra teacher instructed us to chant this mantra before every class. Begin by chanting *Aum* three times to clear the mental cobwebs, reset vibrational energy and create a space for your practice.

Aum, Aum, Aum

Sahana vavatu

Sahanau bunaktu

Sahaviryam karavavahai

Tejas vinav ahditamastu

Mavidvishavahai

Aum shanti shanti shanti

This mantra is directed to Lord Brahma, guardian of the creative spirit in all of us. As we undertake the practice of yoga, the rebirthing of our Self, we ask for several things. First, may all sentient beings everywhere feel safe and shrouded in protection from both external violence and internal torment. If we, as individuals, can ever provide protection or nourishment for another living being, let us not hesitate to act.

Second, may all sentient beings feel nourished, not only with the external needs of food, water, and shelter but also the deeper needs of spirit and soul. Let us work together with courage, strength, and determination so everything we do—our studies, our practice, and our relationships—may be bright and effective. May all the qualities we strive to cultivate in our practice—honesty, integrity, and compassion—weave themselves into the fabric of our lives so we may begin to truly live our yoga.

Finally, let us not bring hatred or dispute amongst each other and certainly not among systems of yoga. If the practice is sincere all roads lead to the same destination: ultimate freedom of body, mind, and heart. *Aum*; peace of the past, peace of the present, and peace for the future.

THE SEAT

The seat is yoga's most humble and holy posture. It begins as a simple crossed-legged position but evolves into some of yoga's most advanced poses: *padmasana*, *siddhasana*, and *swastikasana*. In fact, all of yoga's *asana*s are designed to facilitate evolution of the seat. They remove congestion from your body so you can sit still for long enough to meditate. That's what it's all about: becoming comfortable enough with yourself, inside and out, to transcend your physical, mental, and emotional confines. It is a fantastic journey that begins and ends in the seat.

The seat is a great place to start your practice. It allows you to connect with your breath and your *bandha*s, and is also the traditional *asana* for *kirtan* chanting (call and response). *Kirtan* is a form of *pranayama* that regulates the breath and calms the mind, and we often begin with five to twenty minutes of this practice. Sitting upright for twenty minutes of chanting is a wonderfully grounding experience, unless you spend the whole time thinking about how much your back hurts. Pain makes you fidget and if you're fidgeting you're not focused. Focus requires stillness. To be still in your seat, physically and mentally, you have to be comfortable.

Warm Up Poses

EDDIE:
The seat is the setting for the jewel of your being. It allows you to present yourself to your Self.

Why is the seat so uncomfortable? For most of us, sitting on the floor is uncomfortable because our bodies are accustomed to chairs. Chairs have changed the spinal pathology of the Western world. They shorten the psoas, close the front of the pelvis and stiffen the hips and legs. Most of the stuff we do in chairs, such as working on computers, causes us to hunch over and move our shoulders toward our chest. It rounds the upper back and contributes to a chronic shortening of the front body. But chairs are completely unavoidable; we eat, drive, learn, work, and sometimes sleep in them. Almost everything in the Western world is done in a chair or on a couch. The solution, of course, is yoga.

Warm Up Poses

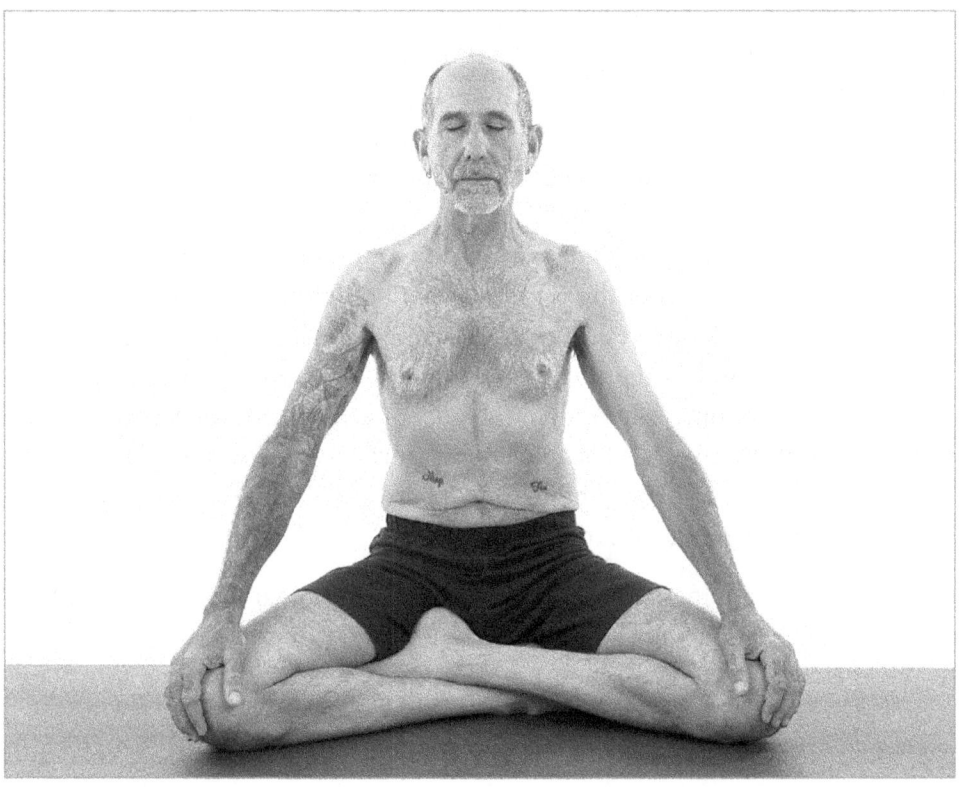

4.a The Seat

EDDIE:
We have made a lot of progress in this world, but progress has side effects. The side effect of furniture is comfort and comfort brings atrophy. The side effect of modern life is stress and stress brings disease. Yoga is the antidote to both of these toxins.

Sukhasana
sook·has·ahn·nuh | *easy pose*

1. Sit on the floor. Bend your knees and bring your feet toward your pelvis. Cross your legs just above the ankles and relax your knees.

Warm Up Poses

2. If your knees are off the ground, come out of the pose and put props under your sit bones. Use as many props as you need to bring your hips higher than your knees and to address any discomfort.

3. Close your eyes and press evenly into both sit bones.

4. Bring your shoulders directly over your hips. Soften your shoulders to lift your chest. Maintain space in your back body.

5. Stay here and breathe. *(4.a)*

STEP 1: Start in a simple seated position. Sit up straight and look closely at the relationship between your pelvis and knees. If your hips are stiff, sitting cross-legged on the floor pulls your knees off the ground; your legs cannot externally rotate in relation to your pelvis so they go up instead. Your knees might be an inch or two off the ground or they may be closer to your elbows than your navel—and that's totally fine. That's how Eddie was when he started doing yoga 30 years ago. He was really, really stiff.

Stiff hips may also pull your sacrum down, forcing you to sit on the back of your sit bones instead of the center of your sit bones. Sitting on the back of your sit bones may injure your lumbar discs; your hips are recruiting flexibility from your spine, and in the long run your spine will not appreciate it. It also creates a corresponding rounding in the upper back that makes it difficult to sit upright. This stiff-person seat is not very comfortable—knees are up, lower back is rounded and upper back is hunched forward—and we don't want you to be uncomfortable. We want you to be happy.

STEP 2: To find happiness, elevate your sit bones until your hips are higher than your knees. Elevating your hips allows your legs to externally rotate in relation to your pelvis. Putting the rotation in your hip socket takes the pressure out of your knees, ankles and lower back. We like to use thick blankets but you can use whatever you have available: bolsters, blocks, books—anything solid and stable. Stack these props under your sit bones until your knees are below your leg crease, which is the line in your groin where your hip meets your upper thigh. This should create a gentle slope from your hips to your knees so that a marble placed on your upper thigh would roll toward your knees instead of your groin.

Once you have established a comfortable height, sit for a moment to see if anything else comes up. If your ankles, knees, or lower back start to hurt, get more props and take your pose higher. Don't judge yourself for using props, even if you use a lot of them. If you feel discomfort in one of your knees try putting a folded blanket under it. If you feel discomfort in both of your knees put more props under your sit bones. Experiment to find what works for you. Use as many props as it takes to sit comfortably. Props can be very effective tools when they are used intelligently as part of a steadily ascending practice that maintains the foundations and listens closely to indications of pain.

STEP 3: Once you are comfortably seated close your eyes and let your awareness fall to your sit bones. Take a couple breaths and see if you can discern which side of your pelvis is heavier. The goal is to have your sit bones evenly weighted but we rarely begin with perfect alignment. Soften your internal judgment and expand your internal awareness. See if your weight falls more to the left or right and if it balances more to the front of your sit bones or the back. This is very subtle work. It may take months or years to identify your patterns, but beginning this journey is a huge part of developing a personal practice. It helps you figure out which hip is tighter, and then which shoulder carries more stiffness, and will eventually unravel all the asymmetries of your body and mind.

STEP 4: Bring your shoulders over your hips and align your sternum directly over your pubic bone. Press your sit bones down and lift your chest, but do not lift your chest by compressing your back body; that action will compress your kidneys. Allow your shoulders to fall away from your ears and move toward your back body. Place your hands on your thighs.

STEP 5: Stay there and breathe. If you are squirming in your seat after just a couple minutes, you haven't really found it yet. Learn to look at yourself and find clarity in your alignment. The alignment of your body affects and influences the alignment of your mind. Keep searching for center. Finding center in your anatomy will help you find center in the rest of your life.

Visit your seat on a regular basis and alternate your legs to reveal patterns on both sides of your hips.

Anjali Mudra
aun·jaw·lee moo·drah | *open or folded hands*

Anjali means "folded or open hands" and a *mudra* is a symbolic way of holding the body. Patanjali, the great Indian sage and oldest known teacher of yoga, means "one who falls into open or folded hands." Receiving the wisdom of yoga means opening your mind to its infinite possibilities, and you can begin this work with the simple placement of your hands.

1. Bring your palms together in a "prayer" position.
2. Align your fingertips, the base of your palms, and the knuckles of your inner triads.
3. Allow the center of your palms to separate.

Warm Up Poses

NICKI: Wipe the slate clean. Make room in yourself to receive these teachings, and let them grow in fertile ground.

This slight separation creates a sacred space between your palms, protected within the symmetry of your hands. This small space is symbolic of the internal space necessary for these teachings to fall into your being. Allow that space to be reflected in your mind, even if it means forgetting everything you already know about yoga. Cultivate a beginner's mind. It's a difficult thing to maintain, especially if you already know a lot about yoga, but it is an essential part of this work.

MARMA
maar·mah | *killing points*

*Marma*s are energy points within your body. They are similar to acupressure points in Chinese medicine and many healing modalities recognize them as a bridge between the external body and internal organs. *Marma* points are also called "killing points" because they identify areas of disease. Sensitivity in a particular *marma* is your body's red flag, indicating internal congestion that may eventually lead to your demise. They're your canary in the coal mine. It is a recurring theme: pay attention to pain and follow your pain to find freedom.

We begin almost every practice by stimulating four *marma* points: the neck, shoulders, wrists and ankles. These four *marmas* are believed to promote full-body flexibility, and it starts with your neck. Your neck is the bridge between your body and mind; the physical avatar of your metaphysical connection to the universe. It is home to essential parts of your lymphatic system, the internal locomotive of cleaning and filtration. It desperately needs to stay open but for many of us it is stiff, stressed, and congested.

Your neck is not designed to be stiff. The cervical spine—the seven vertebrae that make up your neck—supports an astounding range of motion. Your head moves up, down, left, right, and everything in between, all on the collective flexibility of your cervical vertebrae. It's an amazing structure. These *marma* exercises are a fantastic way to safely liberate your neck and develop the requisite flexibility for more advanced *asana*s. It is also a lovely way to start your day. But as with all things in yoga, proceed with intelligence. Never move toward sharp or burning sensations. Use your breath to remain connected to your experience. Be receptive so you may interpret even the subtlest feedback from your body.

1. Begin in your seat. Rest your hands on your thighs and close your eyes.
2. Press into your sit bones and lift your head to neutral.
3. Exhale and release your head toward your right shoulder *(4.b.1)*.
4. Inhale to center.
5. Exhale and release your head toward your left shoulder.
6. Inhale to center and repeat 3-4 times. Stay with your breath.
7. Pause in the center and then exhale to release your head forward. Keep your chest lifted *(4.b.2)*.
8. Inhale to return to center and exhale to release your head back. Keep your chest lifted *(4.b.3)*.
9. Inhale to center and repeat 3-4 times. Stay with your breath.
10. Pause with your chin at your chest, and then inhale as you roll to the right and back. Exhale to the left and forward. Keep your body completely still as you roll your neck. Complete 5-10 circles.
11. Pause with your chin at your chest and then switch sides, again completing 5-10 circles.
12. Bring your head to neutral and breathe.

Warm Up Poses

STEPS 1-2: Lift your head to neutral and feel its weight at the top of your spine. Press your sit bones down to sit up nice and tall, and then exhale and tilt your head to the right. Let the weight of your head bring your right ear close to your right shoulder. Do not push or force your head toward your shoulder; it's already very heavy, you just have to learn to let it go. Allow your tension to recede and let gravity do its thing.

Warm Up Poses

Use your internal awareness to determine if your head is tilted forward or back. Observe your patterns without judging them, and then adjust your head to bring your ear directly in line with your right shoulder. Soften both shoulders and relax your jaw. This exercise is focused on the *marma* points in your neck but it's easy to recruit flexibility from the rest of your spine. Keep everything below your neck completely still; don't let your body wiggle away from the opening. Your sit bones should be equally weighted and both sides of your waist should be equally extended.

STEPS 3–6: Inhale as you lift your head to neutral, and then exhale as you release your head to the opposite side (left). Breathe, soften, and try to let go. Be receptive to any differences between left and right. Spend a few breaths exploring each side and then begin to move with your breath. This is *vinyasa*, where breath and movement are seamlessly combined. Inhale up to center, exhale as you release to the right, inhale back up to center, exhale as you release to the left, and continue.

STEPS 7–9: After a few breaths to the left and right, switch directions; inhale to center and exhale as you release your head forward. Drop your chin toward your chest and pause, and then inhale and return to center. Keep your chest lifted and exhale as you release your head back. Lift your face, stretch your throat, and release your head back as much as is comfortable—do not force it. The lift of your face must be supported by a corresponding lift of your chest; if your chest is dropped, the back of your neck will be compressed. On your next inhale lift your head back to center. Initiate the lift from your chest, not from your chin or jaw. Try to make it a fluid movement.

STEPS 10–12: Exhale forward and pause, and then begin to roll your head in a circle. Inhale as you roll to the right and back, and exhale to the left and forward. Move slowly. Visualize a little pencil sticking straight out of the top of your head and use it to draw a circle in the air above you. Start with small circles and explore increasingly larger ones, but only go as far as is comfortable. You will likely find some flat areas in your circles, and that's fine. Don't judge those areas or rush to correct them, just watch them closely and begin to see your patterns. After a few rounds, pause with your head down and begin to roll in the opposite direction. Keep breathing and observe any changes that arise with the new direction.

Pause with your chin toward your chest, and then inhale to bring your head to neutral. Keep your eyes closed and keep breathing. The next *marma* is for your shoulders.

1. Find your seat.

2. Inhale and lift your shoulders up and back.

3. Exhale and roll them forward and down *(5.b.4)*.

4. Keep your hands still.

5. Pause and then reverse the direction.

Lift your shoulders up toward your ears, roll them forward and down, and then roll them back up toward your ears to make a circle. You can make little circles or big ones and move quickly or slowly, as long as you pay attention to what you are feeling. Yoga is research. Please learn to listen. Keep your spine lifted and your body still to direct the action more precisely into your shoulders. Your arms will certainly move a little bit but try to keep your hands still. Don't let your wrists contribute their flexibility to this exercise, keep it focused on your shoulders.

After a few rounds, pause and reverse the direction: inhale to roll forward and up and exhale as you roll back and down. The wrists are next.

1. Return to center and open your eyes.

2. Bend your elbows and bring your hands to eye level.

3. Interlace your fingers and press the tips of your thumbs together *(4.b.5)*.

4. Roll your right wrist up and forward and then the left.

5. Pause and reverse the direction.

STEPS 1–3: Bend your elbows and bring your hands to eye level and then interlace your fingers. Press the webbing between your fingers firmly together. Push the tips of your thumbs together and bend your wrists to 90° so the tops of your interlaced hands form a relatively flat surface. Place your wrists directly over your elbows and keep your forearms parallel. Apply a small amount of backward pressure, as though your wrists are trying to pull away from each other but your finger webbing keeps them glued together.

STEPS 4 & 5: Roll your right wrist up and forward as the left wrist goes back and down, and then roll your left wrist up and forward as your right wrist goes back and down. These actions should move your wrists in little circles. Keep your hands flat and your elbows directly under your wrists. Don't allow the webbing of your fingers to separate. If you follow these actions precisely, the rotation will be primarily in your wrists. Pause and then reverse the direction before moving on to your ankles.

Warm Up Poses

1. Release your hands and lean forward.
2. Uncross your legs and place your right lower leg on top of your left thigh, just above your left knee.
3. Wrap your right hand around your lower right shin, just above your ankle, and squeeze it to make your foot relax.
4. Hold your right toes with your left hand and roll your foot forward and down *(4.b.6)*.
5. Reverse the direction: roll your right foot up and back.
6. Release your right foot and slap the sole several times. *(4.b.7)*
7. Switch sides.

STEPS 1–3: If you are on a very tall stack of props, shift forward to sit on the floor. Uncross your legs and place your outer right shin on top of your lower left thigh, just above your left knee, so your right foot hangs freely. If this bothers your left knee at all, straighten your left leg. Wrap your right hand around your lower right shin, just above your ankle, and squeeze it to make your foot relax. The goal is to separate your foot from the muscles of your calf, and to do that you have to apply a decent amount of pressure just above the ankle joint.

STEPS 4–7: Interlace your left fingers with your right toes and use that grip to roll your right foot forward and down in a circular motion. Keep a tight grip on your lower right shin so the movement of your foot comes from the action of your left hand, not from the muscles of your right leg. Your right knee should stay relatively still. Now roll your ankle backward. Pause, release your left hand, and slap the sole of your foot several times. Switch sides and repeat.

We begin almost every practice by stimulating these four *marma* points. They are very simple movements but they provide an excellent benchmark for personal evolution. They allow you to monitor your day-to-day variation, which is influenced by an infinite number of variables: what you ate or drank yesterday, how you slept, your mental and emotional state, etc. The poses do not necessarily change but you may change immensely, and that feedback should influence your practice on a daily basis. Consistency is important but don't hold yourself to the same standards every day. You are not the same person every day. Remember, you are far more important than any pose, sequence, or routine.

Warm Up Poses

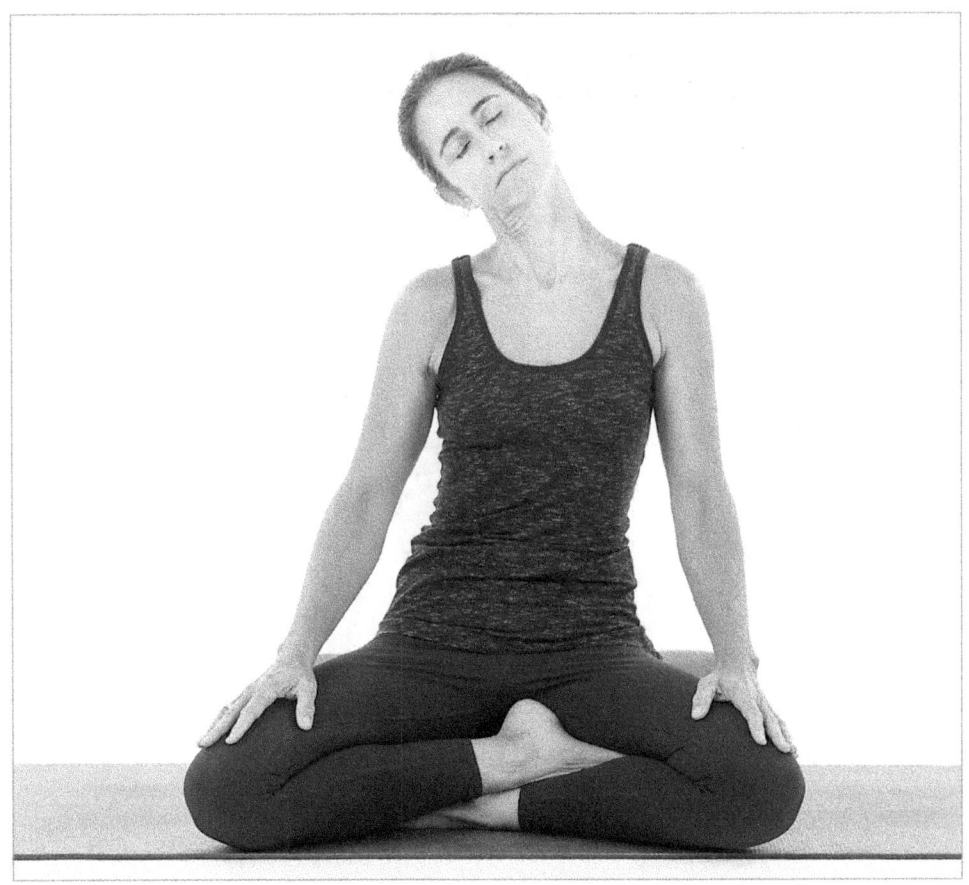

4.b.1 Neck Marma

Warm Up Poses

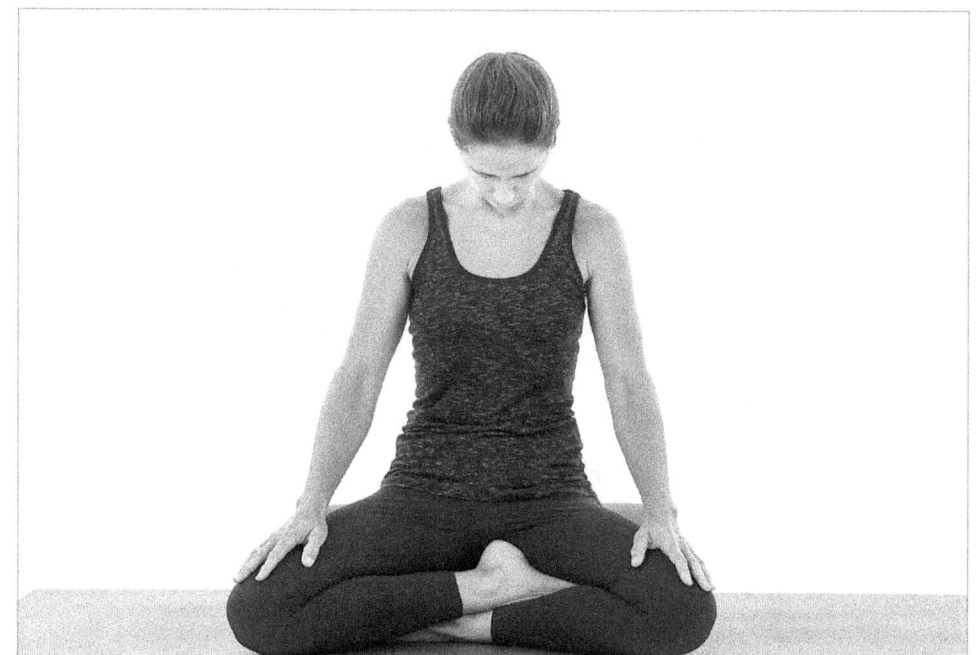

4.b.2 Neck Marma

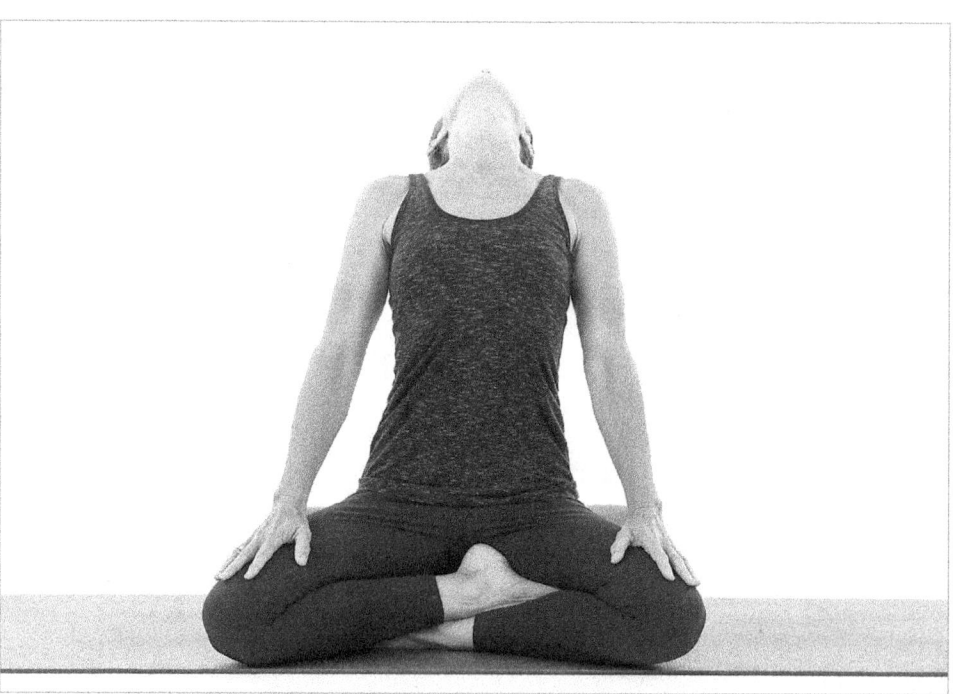

4.b.3 Neck Marma

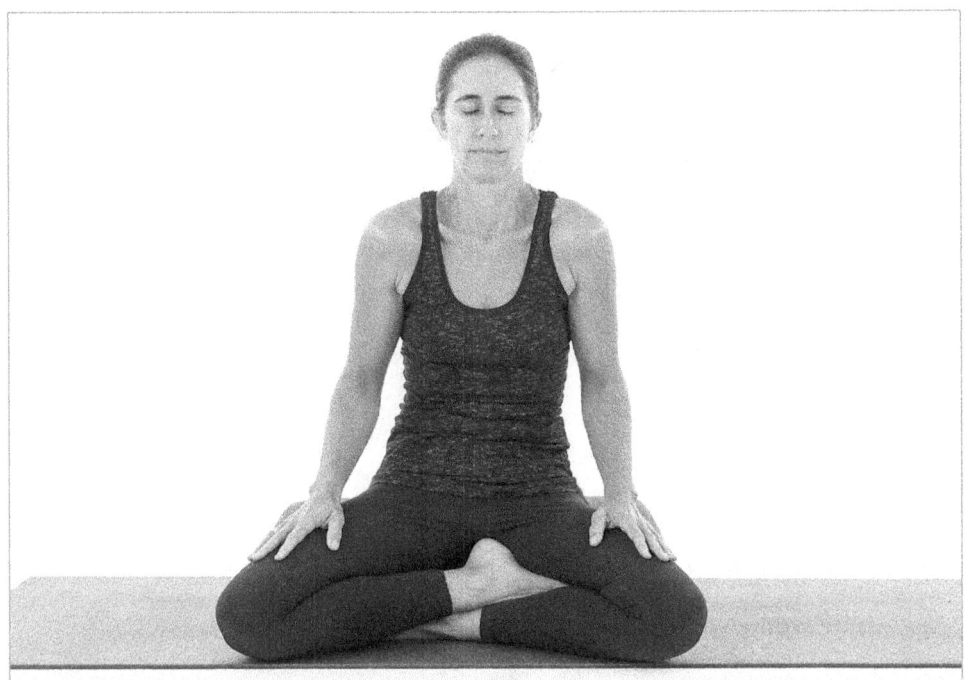

4.b.4 Shoulder Marma

Warm Up Poses

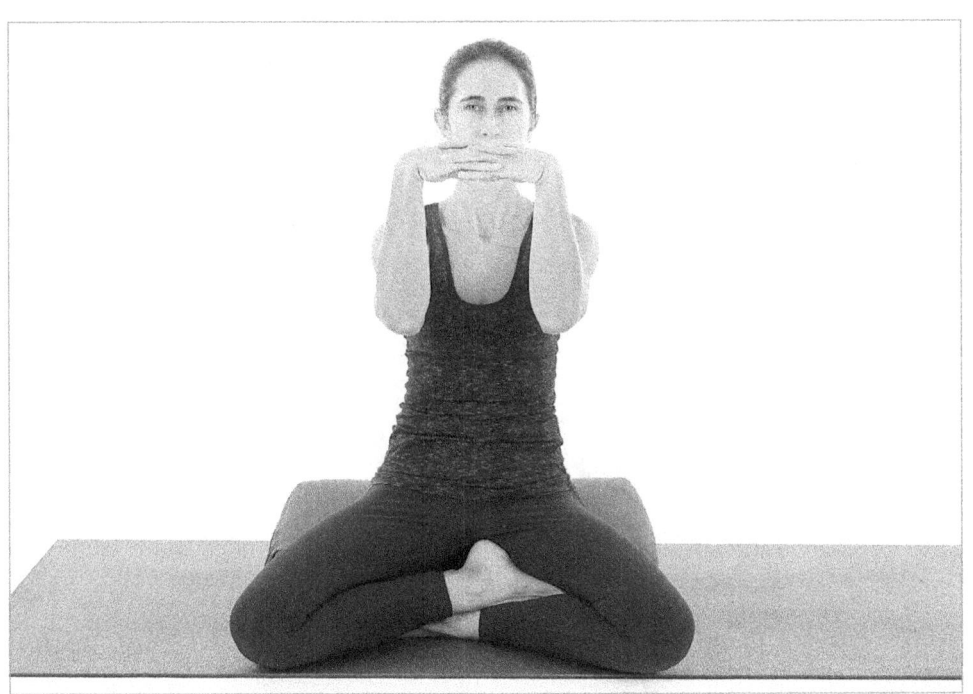

4.b.5 Wrist Marma

Warm Up Poses

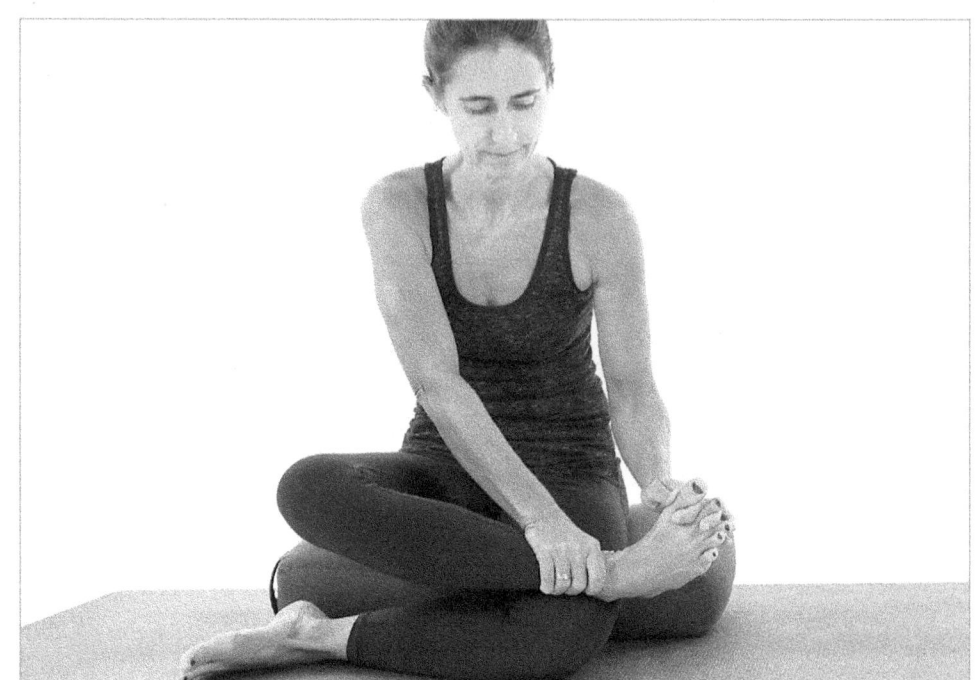

4.b.6 Ankle Marma

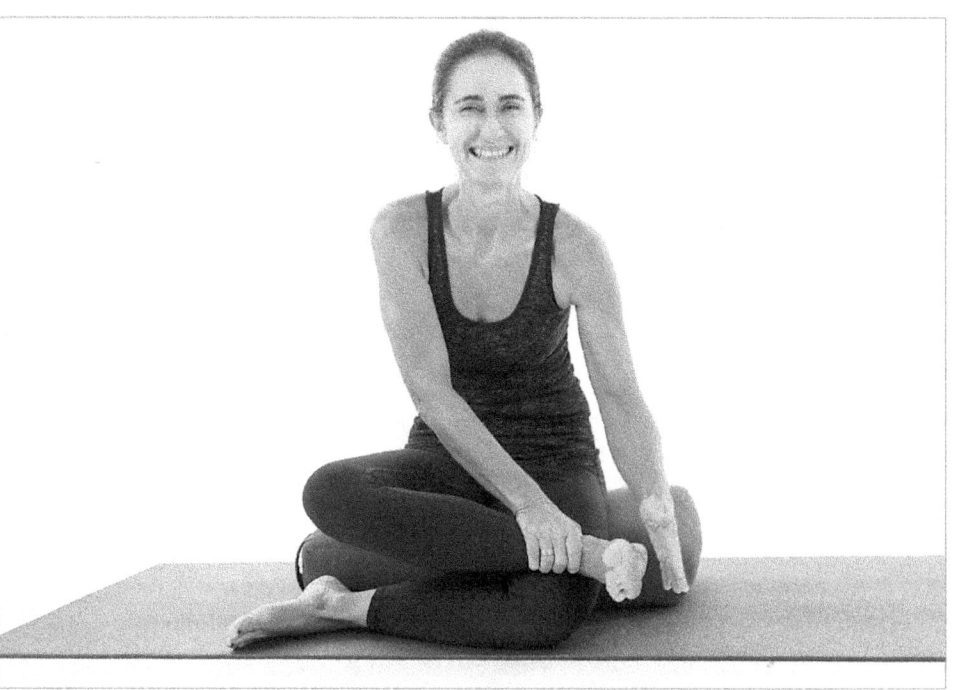

4.b.7 Foot Slap

VAJRASANAS
vaa·draas·ahn·nuh | *thunderbolt pose*

Vajra means thunderbolt and it is a fitting name for the *vajrasana*s; the first time you do them, it may feel like there's lightning striking your feet. We'll introduce three of the five variations: the first opens the bottoms of your feet, the second opens the tops of your feet and ankles and the third opens your arches. All of them may seem daunting at first, but if you give them your time and attention the physical sensations change quickly. The *vajrasana*s are a perfect candidate for a short, simple personal practice, with one-minute timings for each variation. After a few weeks, you'll probably start to want more.

The primary contraindication for the *vajrasana*s is pain in your knees. Do not sacrifice your knees. If any of these poses cause pain or discomfort in your knees, put a comfortable prop between your heels and your sit bones (blankets and bolsters work well). Increase the space between your heels and hips until the pain goes away. If you have had knee surgery, start with a large, supportive bolster and slowly work your way down. If there is a lot of pain in your toes, specifically your big toe bones, you can place a blanket under your knees to alleviate some of the discomfort. But if the pain is in your feet, it's neither surprising nor dangerous. That pain is what Guruji called sweet pain; it's the pain on your path to freedom.

First Vajrasana

1. Start on hands and knees with your toes curled under.

2. Bring your feet and knees together, and walk your torso back until your hips are over your heels.

3. Lean forward and put your head on the floor. Tuck your chin toward your chest and look at your feet. Reach back with both hands and grab all your toes, especially your little toes, and pull them forward to point at your knees. Keep your big toes and big toe bones pressed together.

4. Use your index fingers to press your outer heels together until your inner ankle bones touch.

Warm Up Poses

NICKI:
When we mention timings for a particular pose, start your timer when you are fully in the pose. Don't include the setup—if you include the setup, you may only be in the active part of the pose for 15 seconds, and that's rarely enough.

5. Keep your inner ankles together and sit up onto your heels. Once you are up, the weight of your torso will keep your feet together.

6. Place your hands on your thighs, lower your chin toward your chest, and soften your jaw *(4.c.1)*.

Warm Up Poses

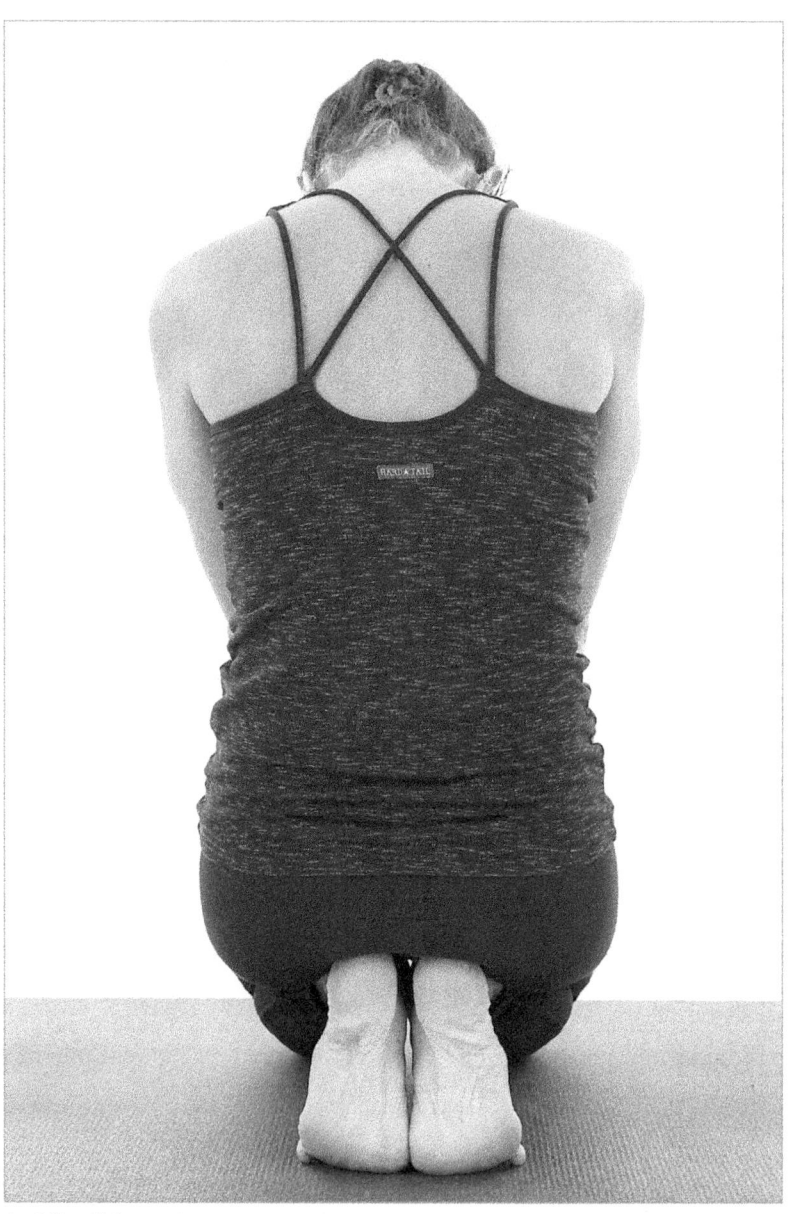

4.c.1 First Vajrasana

7. Lean back to put your shoulders directly over your hips. Soften your front body, move your bellybutton toward your spine, and extend your tailbone toward your knees *(4.c.2)*.

8. Take *jiva bandha* and breathe.

The *vajrasana*s push you forward because leaning forward takes the pressure out of your feet. Removing the pressure removes the thunderbolt, but that sensation in the sole of your foot is exactly the kind of pain you need to chase out of your body. You need the full weight of your torso to create leverage into your stiff feet, so do yourself a favor and lean back. Lean back until your shoulders are directly over your hips, and release the weight of your entire body. Drop your head, soften your ribs toward your spine, and extend your tailbone toward your knees. Take your belly button toward your back so the line from your head to your tailbone resembles the letter "C." Soften your entire body to make your seat heavier, and don't let the tension in your feet creep into your face and jaw.

This work in the torso is consistent in all three *vajrasana*s.

Warm Up Poses

NICKI:
There should not be any pain in your knees. If there is pain in your knees, modify the pose. Put a bolster under your hips and elevate your pose until the pain is gone. If there is extreme pain in your feet and toes, place a block or folded blanket under your knees *(4.c.3)*.

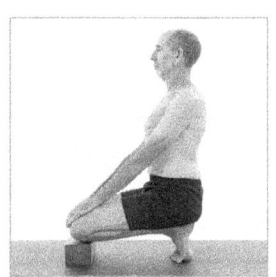

4.c.3

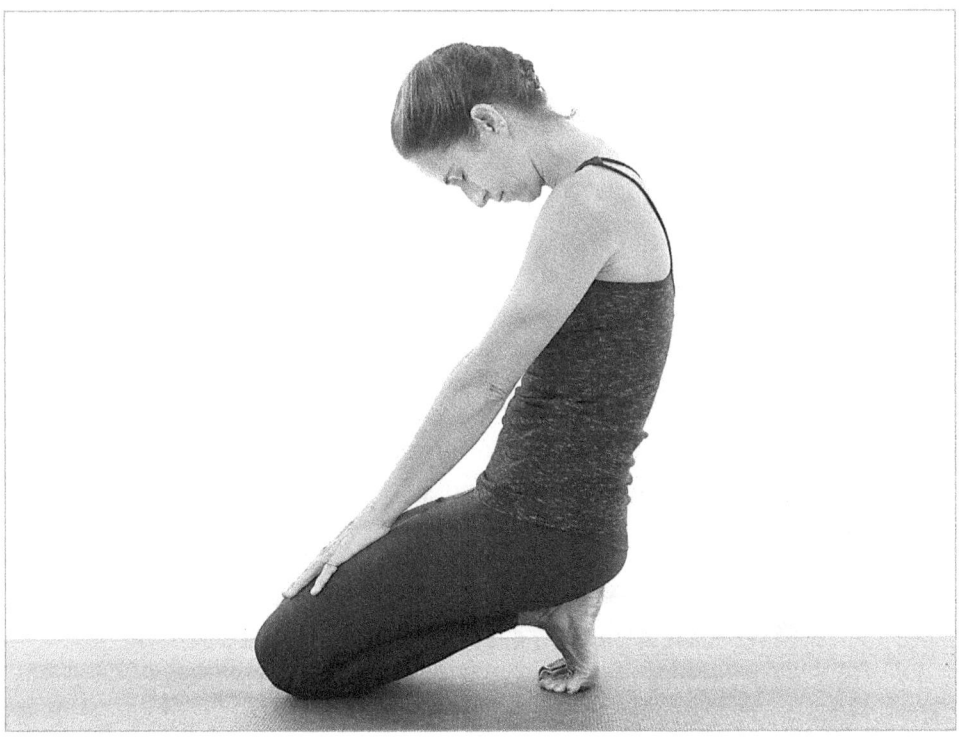

4.c.2 First Vajrasana

Second Vajrasana

From the first *vajrasana*:

1. Inhale, lean forward and put your hands on the mat in front of you.

2. Keep your big toes pressed together, lift your feet, and point all ten toes straight back.

3. Place the tops of your feet on the mat and reach back with both hands to press your inner ankle bones together. Try to get your heels inside your sit bones.

4. Lift your torso and place your hands on your thighs. Slide them toward your knees and straighten your arms. If you feel wobbly, keep your hands on the mat for stability.

5. Lower your chin toward your chest. Set your shoulders over your hips and relax your front body.

6. Lean back and breathe *(4.c.4)*.

Third Vajrasana

The third *vajrasana* has two sides. From the second *vajrasana*:

1. Inhale, lift your head and return to hands and knees on the mat.

2. Move your right knee back about two inches so your left knee is in front of your right *(4.c.5)*.

3. Point your left toes to the right and your right toes to the left, with the tops of your feet on the floor.

4. Lift your right foot and place your instep onto the sole of your left foot, as close to your left heel as possible. Your instep is the high bony ridge at the top of your foot, close to your ankle.

5. Sit back onto your heels and bring your thighs together. Your left knee should be a couple inches in front of your right knee, and your right heel should be just to the inside of your right sit bone *(4.c.6)*.

Warm Up Poses

NICKI:
Use a timer in these poses. One side may be very different from the other, and you need to cultivate balance.

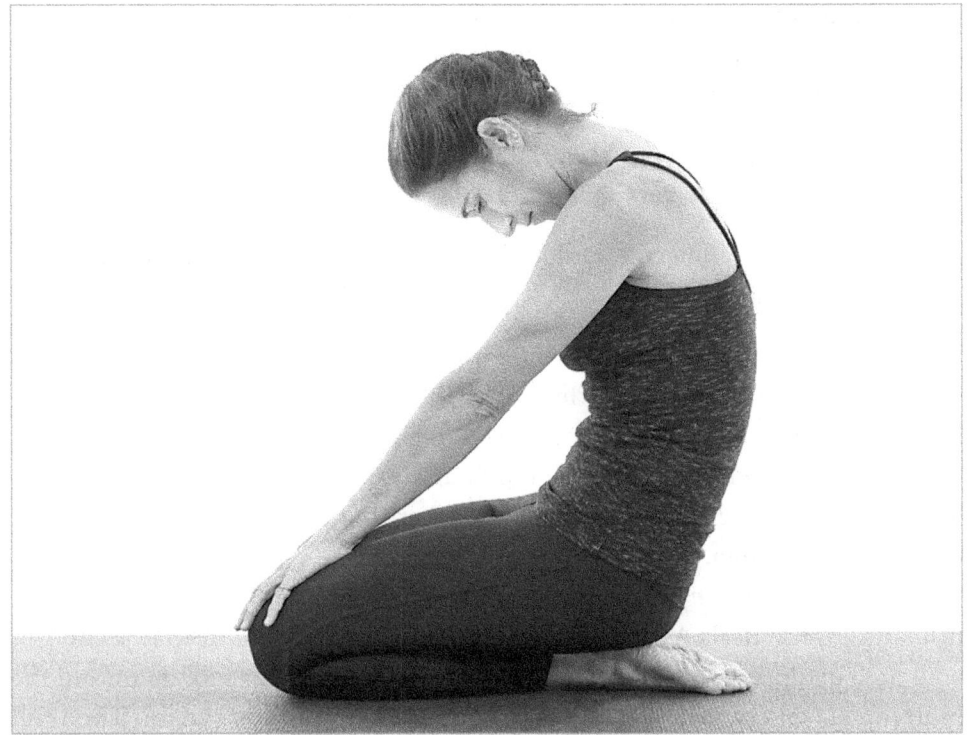

Warm Up Poses

4.c.4 Second Vajrasana

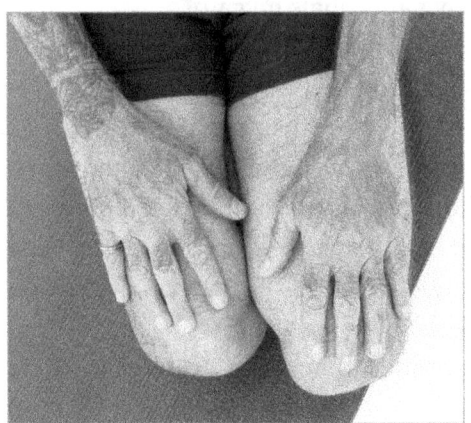

4.c.5 Third Vajrasana

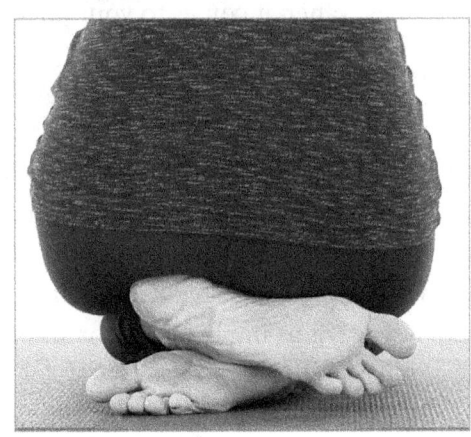

4.c.6 Third Vajrasana

6. Place your palms on top of your knees and wrap your fingers around the front of your knees. Straighten your arms, relax your hands, and soften your gaze.

7. Lean back, drop your chin toward your chest and take your belly button toward your spine.

8. Inhale and come forward to hands and knees. Repeat on the opposite side.

Warm Up Poses

You can probably feel it but just in case it's not obvious: the third *vajrasana* uses your right instep to open your left arch. The congestion in your left arch will actively push you forward so we want you to lean back. Let every ounce of your weight trickle down into your right arch and examine the sensation you find. The *vajrasana*s will erase the pain that lives there but practice implies repetition; once is never enough.

The third *vajrasana* always starts with the back of your arch: the lowest part, just inside your heel. As it matures—i.e. once the stiffness in that section of your arch dissipates—you can experiment with moving your foot up toward the middle and front of your arch. Be patient and sensitive to your knees. If you feel any pain or pressure in your knees, put something between your heels and your sit bones. When it comes to your knees, any pain equals no gain.

SIMHASANA
sim·haas·ahn·nuh | *lion pose*

Simhasana is a powerful detoxifying pose. The *marma* points for your kidney, liver, and spleen intersect on your inner shins, just above your ankles. *Simhasana* applies pressure to this point, and if you feel a strong sensation there these organs may be congested. Congestion in these organs of digestion and filtration can have serious implications for your health and longevity.

Simhasana is contraindicated for pregnant women and women who are trying to become pregnant (soon). The *marma*s for the female reproductive organs are just below the *marma*s being stimulated in *simhasana,* and it is easy to accidentally stimulate them instead. Aside from pregnancy, the primary contraindication for *simhasana* is pain in your knees and addressing it requires the same work as the *vajrasana*s: place a prop between your heels and your sit bones until the pain disappears.

Warm Up Poses

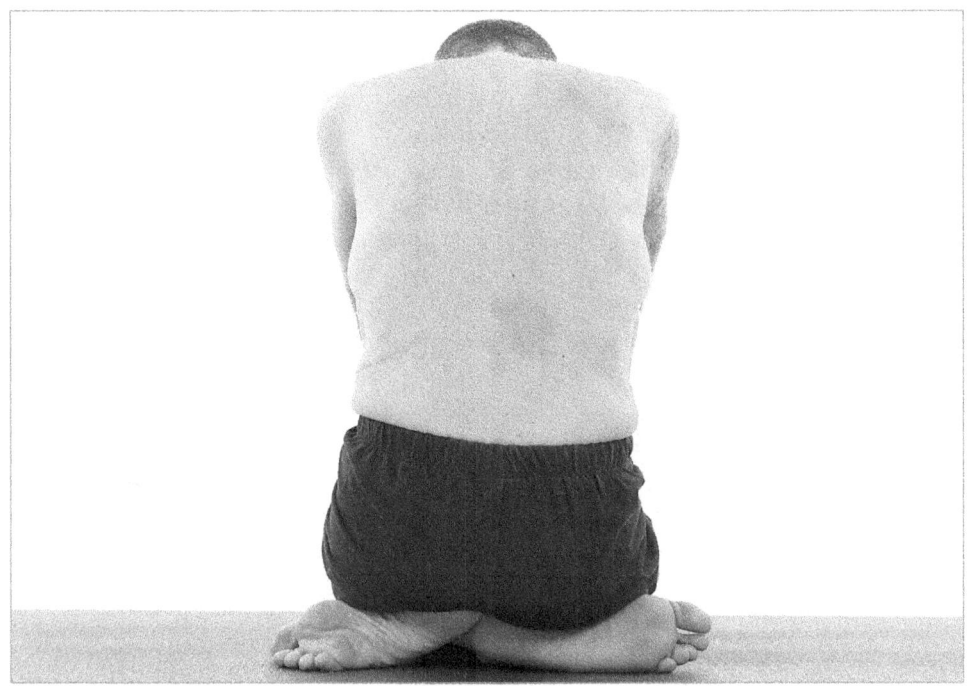

4.d.1 Simhasana

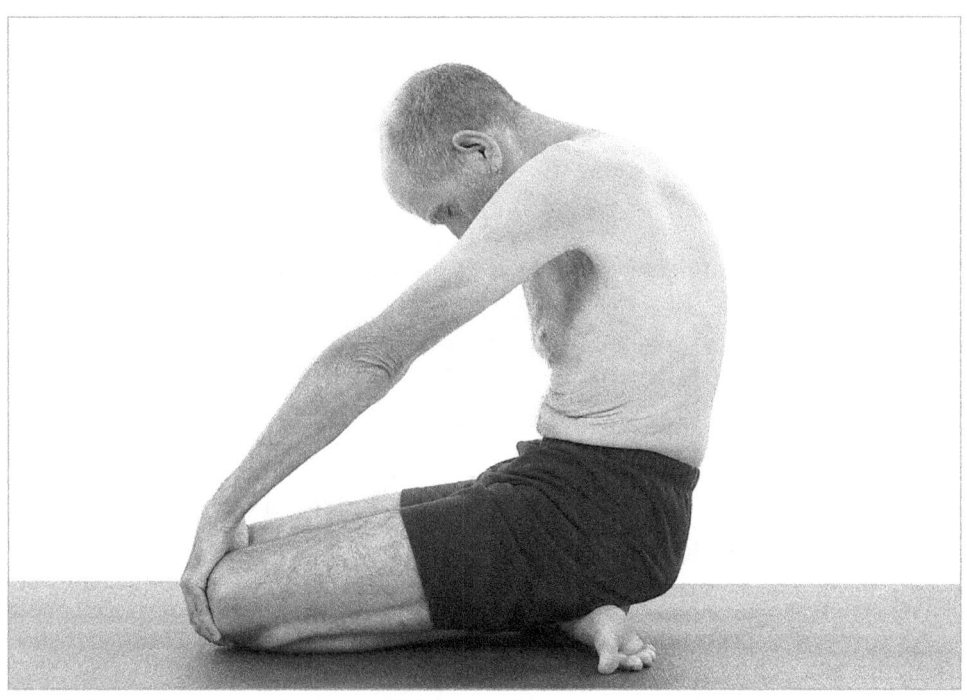

4.d.2 Simhasana: the spine rounds to create a "C" shape, similar to the vajrasanas

Warm Up Poses

1. Start on hands and knees with the tops of your feet on the mat. Point your right toes to the left and your left toes to the right, just like the third *vajrasana*.

2. Lift your right lower leg and cross it over your left calf, just above your ankle bones. The front of your right shin should be just above your left ankle, on the back of your left inner calf.

3. Slowly sit back onto your heels. Your right heel should be just to the inside of your left sit bone. You should be able to see the bottoms of your big toes peeking out on either side of your hips *(4.d.1)*.

4. Place your palms on the top of your knees and wrap your fingers down the front of your knees. Straighten your arms and press your torso back, toward the sensation in your inner left ankle. If this challenges your balance, keep your hands on the mat outside of your hips.

5. Drop your chin toward your chest. Bring your ribs and belly button toward your spine and shift your tailbone toward your knees. Soften your jaw and round your back so your entire body is shaped like the letter "C" *(4.d.2)*.

6. Inhale and come forward to switch sides.

UTTANASANA
oot·tah·naahs·ahn·nuh | *intense pose*

Uttanasana is a standing forward bend. It may seem to be an easy pose at first, especially if your legs are lazy, but laziness will never serve you—not in yoga, nor in life. Learn to hold this pose accurately and to hold it for a few minutes, and it always becomes intense.

The primary contraindication for *uttanasana* is pain in your lower back, and it usually applies to people with stiff legs. Stiff hamstrings will cause the forward-bending action to pull on your lower back instead of your legs. Pulling on your lower back puts forward pressure on your intervertebral discs and pushes them into the exact place they are most at risk of injury. If that is your reality, do box on the wall instead.

Doing box on the wall doesn't mean you'll never do *uttanasana*, it simply means you need to approach your hamstrings from a different angle. When they've opened up a bit, after a few weeks or months of box on the wall, try *uttanasana* again. If you can feel the stretch in your legs and there's no pain in your back, stick with *uttanasana*. If not, go back to box on the wall. These things take time. Be patient, and always listen to your pain.

Do not bend your knees in *uttanasana*. Bending your knees forces the stretch higher up your hamstrings into the muscle attachment at the bottom of your sit bones. Muscle attachments are white tissue and white tissue is not supposed to stretch—it can't bounce back like muscle tissue. Stretching this white tissue creates a nagging pain right underneath the sit bones (often called "yoga butt"), and the pain that lives in those stiff hamstrings never gets released.

It might make sense to bend your knees if doing *uttanasana* "properly" meant getting your hands on the floor, but *uttanasana* isn't about getting your hands on the floor. *Uttanasana* is about opening your hamstrings, and you'll never open your hamstrings if you stretch your tendons instead.

If you need to bend your knees to get your hands on the floor, you should not be doing traditional *uttanasana*. Keep your legs perfectly straight and use props to decrease the bend (we'll provide instructions below) or do box on the wall instead. Box on the wall protects your lumbar discs while opening your legs and developing the ability to rotate your pelvis.

Please note that *uttanasana* is not the same thing as *dwi* position of *surya namaskar a* (the initial forward fold). *Uttanasana* is typically held for several minutes but *dwi* position is only a single *vinyasa*. It's really only half a breath: you begin the exhale standing upright and end it folded forward, so you're only there for a few seconds. *Dwi* is a transition into *trini* so it's okay to bend your knees to put your hands on the floor. You're not staying there long enough to hurt yourself.

We usually approach *uttanasana* from the *vajrasana*s, *simhasana*, or a similar seat. You may need more than one step to get from a seat to *uttanasana*, but over time your transitions will become more fluid. Taking fewer steps between each pose helps maintain your internal focus.

From your seat:

1. Curl your toes under, straighten your legs, bend forward and bring your hands to the mat in front of you.

Warm Up Poses

NICKI:
The "*utt*" in *uttanasana* means "intense." It is one of my favorite names of a pose, and that should tell you a little bit about me and my personality.

Warm Up Poses

NICKI:
People often look at this pose and think, *I don't want to do that, it's too easy*. But after a couple minutes of holding the pose accurately, they may start to think, *I don't want to do this, it's too hard*! This is the foundational work, and it's not necessarily easy but it's extremely important. Assimilate this work into your anatomy and your practice will fly; rush past it and your practice will flounder.

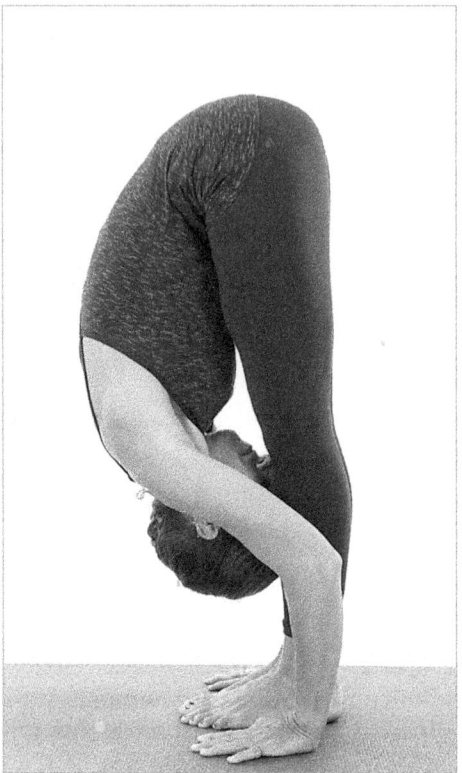

4.e.1 Uttanasana with a long torso, short legs

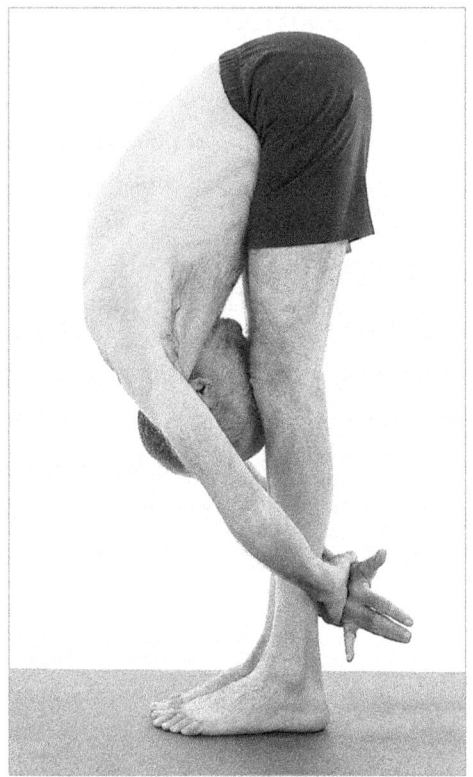

4.e.2 Uttanasana with a short torso, long legs

2. Move your feet together until your big toe bones and your inner heels are touching.

3. Organize your feet and place your ankles directly over the center of your heels.

4. Lift your kneecaps by fully engaging both quadriceps.

5. Internally rotate both legs.

6. Lean forward until your sit bones are directly above the outer edge of your heels.

7. Bring your ribs toward your spine and look at your knees. Let your head be heavy *(4.e.1 and 4.e.2)*.

STEPS 1–3: Place your hands on the floor or on a prop in front of you, soften your spine, and look at your feet. Move your feet together until your big toe bones and inner heels are touching—meaning there is absolutely no space between them. Lift all ten toes and spread them, moving your big toes toward each other and your little toes away from each other. Press firmly through your big toe bones and lift your inner arches. Place your ankles over the center of your heels to align them directly under your knees and hips.

STEP 4: Contracting the front of your leg allows you to penetrate your hamstrings; it's the magnificent natural geometry of your body. Engage your quadriceps as much as possible, enough to reveal little dimples just above your kneecap. Those dimples are just the beginning; eventually you can connect with your quadriceps from your knee all the way to the top of your thigh. Keeping them lifted takes time and practice, but you definitely want to begin this conversation with your anatomy. It may be shaky at first because you don't quite speak the same language yet, but don't give up.

STEP 5: Keep your kneecaps lifted and straighten your legs completely. Scan your legs for hyperextension: draw a mental line through the length of your legs, and if your knees are behind the line from your hips to your ankles, they're hyperextended. Micro-bend them until that line is straight. Micro-bending your knees may make it harder to lift your kneecaps, but it is important to use your leg muscles instead of putting pressure on your ligaments. If your knees are in front of the line from your hips to your ankles, they're bent. Straighten them. Straight is straight and bent is bent, learn to see the difference. Once your legs are straight and your kneecaps are lifted, spin your thighs toward each other to internally rotate your legs and lengthen the line from your pubic bone to your inner heel.

STEP 6: Balance your weight between the front and back of each foot. Your hamstrings may try to pull toward your heels but that's the opposite direction of the stretch in your legs. Remember, this is called intense posture. Lean into the stretch by pressing into the knuckles of your toes until you feel a stretch in your lower leg. Do not let your heels lift. Get "plumb" between your hips and feet, meaning that if we dropped a line from your sit bones it would land on the back edge of your heels.

STEP 7: *Uttanasana* is a forward bend, so bend forward. Do not open your chest or try to pull length into your spine: doing a backbending action in a forward

Warm Up Poses

EDDIE:
Once you have the alignment, simplify the pose by softening your mind. Release any tension in your neck and jaw. Breathe freely. Let your head be heavy and surrender your spine to gravity. Lean forward and know that you are God.

Warm Up Poses

bend puts upward pressure on your tailbone, and if you are flexible, that pressure can destabilize your sacrum. Keep your legs perfectly straight and relax your torso completely. Look at your knees to lengthen the back of your neck and soften your lower floating ribs toward your spine. Use *mula* and *uddiyana bandha* to move your sit bones closer together and keep your tailbone tucked toward your pubic bone. Cultivate an even bend through the length of your spine so the line from your tailbone to your occiput is perfectly arched, like a rainbow.

Stay in *uttanasana* until your legs are fully awake. When they're really asking you to bend, place your hands on the mat or a block in front of you and bend your knees to the floor. Lie forward onto your thighs and rest in *balasana* (child's pose).

Box on the Wall

If *uttanasana* or *adho mukha svanasana* (downward dog) cause pain in your lower back, practice box on the wall instead; it allows you to penetrate your hamstrings without jeopardizing your lumbar discs.

1. Place your hands on the wall at shoulder height and shoulder-width apart.

2. Point your middle fingers straight up and arrange your hands in the shape of the inner triad.

3. Turn the eyes of your elbows to face each other without distorting your hands.

4. Walk away from the wall until your arms are fully extended, and then look down.

5. Bring your feet directly under your hips and separate them to your hips' width. Organize your feet and lift your inner ankle bones.

6. Lift your kneecaps and internally rotate both legs.

7. Engage *mula* and *uddiyana bandha* and lift your sit bones to stretch your hamstrings.

8. Press into your inner triads and reach through your arms. Lengthen your armpit chest.

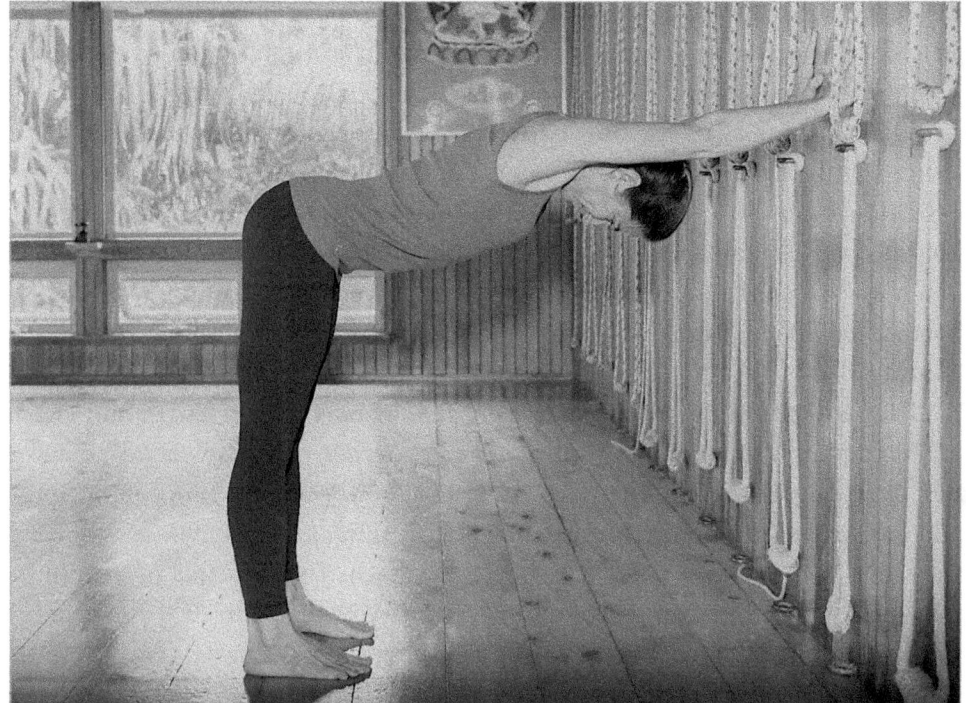

4.f Box on the wall

Warm Up Poses

9. Soften your lower floating ribs toward your spine. Use the action of your arms and legs to lengthen your waist: reach your arms toward the wall and reach your legs away from it *(4.f)*.

10. To come out, walk toward the wall and stand up.

With enough practice, this pose will release your lower back from the strong grip of your hamstrings and hips. It rebuilds the natural curve in your lumbar spine and removes compression from your intervertebral discs, and it will help keep you walking on your own two feet for the rest of your life. It can also be used to practice the work of the inner triad without the full pressure of *adho mukha svanasana*.

BALASANA
ball·aahs·ahn·nuh | *child posture*

In the beginning, the ebb and flow of *Hatha* yoga can be condensed into two poses: *balasana* (child's pose) and *adho mukha svanasana* (downward dog). At

Warm Up Poses

EDDIE:
What is an effective practice? Where is the middle path? The answer to these questions is different for every individual. There is no formula or set sequence that can unravel the complexity of your being. Yoga is a catalyst for your unique personal evolution, and no two paths should look the same. You are much more interesting than a stagnant prescription of postures. Yoga is alive and the process is organic. It encompasses a lifetime of searching, testing, and listening; it is a marathon, not a 100-meter dash. It requires honesty, compassion, and meticulous attention to detail. It unlocks our potential as human beings and reminds us we are God.

the end, it simplifies again into two poses: *sarvangasana* (shoulderstand) and *sirsasana* (headstand). There is a universe between and among these poses, but both sets encompass the balance between sun and moon; between *ha* and *tha*; between reaching and softening; between *sthira* and *sukha*. They illustrate that the growth gained from strength, length, and extension must be balanced by insight brought from softness, silence, and release. You cannot have one without the other. Sustainability lives in the middle, and to create a lifelong practice you must find the middle path between these two energies. Failing to cultivate balance will make your relationship with yoga short, superficial, and possibly painful.

The Sanskrit root of *balasana* is *bala*. *Bala* means both strength and child, and it implies a unique opportunity to redirect your gaze. We spend much of our lives focused on externally oriented goals, expectations, and obligations, and our psyche has the unfortunate habit of pursuing judgemental, self-limiting thoughts. Sometimes it takes the simple, unattached perspective of a child to become comfortable with who you really are. Try to see yourself without judgment, and don't rush to correct your imbalances or idiosyncrasies. Give yourself time to explore them so you may act with understanding and intelligence. The most important relationship you will ever have is the relationship you have with yourself. After all, you are with you all the time; you came with you, and you'll leave with you. Consider *balasana* an introduction to yourself, and be kind.

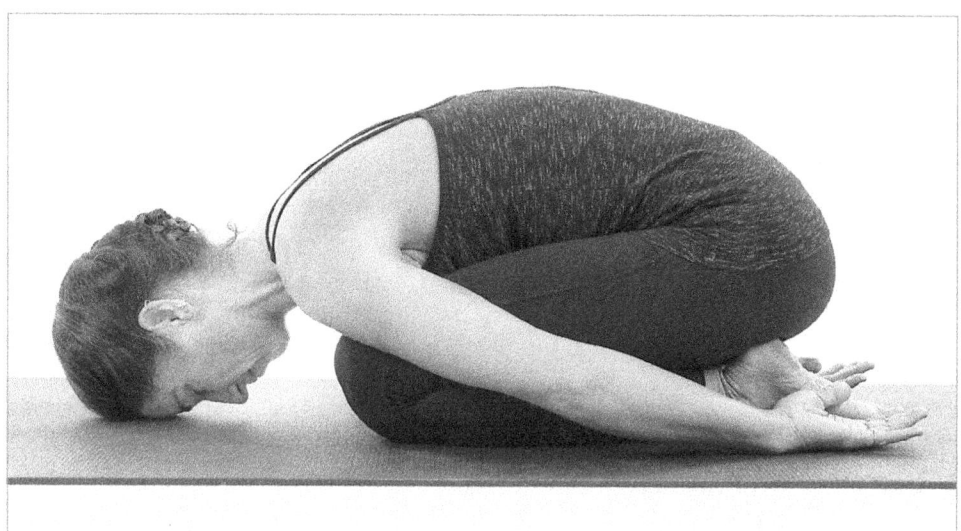

4.g Balasana

Balasana is quieting, nurturing, and introspective. It teaches you to let go, and letting go is a tremendous skill. Stress and tension are pervasive. Most of us are held upright not by our own strength but by the currents of stress and tension coiled tightly around our body and mind. We eat, sleep, and breathe in the structure of our anxiety. It is a powerful restriction. Relaxation is the antidote, and *balasana* is your training wheels. It is a safe place to be wobbly and unsure, to explore letting go without the fear of falling down. Encourage stillness by making the pose extremely comfortable. Use props as necessary: put a bolster or blanket between your heels and hips if they do not meet, or between your belly and thighs. Study yourself in *balasana* and find what it takes to cultivate silence and stillness. Familiarize yourself with the process of letting go so you can utilize that process in more difficult poses.

From *uttanasana*, *adho mukha svanasana* or any upright posture:

1. Bend your knees and bring your hands to the mat.
2. Place the tops of your feet on the mat, point your toes back, and bring your big toes together to touch.
3. Spread your knees to the width of your shoulders.
4. Lower your hips to your heels and rest your shoulders on your knees.
5. Tuck your chin toward your chest and relax your tailbone toward your pubic bone.
6. Relax completely *(4.g)*.

STEPS 1–5: Placing your knees too close together puts pressure on your chest, breasts, and heart; placing them too far apart leaves your face pressed into the mat. Find the appropriate spacing for your body that allows your shoulders to rest on your knees, and then let your back be round. Tuck your chin toward your chest, and point your tailbone down to soften your lower back and sacrum. Shift the weight in your head toward your forehead to free your nose and expand the occiput at the base of your skull. Relax your elbows, wrists, and hands. Do not open your chest or lengthen your torso—it's uncomfortable and confuses the energy of the posture. Visualize yourself as a happy, quiet turtle. Be soft, round, and supported.

Warm Up Poses

EDDIE:
The cells you replace in your body, in every moment, are shaping the life you create. Cells made in the presence of stress carry that stress response with them. Yoga gives you the opportunity to release the frenetic energy of cells created in stress and replace them with cells created in a nourishing environment.

STEP 6: Soften everywhere. Unwind the subtle tension that holds your body away from the earth. Picture yourself as a stone slowly sinking into a pool of water with a gentle, supported descent that invites total relaxation. Surrender your entire being to the reassuring embrace of gravity. Soften your belly, lips, elbows and tongue. After a few moments in the pose, your first layer of tension will begin to unwind. Exhale completely and release more. There is always more. That first glimpse of silence, the realization that you can control the invisible tension that strangles your spine and imprisons your psyche, is the seed of yoga.

ADHO MUKHA SVANASANA
aud·ho·moo·kah sva·naas·ahn·nuh | *downward facing dog pose*

Adho mukha svanasana (downward facing dog / downward dog) cultivates the other side of personal realization: reaching, lengthening, and being attentive. It requires that you look carefully at your foundations—the parts of your body touching the earth—and devote yourself to their refinement. The foundations of *asana*, no matter how advanced you become, are always your hands and feet. In *adho mukha svanasana*, building yourself in the direction of yoga means you start with your hands and never forget them.

Adho mukha svanasana is the best place to solidify the inner triad of the hand, one of our most fundamental teachings. The inner triad connects the energetic dots of your upper body; it connects your hands to your shoulders, your shoulders to your spine, and your spine to your sit bones, so the strength exerted in the inner triad extends all the way to the base of your pelvis. It creates a force-line through the length of your spine, and that force-line meets the upward action of your legs to create ascension in the pose. If the inner triad is weak, the force-line may become lost in the tissue of your arms and shoulders and the pose will begin to sink.

Strengthening the inner triad also profoundly strengthens your wrists. Many practitioners are destroying their wrists in the pursuit of yoga, and as teachers we are obligated to address that pain with meticulous attention to this detailed work. If *adho mukha svanasana* causes pain in your wrists, use box on the wall to solidify the work of the inner triad. It is easier and safer to train your hands when they're not bearing the full weight of the pose. Don't stay on the wall forever; use the wall to bring you closer to the pose. Be willing to find your threshold and explore.

Warm Up Poses

EDDIE:
Adho mukha svanasana is central to *surya namaskar*, which is central to yoga. If *adho mukha svanasana* hurts your back, we teach a modification that can be used in conjunction with *surya namaskar* so you can do the pose safely without interrupting the flow of the sequence.

In *adho mukha svanasana* the primary contraindication is similar to that of *uttanasana*: pain in your lower back. Stiff hamstrings will pull on your lower back instead of your legs, and that pull will be most visible in your sacrum. The sacrum of a person with tight hamstrings will be flat, roughly parallel to the floor, and their downward dog will look more like a trapezoid than a triangle. The sacrum of a person with open hamstrings will have an ascending slant, one that creates the triangle at the top of the pose: the sacrum forms one side and the top of the legs forms the other. The flat-sacrum person is at risk of injuring their lower back and probably shouldn't spend a lot of time in this pose; do box on the wall instead, until your hamstrings are open enough to let your pelvis rotate forward.

Finally, many students are taught to pull their shoulders down when their arms are extended in *adho mukha svanasana*—i.e. roll their shoulders down their back—and we disagree. Anatomically, the shoulder blade must lift when the arm extends; pulling the shoulders down separates the arm from the torso and prohibits it from fully extending. If your arms are not fully extended, the action of downward dog cannot reach your spine and is thus ineffective. To do this pose effectively, don't think about rotating your arms or pulling your shoulders down your back. Think about pressing into your inner triads and reaching your arms more than you ever have before.

Start on hands and knees at the front of your mat:

1. Place your hands exactly shoulder-width apart and align your shoulders over your wrists.
2. Point the middle finger of each hand straight forward and evenly spread the rest of your fingers. Keep your pinkie and thumb in line with your palm.
3. Press the inner triad of your hands into the mat.
4. Turn the eyes of your elbows to face each other without disturbing the work in your hands.
5. Walk your knees back until they are under your sit bones *(4.h.1)*.
6. Inhale and look forward without disturbing the organization of your hands and arms.

Warm Up Poses

NICKI:
We must pay attention to pain, first in ourselves and then in our students, and follow the lines of yoga until the pain has been erased.

7. Exhale, lift your hips and straighten your legs. Let your head come back last.

8. Inhale, reach your arms forward and lengthen your armpit chest.

9. Exhale, lift your sit bones, engage your legs, and descend your heels.

10. Look toward your navel and soften your lower floating ribs toward your spine *(4.h.2 and 4.h.3)*.

Warm Up Poses

EDDIE:
In every pose, it's important to ask yourself, "Which way is my skin being pulled?" Your skin is the largest organ in your body and it is intimately connected to your nervous system. It is the periphery, and you can use it to determine what's going on underneath the surface. In downward dog, move the skin of your hand in the direction of your index finger knuckle because the skin is indicative of the action within.

STEPS 1 & 2: Place your hands exactly shoulder-width apart; placing them too far apart narrows your shoulders and putting them too close together pushes your shoulder blades apart. Point the middle finger of each hand straight forward and spread the rest of your fingers evenly so there is an equal amount of space between each finger—including the pinkie and thumb. Center your weight in the inner triad to shift pressure away from your outer wrist. Make your wrist creases parallel with the front of your mat, unless that distorts the inner triad of your hand; the work of the inner triad is paramount.

STEP 3: Turn the eyes of your elbows (the inner elbow, where blood is drawn) to face each other and make your arms perfectly straight. Be conscious of hyper-extension; draw a mental line from your shoulders to your wrists and put your elbows in the middle of that line. And remember: finding "straight" may mean adopting a permanent micro-bend to avoid overstretching your ligaments. Try to visualize your bones; looking at your muscles can distract you from the true shape of your skeleton. Once you have set your arms, review steps 1 & 2 to stabilize your foundation before moving further into the pose.

STEP 4: Bring your shoulders directly over your wrists without disturbing the organization in your hands. Walk your knees back until they are under your sit bones, behind your hips. This pose is designed to lengthen your spine, and your hands and feet need to be far enough apart to facilitate that length.

STEP 5: Inhale and look forward. Keep the organization of your hands and arms perfectly still.

STEP 6: Exhale, curl your toes under and straighten your legs. Lift your hips and let your head come back last, giving you one last opportunity to check your foundations as you move into the pose.

Warm Up Poses

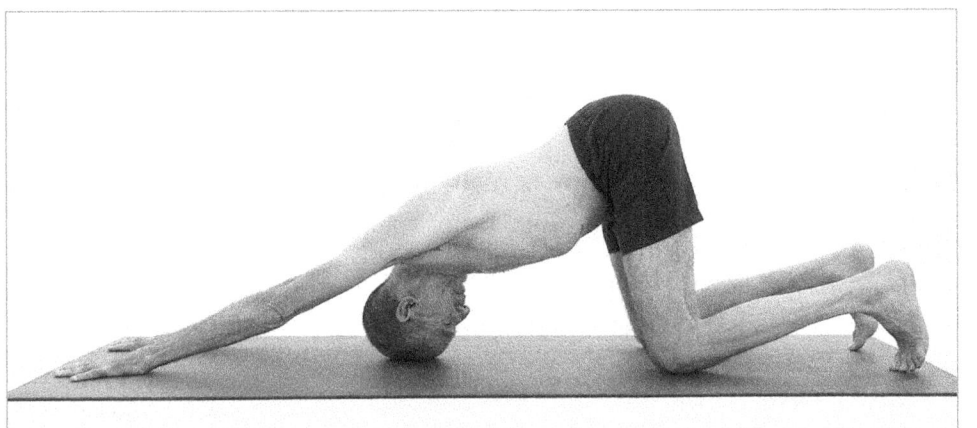

4.h.1 Setting up for adho mukha svanasana

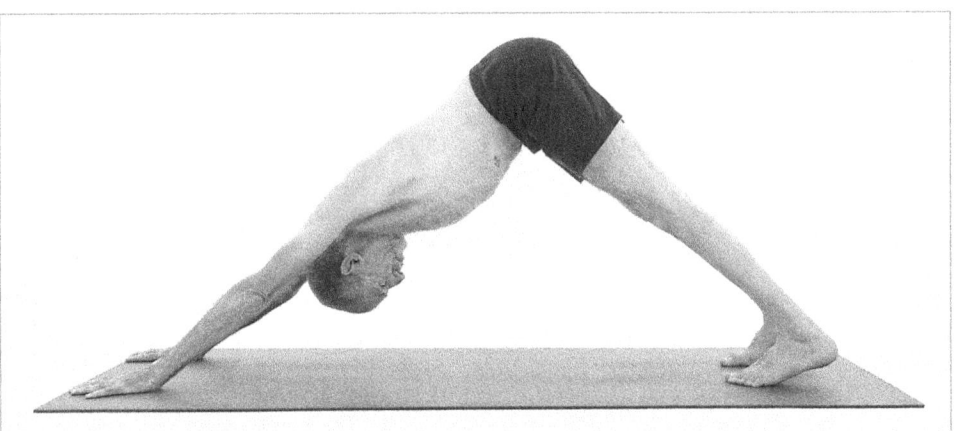

4.h.2 Eddie in adha mukha svanasana

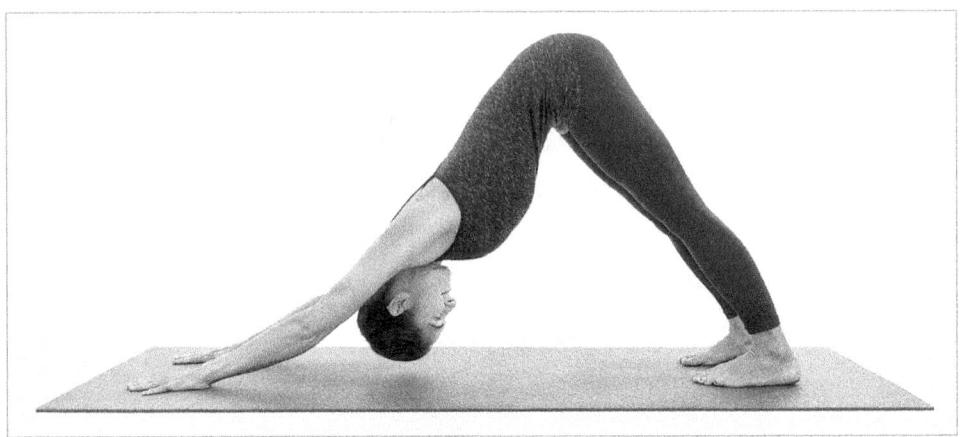

4.h.3 Nicki in adho mukha svanasana

EDDIE:

Downward dog should strengthen and extend the natural curves of the spine. It should not reverse the natural curves of the spine so don't let your chest sag toward the floor. This pose is about extension and ascension. Go up. There is a universe in this pose. There is health and youth in this pose. Become familiar with *adho mukha svanasana*; spend time with it every day and watch your capacity develop.

STEP 7: Inhale and extend your arms forward like you're trying to reach something just beyond your fingertips. Press into the knuckles of each hand, and make your wrists light to put the work more into your forearms than in your wrists. Explore lifting your pinkie fingers off the mat to pressurize the inner triad. Straighten your arms more than you ever have before (remaining conscious of hyperextension) and lengthen your armpits.

Warm Up Poses

STEP 8: Exhale as you lift your sit bones and reach your heels toward the mat. Lift all ten toes to engage your feet, and lift your inner ankle bones to put your ankles directly over the center of your heels. Press your big toe bone straight down into the mat in the same way that the inner triad reaches forward. Straighten your legs and lift both kneecaps. Engage the tissue from your kneecaps to the top of your thigh and extend the inseam of your legs into the space behind you. Tilt your pelvis just enough to honor the natural curve of your lumbar spine (lower back) but keep your tailbone curled toward your pubic bone. Engage *mula* and *uddiyana bandha*. Lift your sit bones and descend your heels.

NICKI:
This pose will open your armpit chest; the area where your chest connects to the underside of your arms. It is one of the bodily seats of health, along with the groin, because that's where most of your lymph nodes are. This pose banishes stagnation and disease by bathing the lymphatic system in fresh blood, and it all starts in your hands. If the knuckle of the index finger is pulled off the floor, your shoulders are closed. If the knuckle is pressing into the floor, and the ribs are moving toward the spine, the armpit chest is opening.

STEP 9: It is important to prevent your front body from collapsing toward the mat. Move your lower floating ribs toward your spine to integrate your diaphragm with the bowl of your pelvis. Lengthen your back body, waist, and front body equally. Once you have gotten to this step, use your breath to reinforce the actions of steps 7 & 8: inhale to extend your arms and exhale to engage your legs. When you are ready to come down, bring your knees to the mat and rest in *balasana*.

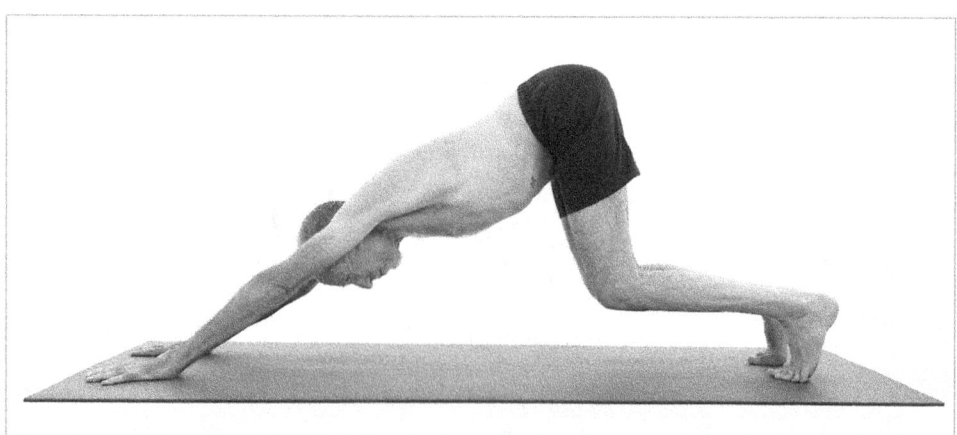

4.h.4 Modification to address back pain in adho mukha svanasana

MODIFICATION: If downward dog pulls on your back, use this modification:

Once you are in the pose (STEP 7), lift your heels and bend your knees to the height of your ankles. Bending your knees takes your hamstrings out of the equation and allows you to extend your spine. Keep your knees bent as you lift your sit bones, extend your arms, and open your armpit chest. Look at your navel and breathe *(4.h.4)*.

Balasana and *adho mukha svanasana* are complementary poses. They are an excellent starting point for *asana* practice as they prepare you for both physical exertion and total release. They are two sides of the same coin; they are the balance of *Hatha* yoga.

SAMASTITI
sa·ma·stee·ti·hee | *equal standing*

Sama means even and *stiti* means steadiness or strength. *Samastiti* means "equal standing" and it plants the seed for the eighth limb of Ashtanga yoga, which is *samadi*. *Samadi* is pure enlightenment, a true equanimity of being, and the culmination of all our mental and physical practices.

The lotus is a symbol of divinity, rising pure and clean from the stagnant, murky pond that symbolizes our consciousness. Almost all Indian deities are represented as seated or standing on a lotus flower as they have transcended the muddy waters of life and attained purity of being. Stepping into *samastiti* connects you to that spiritual lineage by placing your feet in the same place all great teachers have stood. It presents an opportunity to acknowledge and give thanks to all your teachers, and your teachers' teachers, who have graciously left their footprints for you to follow. Joining your lotus flower feet in *samastiti* aligns you with the divine, reminding you of your individual divinity and the divinity of all earthly beings.

Samastiti will help you discover how you manage balance. Balance is not absolutely still; it is constantly adjusting and actively reaching for the center of your being. You may rock side to side or forward to back; watch yourself and observe your patterns. Over time your adjustments will become more subtle as you become more familiar with center, and your oscillations away from center will be smaller and smaller. That is the beauty of this work. You already know the answers. You already possess the balance. It is written in the core of your being. You've just forgotten it, and the practice of yoga is here to help remind you.

Warm Up Poses

NICKI:
It is said that all yogis have lotus flowers for feet.

Warm Up Poses

1. Stand at the front of your mat. Join your feet by bringing your big toe bones and your inner heels together to touch.

2. Organize your feet, lift your inner arches and set your ankles directly over your heels.

3. Lift your kneecaps and straighten your legs.

4. Soften your shoulders away from your ears and expand your chest *(4.i.1)*.

5. Bring your palms to *anjali mudra*, close your eyes, and explore your balance *(4.i.2)*.

STEPS 1 & 2: Bringing your feet together creates a *mudra* similar to *anjali mudra*; it facilitates a physical and symbolic unity of right and left, east and west, conscious and subconscious. It is similar to the circular energetic current created through *jiva bandha*, and it contributes to your vibrational and energetic unity.

STEP 3: Lift your toes and spread them, reaching your big toes toward each other and your pinkie toes away from each other like petals on a blossoming lotus flower. Keep your feet together, spread your toes and organize your ankles. Some of this effort may speak to your hands instead of your feet, and that's an important thing to understand: you have a greater neuromuscular connection to your hands than your feet. You are not alone; we all start this way. Yoga will teach you to expand your mental and physical awareness, and in this pose, that means cultivating an ability to talk to your feet while keeping your hands quiet. Train your hands to soften and your feet to wake up.

STEP 4: Lift your kneecaps, spin your thighs toward each other and drop your tailbone. Internally rotating your legs tends to make your pelvis tilt forward, so engage *mula bandha* and extend your tailbone toward your heels. Lengthen your lower back, soften your shoulders and lift your chest. Soften your lower floating ribs toward your spine and maintain space in your back body.

STEP 5: Place your palms in *anjali mudra* and close your eyes. Bring your awareness to the foundation of the pose: your feet. Can you tell which one carries more weight? Try to discern the difference between each side before you move to correct it; you must learn how to look before you can see. Begin to develop equal weight in your feet, from front to back and left to right, and watch for changes in the rest of your body. It is normal to feel wobbly but resist the urge to open your eyes. Stay in the pose and find stability from the inside out, not from the outside in.

TADASANA
ta·daas·ahn·nuh | *mountain posture*

Samastiti is also known as *tadasana*, which means mountain posture. From Step 4 of *samastiti*:

5. Release your hands to your side and face your palms toward your body.

6. Press the fingers of each hand firmly together to make your hands sharp.

7. Extend your hands toward the ground. Soften your wrists and keep the base of your palms open.

Warm Up Poses

EDDIE:
Your yoga practice has a strong effect on the ripples that shape this universe.

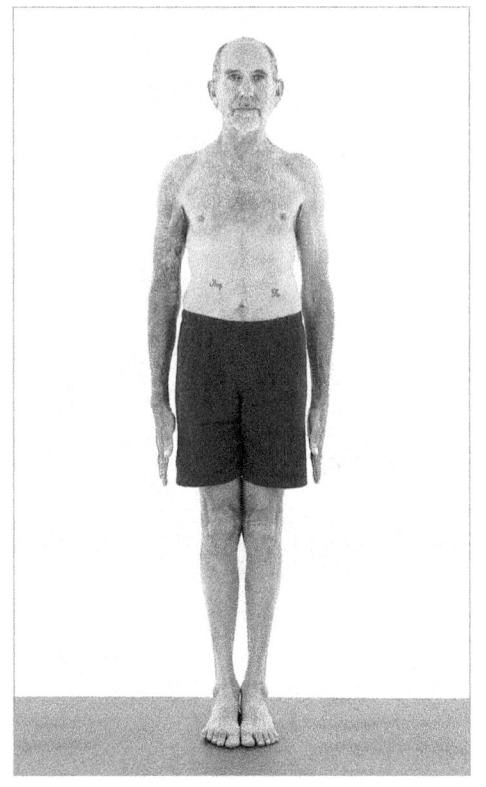

4.i.1 Samastiti

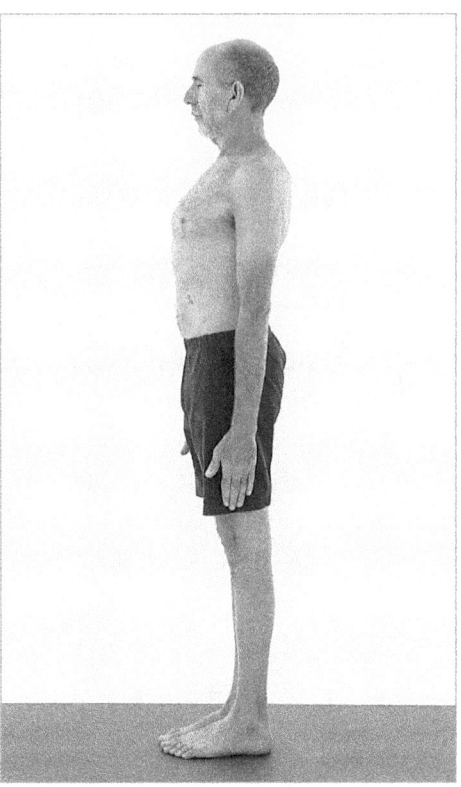

4.i.2 Finding balance in samastiti

8. Cultivate the stillness of a mountain. Mountains do not sway, rock, or fidget; they are rock solid. Develop stillness in the center of your being.

URDHVA HASTASANA
erd·vuh haas·tas·ahn·nuh | *upward-facing hand pose*

Warm Up Poses

Urdhva hastasana is one of the most basic standing poses. *Urdhva* means up and *hastas* are your hands. There are three different hand and *dristi* positions that are usually done sequentially. From *tadasana*, with your hands at your side:

1. Press the fingers of each hand firmly together to make your hands sharp.

2. Inhale and lift your arms overhead. Bring them to shoulder-width apart and face your palms forward.

3. Reach your arms up and soften your ribs toward your spine. Stay here one minute.

4. 2nd position: Drop your head back and look up. Lift your spine and keep breathing. Stay here 30 seconds.

5. 3rd position: Keep looking up and turn your palms to face each other. Stay here 30 seconds *(4.j)*.

6. Exhale and release your arms to your sides. Return to *tadasana/samastiti*.

STEPS 1–3: Set your hands in line with your shoulders and straighten your elbows. Spread the skin on your palms and reach your fingertips toward the ceiling. Reach your shoulders up as well; your shoulder blades must lift to fully extend your arms. Stiff shoulders may make your ribs flare forward and your butt stick out. Soften your ribs toward your spine, internally rotate your legs and drop your tailbone to keep your pelvis neutral. Stay here and breathe.

STEPS 4 & 5: The second and third positions are usually held for 30 seconds each, after holding the first position for 1 minute or more. Keep your arms fully extended for the duration of the pose.

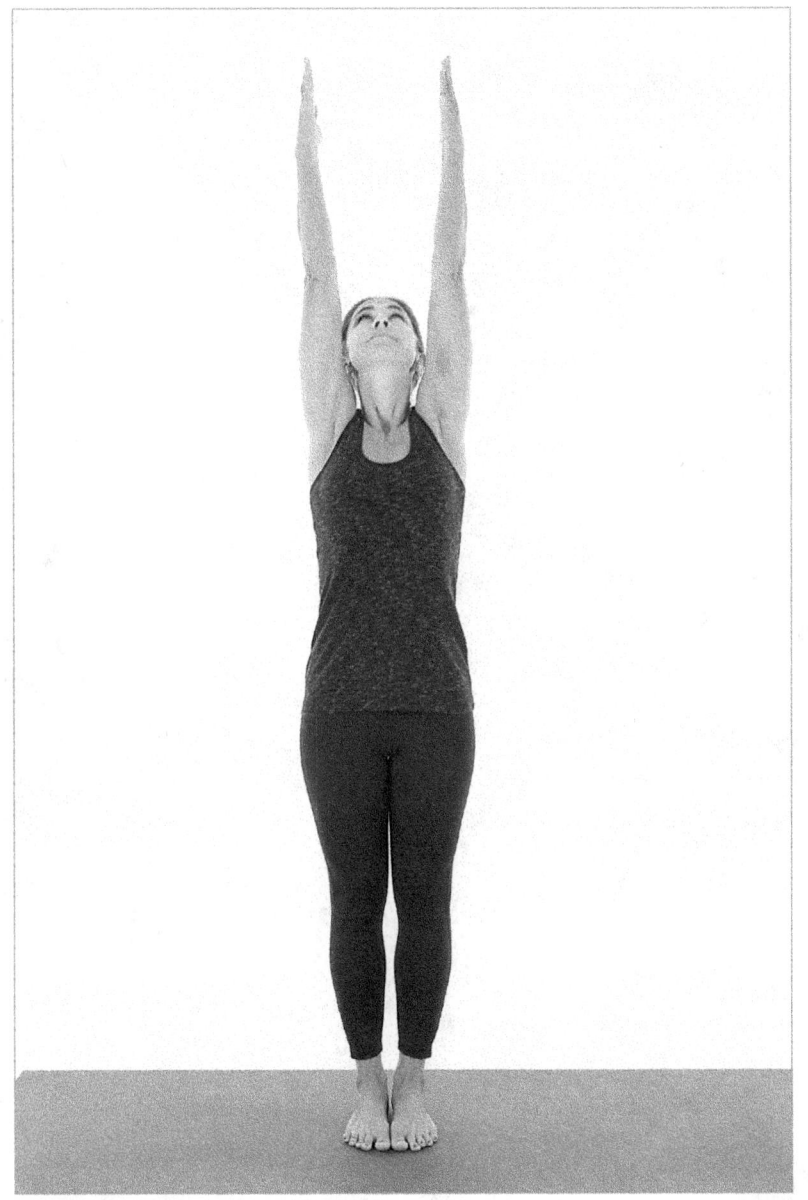

4.j Urdhva hastasana

Warm Up Poses

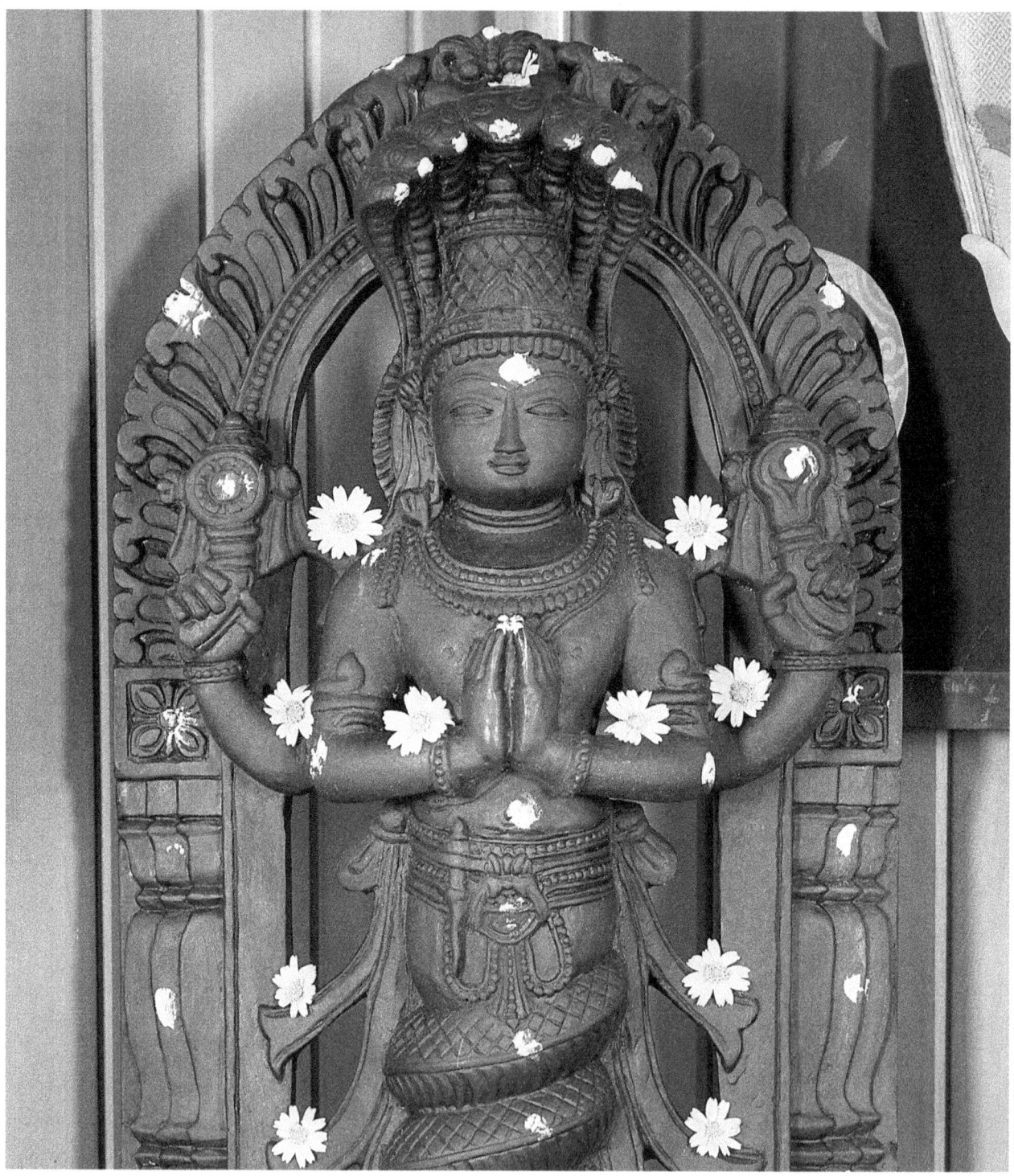

SURYA NAMASKAR A

soor·ya na·ma·scar A | *sun salutations A*

In the Ashtanga tradition, *surya namaskar* begins with the Invocation to Patanjali. Guruji loved this chant, and reciting it brings his loving energy into our practice. It connects us to yoga's broad collective consciousness and to a lineage that stretches all the way back to Patanjali himself.

INVOCATION TO PATANJALI

Stand in *samastiti* with your palms in *anjali mudra*. Close your eyes and settle into *ujayii breathing*.

vande guranàm charanàravinde

sandaràshita svàtma sukhàvabodhe

nishreyase jàngalikàyamàne

samsàra hàlàhala mohashàntyai

àbàhu purushàkàram

shankhachakràsi dhàrinam

sahasra shirasam shvetam

pranamàmi Patanjalim

I bow to the lotus feet of the great Guru

Awakening the happiness of the Self revealed

Beyond comparison, acting like a jungle physician

To pacify delusion from the poison of existence.

Taking the form of a man to the shoulders,

Holding a conch, a discus and a sword,

One thousand heads white, to Patanjali I salute.

NICKI:
Surya namaskar is about breath and movement. One thing Pattabhi Jois always taught is blood circulation. People would ask him really deep, profound questions about the postures, and he would just say, "Blood circulation!" It's funny, but it's also true. You need to keep your blood moving. If it starts to stagnate in certain areas, those areas will breed congestion and disease. Use this practice to banish the stagnation from your life.

Surya Namaskar A

EDDIE:
Contain yourself. Some of us are all over the place with our bodies, our minds, and our energy. Yoga is a practice of discipline. Apply yourself, and find stillness and grace in every movement.

Surya namaskar is at the heart of yoga. Guruji described it as a *Hatha* yoga breathing system: the inhale is for expansion and the exhale is for contraction. It is as simple and fundamental as your pulse, and like your pulse, it does not stop. There is no retention or holding of the breath; it is fluid, just like the movements. Breath initiates and completes every movement, and in doing so, it challenges you to be both efficient and accurate. After all, you only have a single breath to get where you are going.

Surya namaskar is a prayer. It cultivates grace, fluidity, and endurance. There are three main things to remember: first, keep breathing. Do not hold your breath. If you need an extra breath at any point in the sequence, take it. Breath is presence, and if you stop breathing you've closed the door on your experience. Your capacity will develop with time and practice, but it will not develop if you strain against your limitations. Be compassionate and understanding. Give yourself every consideration you would give to someone you love.

Second, be meticulous about the alignment of your wrists, elbows and shoulders. This is particularly important in the middle portion of the sequence—*chataranga dandasana* to downward dog—and the key is to keep your inner triads heavy. We see a lot of wrist braces in yoga today and it saddens us. Wrist braces, clenched fists, and all those other anatomical Band-Aids are an insult to yoga because they imply that people who do yoga are bound to injure their wrists. That could not be further from the truth. Yoga will profoundly integrate and strengthen your wrists, and the work is in your inner triad. Train your hands in *adho mukha svanasana* and box on the wall, and when you begin *surya namaskar*, build every movement from the solid foundation of your hands and feet.

Finally, it is extremely important to cultivate your *dristi* in *surya namaskar*. *Dristi* is your gaze and it aligns your internal and external tissue in the direction of the sequence. Your *dristi* determines the orientation of your head, and the orientation of your head influences the energetic direction of each pose and the transitions between them. The movement of your head should be contiguous with your spine and synonymous with your breath. Unnecessary movements will disrupt your mind, and this practice is about focusing your consciousness inside of your movements. Learning to focus your *dristi* simplifies your movements and cultivates grace throughout the sequence.

Surya namaskar is at the core of modern yoga. The three middle poses, in particular, are used as a bridge between static postures, and you may do them many, many times in a yoga class. Injuries are caused by misalignment and repetition in misalignment so take time to ensure the movements in this sequence are perfect, or as perfect as you can manage.

We will begin with a brief introduction to the sequence and follow with a more thorough explanation of each breath and its corresponding actions. Each movement is marked with a Sanskrit number: *ekam* means one, *dwi* means two, *trini* means three, and so forth. In the Ashtanga system, each one of these numbers forms a *vinyasa*: *ekam* is the first *vinyasa*, *dwi* is the second *vinyasa*, *trini* is the third, etc. Remember, this is a breathing system. Each movement is linked to your breath and each breath is married to movement. Whatever you do, don't stop breathing.

Surya Namaskar A

Begin in *samastiti*. Open your eyes and bring your arms to your sides.

> **EKAM:** Inhale. Lift your arms up and over your head, look up, and bring your palms together to touch.
>
> **DWI:** Exhale. Bend forward from your hips, bring your hands to the floor and look at your knees.
>
> **TRINI:** Inhale. Lift your head, look forward and extend your spine.
>
> **CHATWARI:** Exhale. Keep your head lifted and step to the back of your mat—do NOT jump. Keep looking forward, bend your arms, press your elbows toward your ribs and lower your shoulders to the height of your elbows into *chataranga dandasana*.
>
> **PANCHA:** Inhale. Straighten your arms to lift your chest, point your toes straight back and look up into *urdvha mukha svanasana* (upward dog).
>
> **SHAT:** Exhale. Lift your hips, extend your arms and reach your heels to the mat. Let your head come back last into *adho mukha svanasana* (downward dog).
>
> Stay in *adho mukha svanasana* for five breaths. Check your hands, arms, and legs for accuracy. At the end of your fifth breath, exhale completely and look toward your hands.
>
> **SUPTA:** Inhale. Step both feet to your hands and look forward to extend your spine.

EDDIE:
Every movement should be fully encapsulated in breath; begin your breath before you begin the movement and finish the movement before you finish your breath.

ASTO: Exhale. Bend forward from your hips, straighten your legs and look at your knees.

NAWA: Inhale. Keep your heels heavy and rise up. Lift your arms overhead and look up at your palms as they touch.

EXHALE. Bring your arms to your sides, level your gaze, and return to *samastiti*.

EKAM | yay·kum | *one:* Stand in *samastiti* (5.a). Press the fingers of each hand firmly together and spread the base of your palms. Lift your arms as you begin your inhale. Drop your head back to get it out of the way of your upper arms and look up at your hands as they join overhead. Straighten your elbows completely and reach your entire upper body—your chest, shoulders, elbows, and hands—toward the ceiling. Stay strong in your legs and rooted through the center of your heels. At the top of the inhale you are gazing at your thumbs with your palms touching and your arms fully extended *(5.b)*.

DWI | dwhey | *two:* Root your feet to the earth. Exhale and separate your hands as you bend forward at the hips. Gracefully float your arms down and bring your palms to the mat on either side of your feet. Drop your head and round your spine as your hands meet the mat. Gaze at your knees. If your hands don't reach the floor, or if touching the floor hurts your back, bend your knees to protect your lower back. This is NOT *uttanasana*; *uttanasana* is held for several minutes, *dwi* position is only half a breath. You're not here long enough to endanger your connective tissue so it's okay to bend your knees. At the bottom of the exhale you are in a deep forward bend with your hands on the floor, legs straight (unless you need to bend them), spine soft, head heavy, and gaze at your knees *(5.c)*.

TRINI | tree·knee | *three:* Inhale and lift your head to look forward. Lift your palms off the mat but leave your fingertips connected. Keep your legs straight and strong, unless they were bent in *dwi* position. Soften your shoulders and look forward to extend your spine. If looking forward hurts your neck, reach your sternum forward and soften your shoulders away from your ears. Open your chest and put your shoulders on your back to remove the congestion in your upper spine. Allow your throat to extend freely. At the top of your inhale your legs are reaching back and your torso is reaching forward, creating a slight backbend in your upper back. The traditional gaze is *antara dristi*; your face is

Surya Namaskar A

NICKI:
Ekam is different from *urdhva hastasana*. *Urdhva hastasana* is a static posture with the hands separated and the gaze forward; *Ekam* is held for only half a breath and the *dristi* is up at your joined hands. And please join your hands! Keeping your hands wide will make your shoulders narrow; bringing them together will open your shoulders and lengthen your upper back. It contributes to the beautiful upward energy of the pose.

forward but your gaze is directed inward *(5.d)*.

The first three movements of *surya namaskar A* are relatively easy. It's usually the next three movements—*chataranga dandasana*, *urdvha mukha svanasana*, and *adho mukha svanasana*—that are more difficult to maintain. It's absolutely essential to hold these next poses accurately because they pose the greatest risk of injury from misalignment and repetition. Remember: yoga does not cause injury. Injury is caused by misinformation and a lack of attention to detail. Be meticulous, and you will be safe.

CHATWARI | chut·twar·ee | *four:* The end of *trini* position has your head up, gaze forward and spine extended—the perfect setup for *chataranga dandasana*. Now pay close attention because there's a lot going on in the next breath.

Keep your head up and gaze forward in *antara dristi*. Exhale as you bend your knees and step both feet to the back of your mat. Straighten your legs as they reach the back of your mat and shift forward onto the tips of your toes. Simultaneously bend your elbows in toward your ribs as you lower your torso forward and down. Reach your chest, throat, and gaze forward to keep your elbows directly over your wrists, and lower your shoulders to the height of your elbows. Lower your torso only enough to form a right angle in your arms; don't go any lower. Keep your inner triads heavy.

Please do not jump into *chataranga dandasana*. It takes a lot of practice to figure out how far back you need to go to keep your elbows over your wrists, and stepping is more accurate than jumping. It's also essential to keep your gaze forward. In fact, the head barely moves in the transition from *trini* to *chatwari*; it stays upright and forward to guide the energy of the pose. Looking down as you step back takes your pose backward, and moving backward will collapse your shoulders onto your wrists and put pressure in your elbows.

At the end of the exhale your gaze is forward with your chest and throat extended, your elbows squeezing your ribs, and your legs completely straight. There is a slight backbend in your upper back to support the opening in your chest, but your tailbone is reaching toward your heels to lengthen your lower back. Find *mula* and *uddiyana bandha* at the bottom of your exhale, and be as straight and strong as a four-limbed staff *(5.e)*.

This is the most difficult pose in *surya namaskar*. At the end of the exhale your ears, shoulders, elbows, and hips are in a perfectly straight line, and that

Surya Namaskar A

NICKI:
Your gaze is forward at the end of *trini* position and it should stay forward as you move into *chataranga dandasana*. That's how Guruji taught us the pose: with the face forward and throat fully extended. If we looked down, he was not happy. And there's a reason: lifting your head feeds your thyroid gland, extends your chest, and puts your shoulders on your back. It guides the energy of the pose in a magnificent way. But physiology aside, we teach the pose this way because that's what he taught us. We hope to honor him and his teachings in all we do.

takes a lot of strength. Most of us don't come to yoga with that level of strength and awareness so it's absolutely essential to find a modification that meets you where you are. Without modification, the pose can get sloppy and potentially injurious. The most common mistake is over-dropping the torso: you look down at the floor, your body weight sinks backward, your wrists end up under your shoulders instead of under your elbows, and your shoulders collapse toward your wrists. This puts your face just inches above the ground and lifts your pelvis, leaving you in a forward bend instead of a backbend. It's uncomfortable and it can also severely strain your elbows, wrists, and shoulders. That misaligned pose will not move you any closer to *chataranga dandasana* so any effort you exert there is completely wasted. Please don't do that to yourself.

MODIFIED CHATWARI: If you don't have the strength to maintain the fundamental structural alignment of *chataranga dandasana*, don't worry. You're not alone. We see it in almost all of our beginning (and even advanced) students and we offer this modification:

From *trini* position, exhale and step to the back of your mat. Keep your legs straight and shift onto your tippy toes, and then bring your pelvis straight down to the mat as you bend your elbows to 90°. Rest your pelvis on the mat and extend your tailbone toward your heels. Straighten your legs, lift your chest, and keep your gaze forward so only your hands, toes, and pelvis are on the mat. Squeeze your elbows toward your ribs and keep your shoulders at the height of your elbows *(5.e.2)*.

Surya Namaskar A

NICKI: If your face is closer to the mat than your elbows, something is wrong.

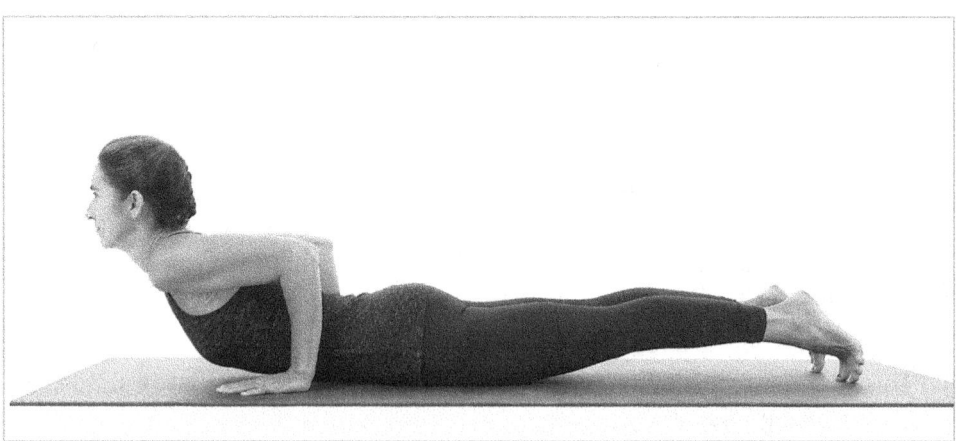

5.e.2 Modified chatwari

This modification creates a structural memory in the direction of *chataranga dandasana*: strong legs, strong arms, and an open chest and throat. Putting your pelvis down accomplishes two things: 1) your arms don't have to support the full weight of your body so you have more mental space to focus on the alignment of your chest, shoulders and pelvis. 2) Your pubic bone moves toward your front body to open your legs and pelvis, which supports the slight backbend in your upper back. As you build strength in your arms and legs, experiment with keeping your pelvis lifted off the mat—while maintaining the foundations of the pose, of course.

PANCHA | pawn·chuh | *five:* Inhale and straighten your arms, roll forward onto the tops of your feet and point your toes straight back. Externally rotate both arms and roll your shoulders back to open your chest. The eyes of your elbows will naturally roll forward with your arms but keep your inner triads heavy. Lead with your sternum to shift forward and up. Internally rotate your legs, straighten your knees, and drop your tailbone toward your heels to lengthen your lower back. Look up and stretch your throat, but only if it's okay with your neck—lifting your head is the last piece of the pose. At the top of the inhale you are in full *urdhva mukha svanasana* (upward-facing dog), with your arms and legs completely straight, your shoulders back, your chest reaching forward and your gaze up in *antara drishti (5.f).*

Pancha position brings up one last thing about *chataranga dandasana*. The real beauty of *surya namaskar* is the intelligence of the sequence itself; each pose leads you to the next in a magnificent way. Studying the architecture of the poses reveals that the upright face and open chest of *chataranga dandasana* set the stage for the beautiful backbending motion of *urdhva mukha svanasana*. Moving toward *urdhva mukha* from the squished *chataranga*—the one with your shoulders barely above your wrists, face down, pelvis up and chest closed—is much, much harder. Each pose is far more graceful and enjoyable if you honor the fundamental structural alignment of the previous one.

SHAT | shat | *six:* Exhale, keep your legs straight, lift your hips and roll over your toes. Reach your heels toward the mat and lift your sit bones into *adho mukha svanasana*. Let your head come back last; the transition from upward facing to inward facing (the gaze in downward dog is at your navel) encompasses the full length of your exhale so your head is the last thing to come into position. Extend your arms and open your armpit chest. At the top of the exhale you are in *adho*

Surya Namaskar A

NICKI:
Yoga always builds sequentially. If you can't do the pose, use props and modifications to align your body to its shape. We call it *netti netti*—a little of this, a little of that; step by step; trial and error. But you have to follow the lines of yoga. Don't alter the lines of yoga to make the pose easier because it will never make the full pose more accessible.

Surya Namaskar A

mukha svanasana with your arms and legs fully extended and gazing at your navel *(5.g)*.

Stay in *adho mukha svanasana* for five breaths. In time this will become the most restful pose in an otherwise demanding sequence. Use it to check your foundations. The transition from *trini* to *chatwari* tends to set your hands wider than your shoulders so take the time to make them perfect. Your inner triads should be heavy when you enter the pose because they stayed heavy through *chataranga dandasana* and upward dog. Keeping the inner triads heavy may seem difficult, especially when there's so much going on, but it will train your arms to take responsibility for their work and profoundly strengthen and protect your wrists.

MODIFIED SHAT. If downward dog pulls on your back, use this modification:

Exhale, keep your legs straight, lift your hips and roll over your toes. Reach your heels toward the mat, lift your sit bones and let your head come back last into *adho mukha svanasana*. Once you are in the pose, lift your heels and bend your knees to the height of your ankles. Bending your knees takes your hamstrings out of the equation and allows you to extend your spine. Keep your knees bent as you lift your sit bones, extend your arms, and open your armpit chest *(5.g.2)*. Look at your navel and breathe.

SUPTA | sup·tah | *seven:* Finish your fifth exhale and look up at your hands. Inhale, keep looking up and step or walk both feet to the front of your mat. Don't jump. Ground your feet between your hands and lift your chest as you look forward. Leave your fingertips on the mat and straighten your arms and legs. If you need to bend your knees to protect your lower back, please do so. The top of the inhale finds you in *trini* position: legs strong, arms extended, shoulders soft, chest open and gaze forward *(5.h)*.

ASTO | ash·toe | *eight:* Exhale and bend forward at your hips. Release the weight of your head and allow your spine to round as you gaze toward your knees. Straighten and internally rotate your legs, and lift your kneecaps. At the end of the exhale you are in a deep forward bend with your palms on the floor and your forehead pressed into your shins—if you can go that far. If you can't, don't worry about it; just bring your head toward your legs, soften your ribs and let the back of your neck lengthen *(5.i)*.

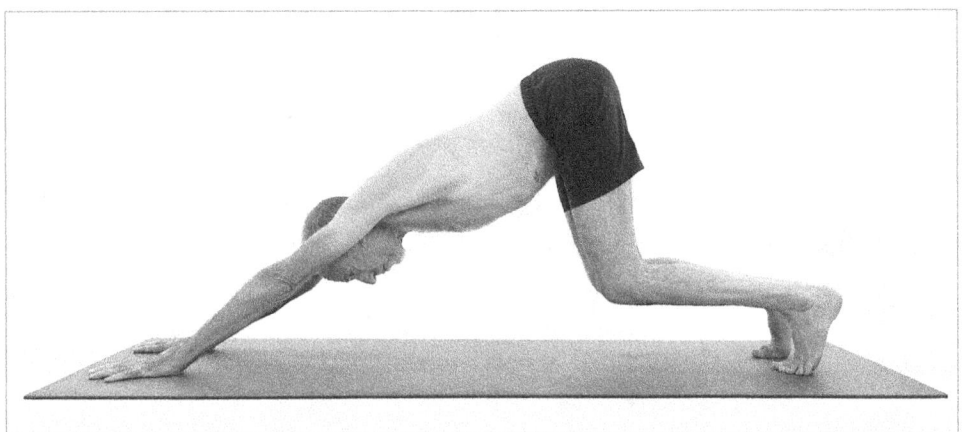

5.g.2 Modified shat

Surya Namaskar A

NICKI: Doing this modification doesn't compromise the integrity of the pose, or the integrity of your practice. It's a modification that gives you access to your spine while protecting your lower back. It moves you in the direction of yoga, not away from it.

NAWA | naah·wah | *nine:* Ground firmly through the center of your heels and keep your kneecaps lifted. Inhale as you lift your torso and simultaneously reach your arms up and to the side in a smooth arc. Lift your head, torso and arms at the same rate. When your torso is upright, drop your head back to look at your palms as they join overhead. At the top of the inhale your arms and legs are fully extended, your palms are together, and your gaze is at your thumbs—just like *ekam* position *(5.j)*.

Exhale and release your palms to your side, returning to *samastiti*. The last position is not counted; you simply return to *samastiti (5.k)*.

That is one full cycle of *surya namaskar A*. It cultivates a profound unity between breath and movement in preparation for more static postures. We typically do five to ten rounds of *surya namaskar A* to begin our practice, but there's really no limit. Eddie did *surya namaskar A* until a single bead of sweat dripped off his nose because that meant he was warmed up enough to do standing poses. Develop your own personal barometer and let it guide you through this fantastic practice.

That concludes the "beginning" postures of a general yoga sequence. We find them highly effective and wonderfully synchronistic and start most of our classes with them. They allow us to move into more static postures, such as lunges and standing poses, with internally developed heat and flexibility and a profound unity of being. You don't have to do the beginning postures in exactly the same sequence or in exactly the same way because your practice should be intelligent enough to reflect your personal needs. Listen to yourself and adjust accordingly.

Surya Namaskar A

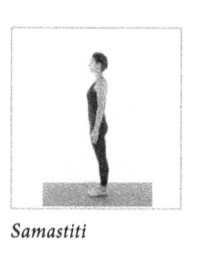 *Samastiti*
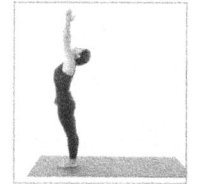 *Ekam*
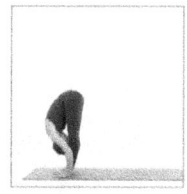 *Dwi*
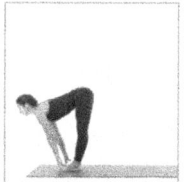 *Trini*
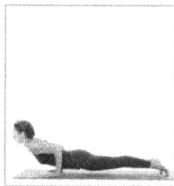 *Chatwari*

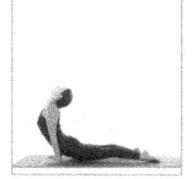 *Pancha*
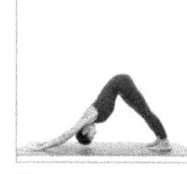 *Shat*
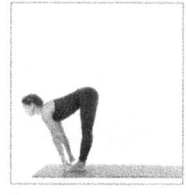 *Supta*
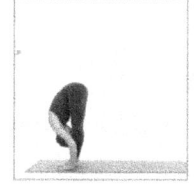 *Ashto*
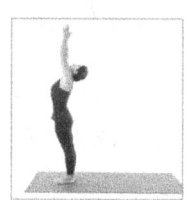 *Nawa*

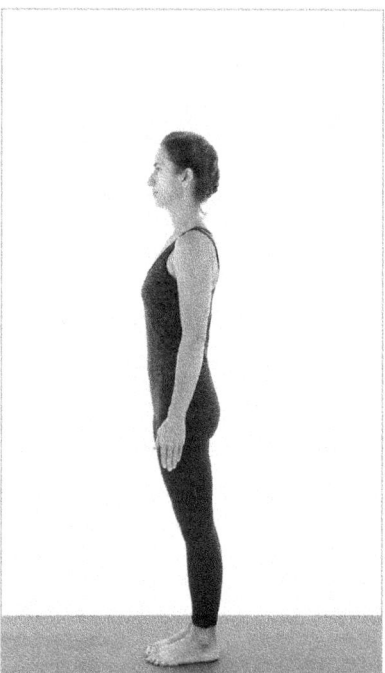

5.a Samastiti

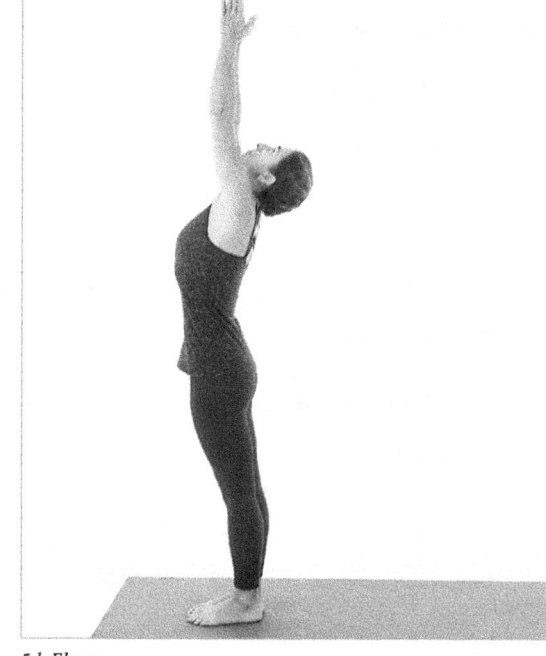

5.b Ekam

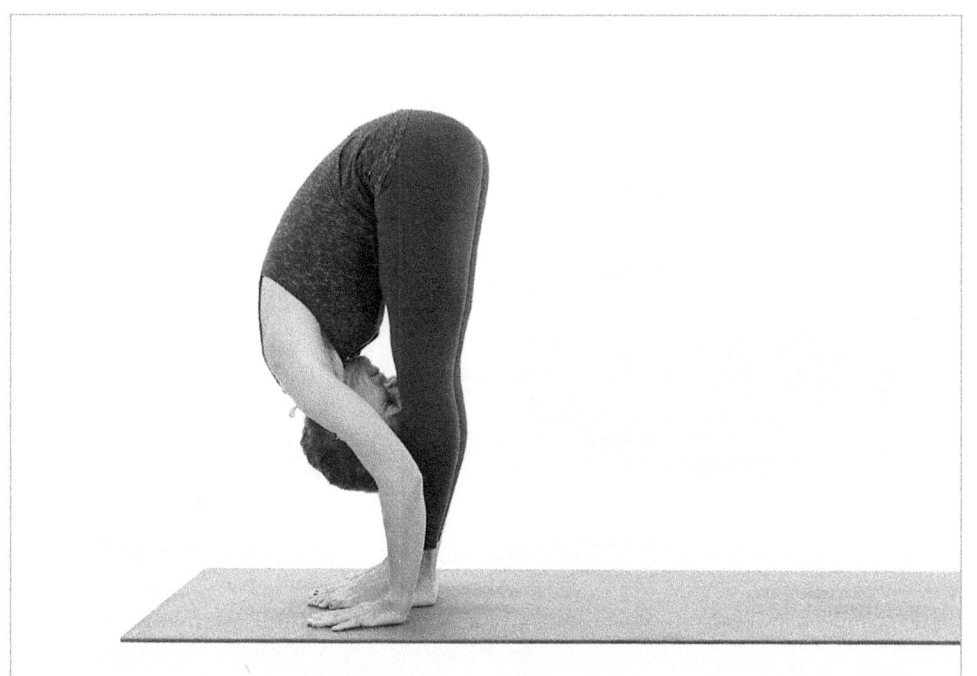

Surya Namaskar A

5.c Dwi

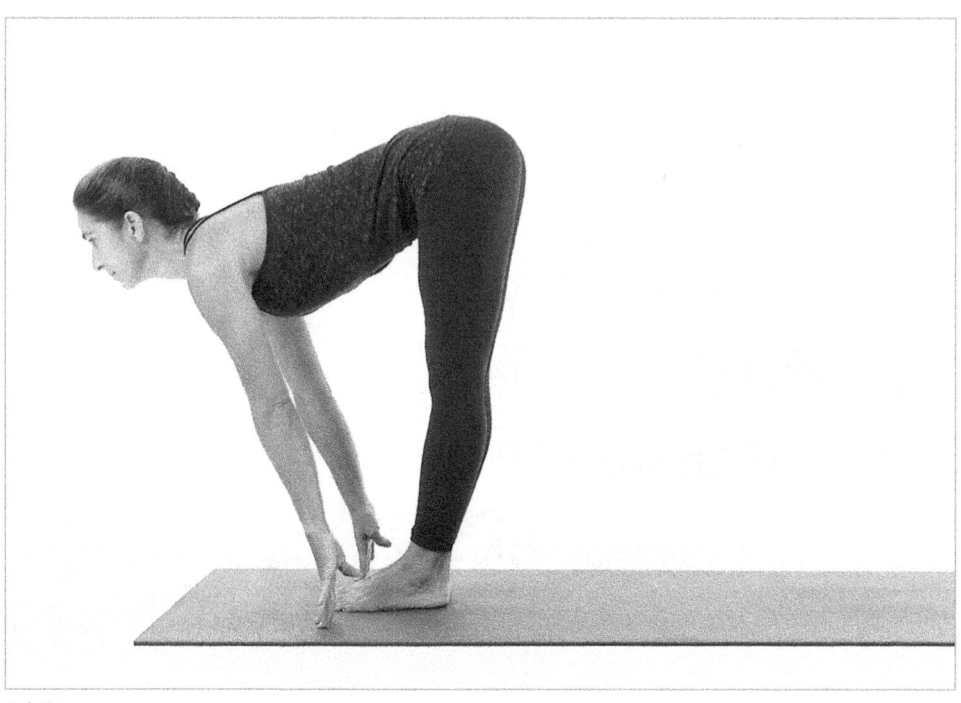

5.d Trini

Surya Namaskar A

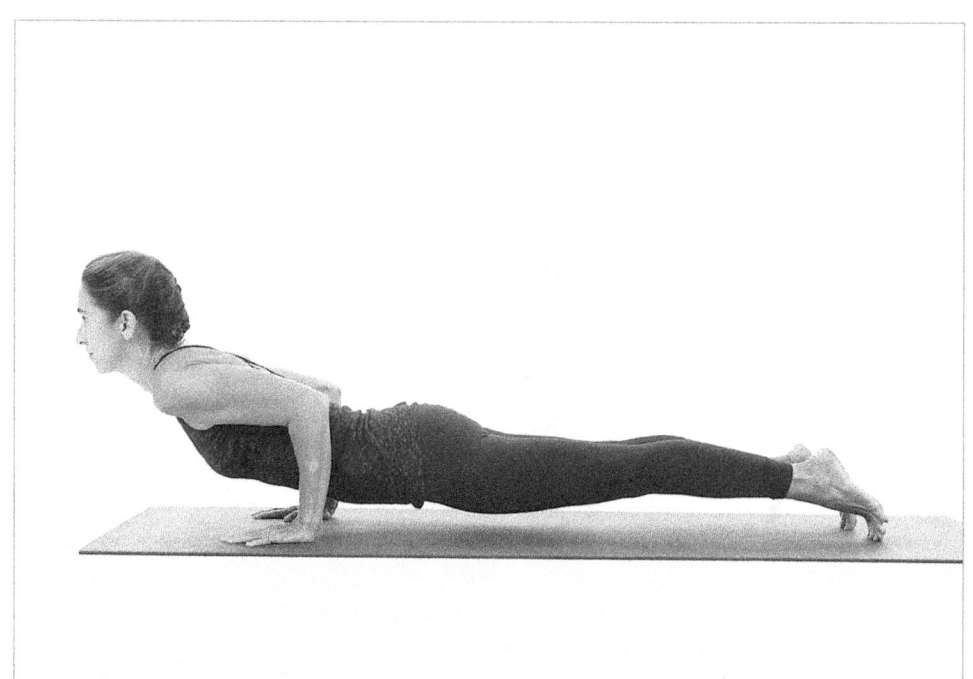

5.e Chatwari

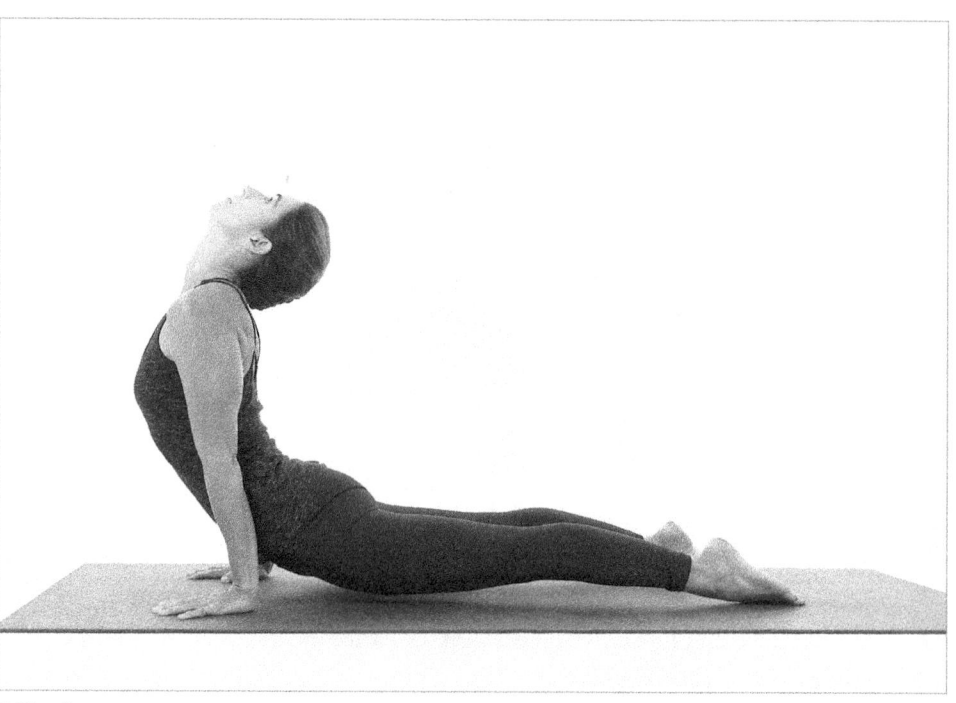

5.f Pancha

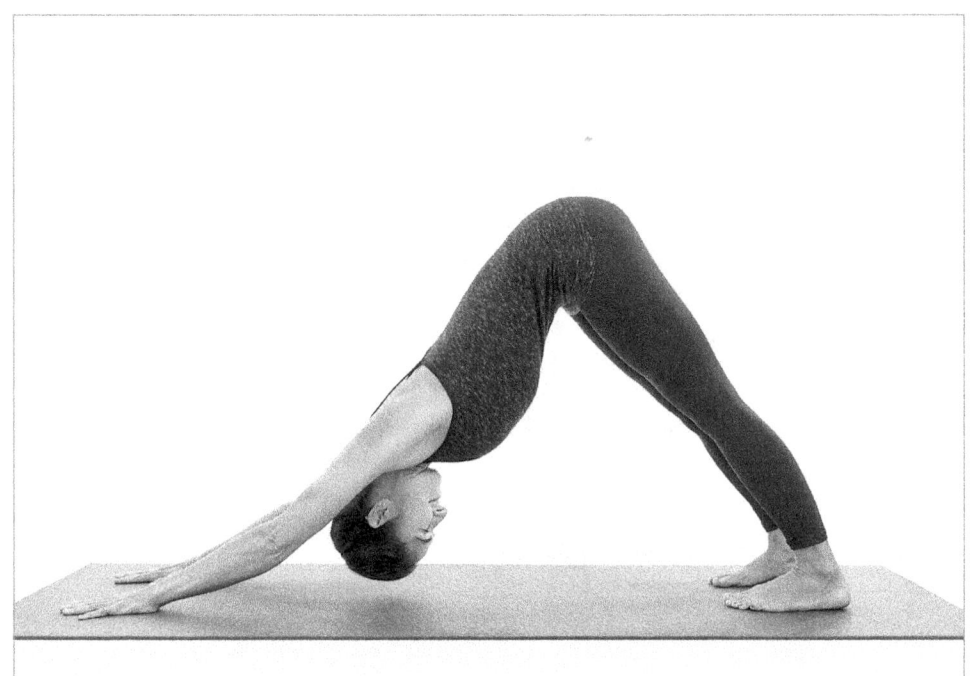

Surya Namaskar A

5.g Shat

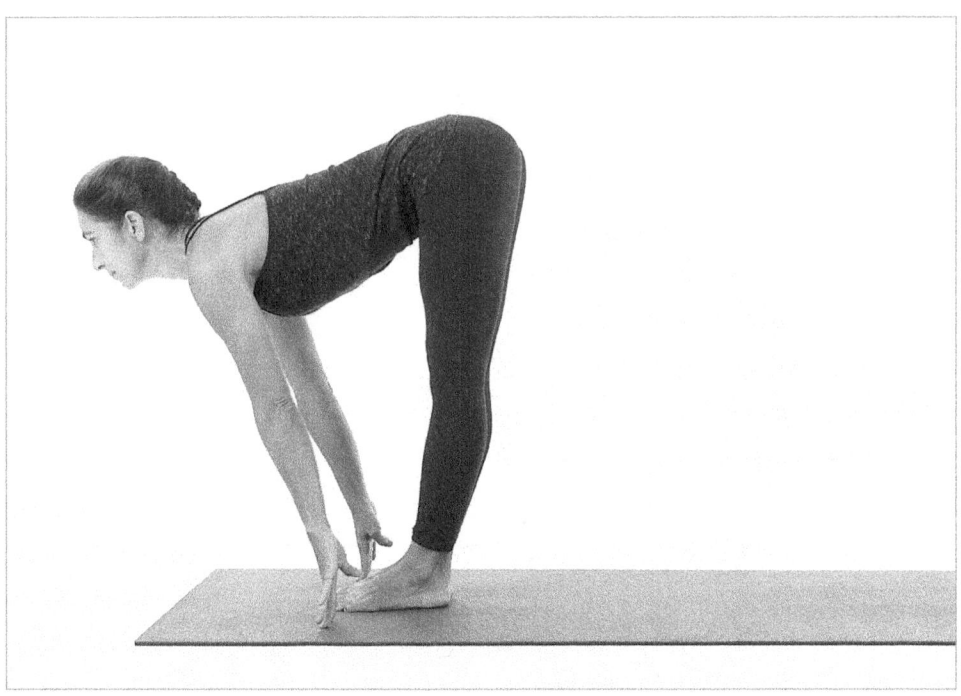

5.h Supta

Surya Namaskar A

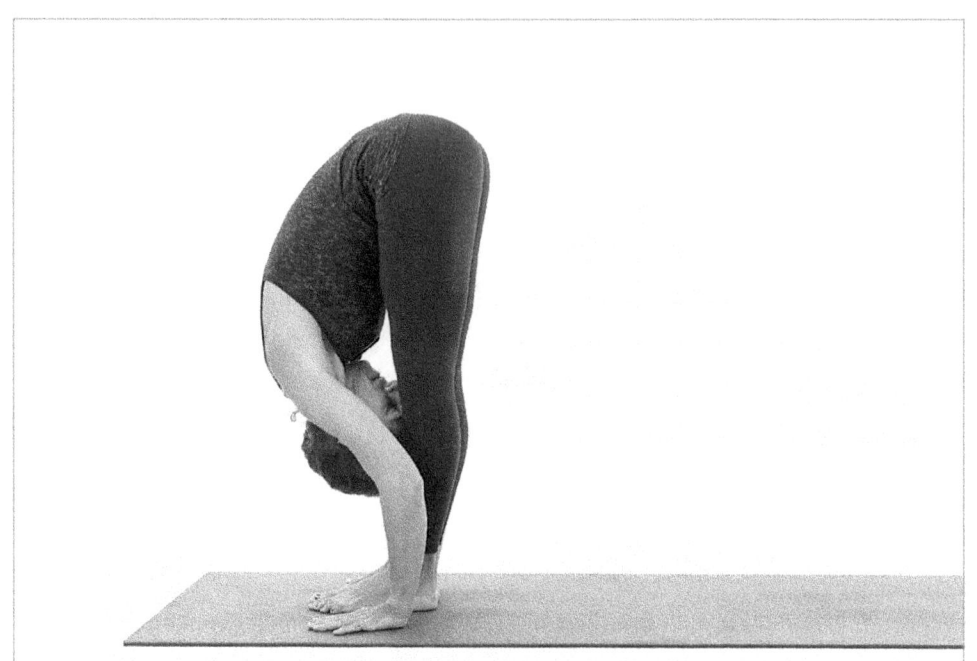

5.i *Asto*

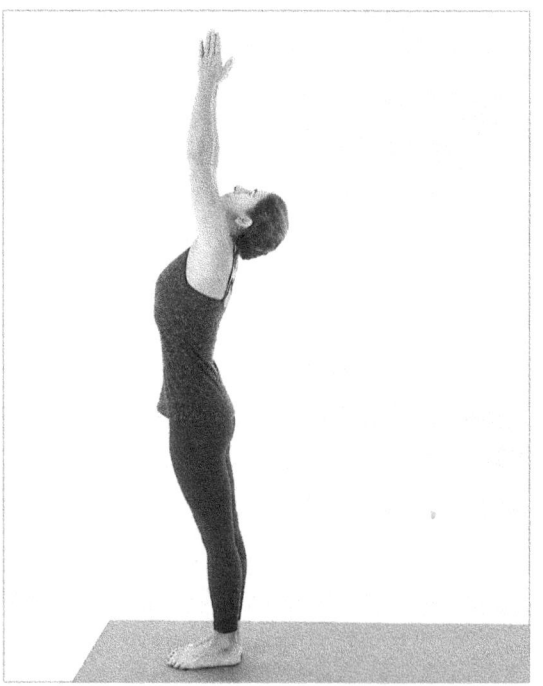

5.j *Nawa*

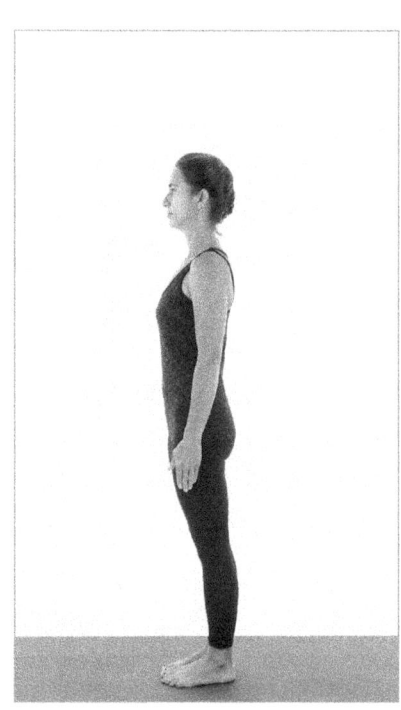

5.k *Samastiti*

LUNGES

We developed this sequence of lunges to address mankind's most common anatomical restriction: stiff legs and hips. There are 10 lunges total (though we often go up to 16 in our classes) but in this section we'll focus on a few foundational ones. Spend about a minute in each lunge, or perhaps longer, and spend the same amount of time on each side. We recommend using a stopwatch for accuracy.

FIRST LUNGE

From *adho mukha svanasana*:

1. Inhale and step your right foot forward between your hands.
2. Bend your right knee to 90° and straighten your left leg. Your hands should be on either side of your right foot.
3. Shift your right heel slightly to the right and organize your right foot. Set your ankle directly over the center of your heel.
4. Push into your right leg without lifting your hips above your right knee. Lift your hands off the floor and take your belly off your thigh.
5. Put your hands down as lightly as possible and ensure there is no pressure in your wrists.
6. Take your right sitting bone closer to your left sitting bone without over-dropping your left hip.
7. Straighten your back leg and make your hips level *(6.a)*.
8. Inhale and lift your hips. Exhale and step back to downward dog.

STEPS 1-3: Shift your heel slightly to the right to make the outer edge of your foot roughly parallel to the long edge of your mat. Notice we said roughly parallel; the back of your foot is narrower than the front of your foot so it's not going to make a perfectly straight line. Lift all five toes on your right foot and spread them. Press firmly through your big toe bone to create a visible depression in the skin between your big toe bone and your second toe bone. That little trough between

Lunges

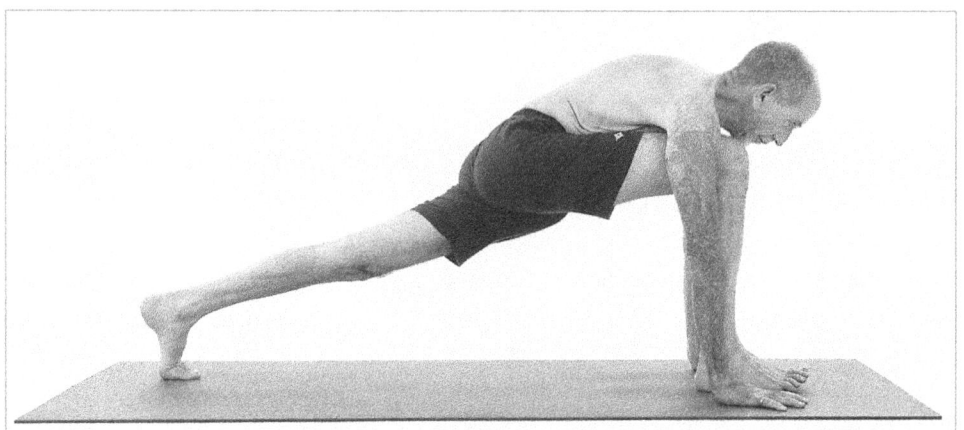

6.a First lunge, hands outside of front foot

your first and second toes is your anchor. Keep it heavy as you lift your inner arch and bring your ankle directly over your heel.

STEPS 4 & 5: Press firmly into your right foot and take your hands an inch or two off the ground. Take your belly off your thigh and use the strength of your right leg to keep your hips at the height of your right knee. Once you're balanced, place your fingertips back on the mat as lightly as possible. There should not be any pressure in your wrists because your legs are doing all the work, but if you do feel pressure, lift up onto your fingertips or knuckles to alleviate any discomfort.

STEP 6: Bring your awareness to your sacrum, tailbone, and right sitting bone. Are they being pulled to the right? They probably are, and you're not alone. When you split your legs and bend one knee, tightness in your front hip will pull your entire pelvis in the direction of your bent knee. It also creates a sideways "C" curve in your spine that shortens the right side of your waist; your hip is too stiff to create the shape of the pose so your spine gets dragged along instead. This is the recruiting we discussed in the Foundations section. In the 1st, 2nd, and 4th lunge, recruiting usually happens between your hips and spine; the pose pulls your right hip forward and to the right from the flexibility of your lower back. It may also distort your right ankle because your ankle is also more flexible than your hips.

At the bottom of your next exhale, take your right sitting bone closer to your left sitting bone without over-dropping your left hip (i.e. letting it go lower than your right hip) or distorting your right ankle. Move your outer right hip toward your inner left thigh, and shift your hips slightly to the left to bring your pelvis in line with your sternum. Move your sit bones closer together, engage *mula* and *uddiyana bandha*, and balance both sides of your pelvis.

STEP 7: Straighten your back (left) leg completely. Initiate the lift from your knee and engage your inner left thigh all the way to your groin. This action is often the hardest to maintain; there's a lot of specific work in the front leg to absorb your attention while the back leg stays out of sight. But keeping the back leg straight forces anatomical integrity into your right hip, which is extremely important. Use the rhythm of your breath to reinforce the action of *mula* and *uddiyana bandha* and use *jiva bandha* to relax your jaw, face, and shoulders. Stay here for one minute.

Inhale and lift your hips and exhale to step your right foot back into downward dog. Take a resting breath between sides and then repeat the lunge with your left foot forward.

Lunges

EDDIE: Channel the strength of *uttanasana* into your left leg and the softness of *balasana* into your right hip.

SECOND LUNGE

All the remaining lunges begin in *adho mukha svanasana* (downward dog) with the thumbs touching. From *adho mukha svanasana*, look at your hands and move them toward each other until your thumbs are touching in the center of your mat. Keep your hands and wrists organized and your inner triads heavy.

From *adho mukha svanasana* with your thumbs touching:

1. Inhale and step your right foot to the outside of your right hand.
2. Exhale and bend your right knee to 90°. Drop your right hip to the height of your right knee.
3. Shift your right heel slightly to the right and organize your foot. Set your ankle directly over the center of your heel.
4. Press into your right leg to alleviate any pressure in your wrists. Straighten your left leg completely.
5. Bring your right sitting bone closer to your left sitting bone while keeping your hips level *(6.b)*.
6. Inhale and lift your hips. Exhale and step back to downward dog.

STEPS 1-3: The organization of your front foot and ankle are consistent with the

Lunges

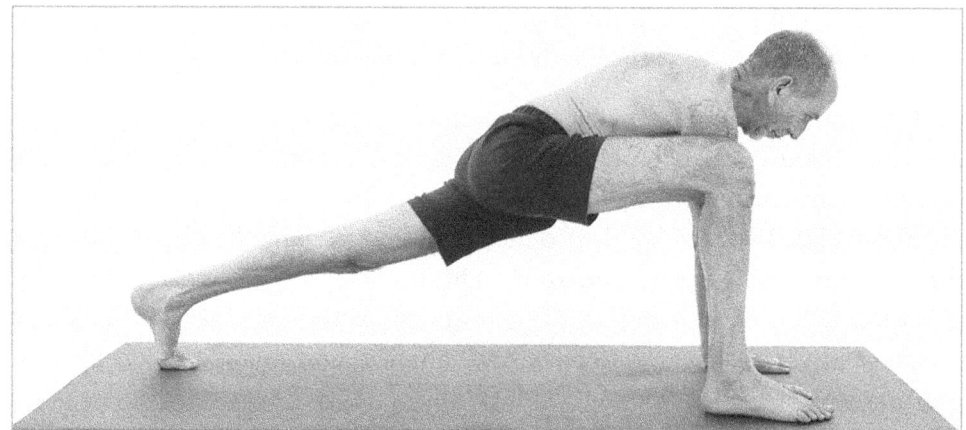

6.b Second lunge, hands inside of front foot

first lunge. The primary difference between the first and second lunge is your torso is now inside of your front leg, allowing you to go deeper into your groin. That extra leverage may also pull your right knee into your right armpit, so soften both shoulders away from your ears and keep your right knee just outside of your right shoulder.

STEP 4: Be conscious of pressure in your wrists. Lift onto your fingertips or knuckles to alleviate the pressure or (more effectively) train your front leg to carry its own weight. Teach the segments of your body to take responsibility for their work; don't allow any part to freeload on another part's flexibility.

STEP 5: Bring your awareness to your pelvis and use *mula bandha* to shift your right sit bone toward your left sit bone. Reach your right outer hip toward your left inner thigh, and be conscious of your body's attempts to wiggle away from the stiffness in your right hip; watch your right big toe bone, your right ankle, and the extension of your left leg. It's the same action as the first lunge: use your awareness to integrate your spine and sacrum so that your hips and legs can take responsibility for their opening. Breathe freely and use *jiva bandha* to soften into the opening in your right hip. Stay here for one minute.

Inhale and lift your hips and exhale to step your right foot back into downward dog. Take a resting breath between sides and then repeat the lunge with your left foot forward.

THIRD LUNGE

The third lunge is a more advanced version of the second lunge. The primary contraindication is pain in your front knee. If you feel pain or discomfort in your front knee, turn your right toes and right knee to the right.

From downward dog with your thumbs touching:

1. Inhale and step your right big toe to your outer right wrist.
2. Exhale, bend your right knee and lower your left knee to the mat. Point your left toes straight back.
3. Shift your right heel slightly to the right and organize your foot and ankle. Keep your right knee tracking forward over your toes. If there is any pain in your right knee, turn your knee and toes to the right.
4. Exhale and come down onto your elbows inside of your right foot.
5. Squeeze your right knee toward your right shoulder.
6. Soften your right hip toward your right heel. Press your right elbow into the mat to make your forearms evenly weighted *(6.c.1)*.
7. Curl your back (left) toes under, and on an exhale, straighten your left leg.
8. Lift your hips until you can see your entire left ankle *(6.c.2)*.
9. Bring your right sit bone toward your left without over-dropping your left hip, and squeeze your right knee toward your right shoulder.
10. Look forward and extend your sternum toward the front of your mat *(6.c.3)*.
11. Exhale and bring your left knee to the mat. If your right knee and toes are pointed out, return both to center before coming out of the pose.
12. Inhale and lift your hips. Exhale and step back to downward dog.

Lunges

NICKI:
If any of these lunges hurt your front knee, turn your toes and knee out to the side. Always point your knees and toes in the same direction.

Lunges

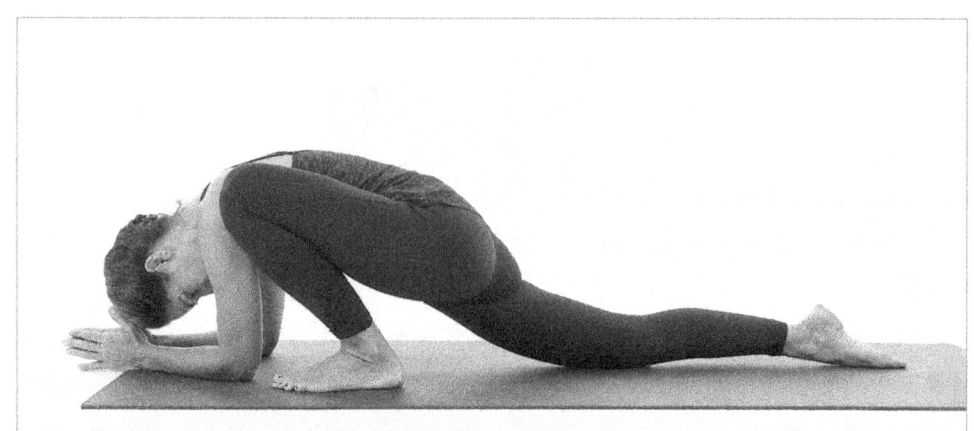

6.c.1 Third lunge setup

NICKI:
Please be very patient with your joints. Don't break your knees to open your hips.

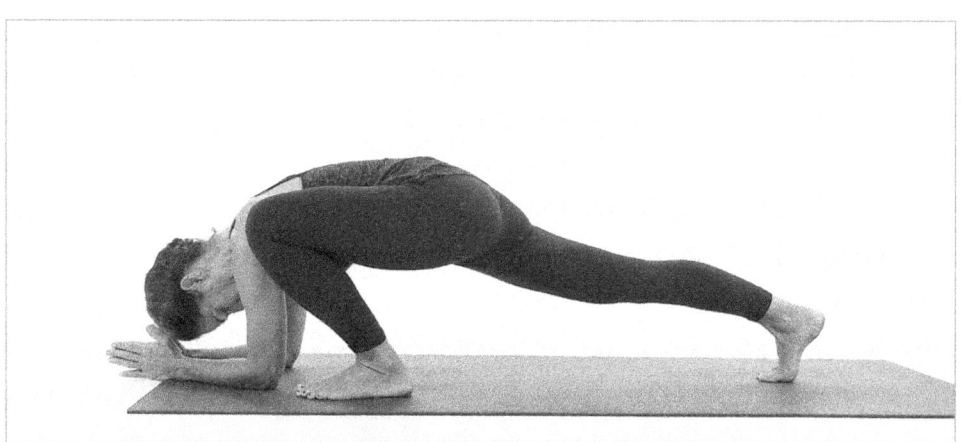

6.c.2 Third lunge, second stage

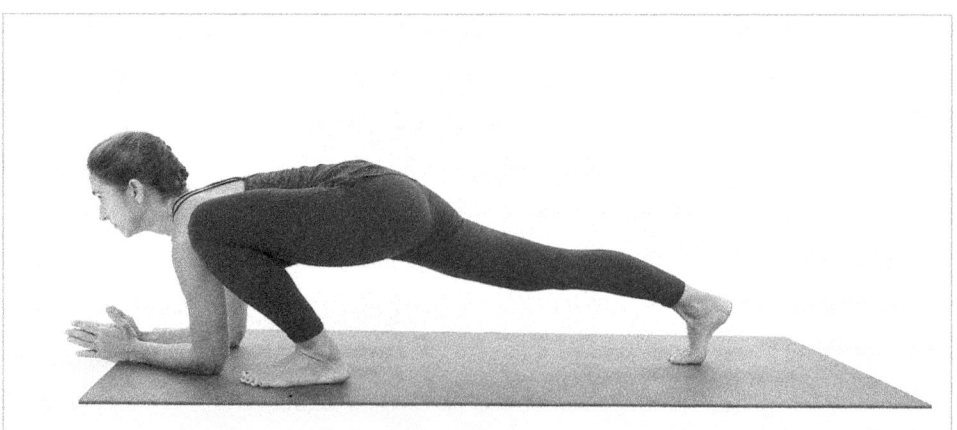

6.c.3 Third lunge, full pose

STEPS 1-3: Set your foundations: look over your left shoulder to check the alignment of your back foot and then look down to organize your right foot and ankle. Keep your right heel heavy on the mat. If there is any pain or discomfort in your right knee, turn your right toes and your right knee slightly out to the right. Always keep your knee and toes pointed in the same direction. Turn them out as little or as much as it takes to alleviate any discomfort in your knee, and as you become more familiar with the pose, you can explore pointing them back toward the front of your mat.

Lunges

STEPS 4 & 5: On an exhale, bend your elbows and bring your forearms to the mat. If one or both of your elbows don't reach the floor, put a block under both forearms. Stiffness in your right hip may pull your knee to the right by recruiting flexibility from your knee and ankle; counteract the stiffness by squeezing your knee toward your right shoulder to keep it pointed in the same direction as your toes (forward). If keeping your knee close to your shoulder hurts your knee, allow them to separate and turn both your knee and your toes out to the right. If you already had your knee and toes turned out to the right (to accommodate discomfort in your knee), make sure they remain pointed in the same direction for the duration of the pose.

STEP 6: Sink your right hip toward your right heel, and keep your right knee hugged into your right shoulder (unless it's turned out to avoid pain in your knee). Stiffness in your right hip may push your weight to the left, making your left forearm heavier than your right. Balance the weight by pressing your right forearm into the mat (or blocks), and simultaneously encourage your right hip to release toward your right heel. Drop your head, soften your jaw, and let your torso get heavy. Try to find a sense of release in your hips. Remember *balasana*, where you explored complete and total release? Cultivate that same sense of softness and relaxation, and channel it into your right hip.

This is the "first" stage of the lunge, and if it's already arduous to maintain, you may want to explore it for a few weeks before incorporating the next step. When you're ready to move forward, stay in this step for 15 – 30 seconds before moving on.

STEP 7: On an inhale, curl your left toes under and straighten your left leg. Engage your quadriceps and internally rotate your entire left leg to reach your left inner thigh toward the ceiling. Initiate the lift from the back of your knee, and keep it perfectly straight for the duration of the pose.

STEP 8: Drop your head and look at your left foot. If you cannot see your entire left foot and ankle, your hips are too low. Lift them until your left ankle is visible and then straighten your back leg more. Soften your right hip, relax your hands, and use *jiva bandha* to soften your jaw.

Lunges

STEPS 9 & 10: Move your right sitting bone closer to your left sitting bone, just like you did in the first and second lunges. Bring your right outer hip toward your left inner thigh, and don't over-drop your left hip—make sure you can see your entire left ankle. If you want more, extend your sternum and look forward. Reach your gaze forward from the entire length of your spine: roll your shoulders back, reach your chest forward, extend your throat and straighten your back leg even more. Stay here for 30 seconds.

To come out, bring your left knee to the mat and straighten your arms. If your right toes are pointed out to accommodate your knee, turn both your knee and toes back to center. Inhale and lift your hips and exhale to step your right foot back into downward dog. Take a resting breath between sides and then repeat the lunge with your left foot forward.

FOURTH LUNGE

The first three lunges address the relationship between the femur (thigh) and the acetabulum (hip socket); more specifically, their ability—or inability—to externally rotate in relation to one another. The fourth lunge changes the orientation to address stiffness in your front body: specifically the psoas, groin, and quadriceps.

The primary contraindication is pain in your knees and we will include specific directions for the front and back knee. There are also additional contraindications for stiff people and flexible people. The lunge leads into a backbend, and if you have a stiff front body (like most of the Western world) it may put pressure on your lower back. If that is your reality, drop your tailbone to extend your lower back and lift your sternum to lengthen your spine. Think about bringing the pose forward and up, and develop length in your lower back by opening the front of your pelvis.

Flexible people are less likely to compress their lower back but they may be at risk for overextending the labrum in the front of the groin. Your labrum is most at risk when your back leg externally rotates and your pelvis tracks away from your front heel. The best way to protect your labrum is to pay close attention to your alignment: keep your back leg neutral by evenly pressing both sides of your back foot (do not let it externally rotate), press into your front heel to support the weight of the pose, track your pelvis straight forward (do not sag into your extended hip), and use *mula bandha* to hold it all together.

From downward dog with your thumbs touching: *Lunges*

1. Inhale and step your right big toe to your outer right wrist.

2. Exhale and bend your right knee. Bring your left knee to the floor and point your left toes straight back.

3. Look over your left shoulder to ensure your left heel is pointed straight up. Press evenly into the big toe and pinkie toe sides of your left foot.

4. Shift your right heel slightly to the right and organize your foot and ankle. If there is pain in your right knee, turn your knee and toes to the right.

5. Bend your right knee and sink your right sit bone toward your right heel. Press your heel into the mat and keep your knee tracking in the direction of your toes.

6. Roll your shoulders back, drop your tailbone and lift your sternum *(6.d)*.

7. Exhale and press the top of your left foot into the mat to straighten your left leg.

8. Sink your right sit bone toward your right heel and fully engage your left leg.

9. Lift your chest, and if it feels right, extend your throat and look up.

10. Release your left knee back to the mat. If your right toes are pointed out, bring them back to center.

11. Inhale and lift your hips. Exhale and step back to downward dog.

Lunges

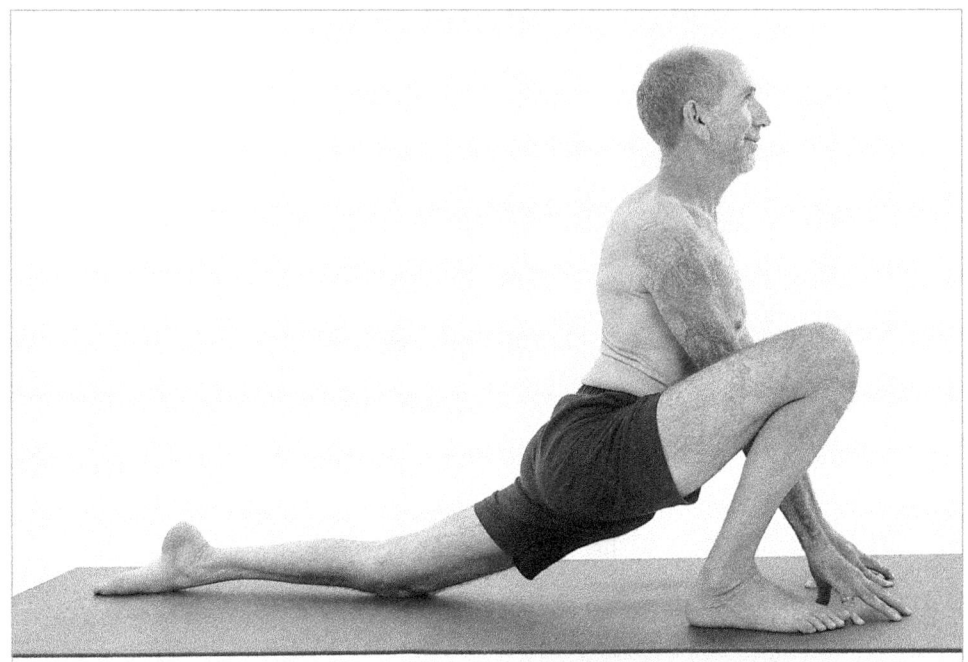

6.d Fourth lunge

STEPS 1-3: Point your left toes straight back and balance the weight between your big toe and your pinkie toe, so your left heel points straight up instead of sickling to the right or left. And yes, we want you to actually turn your head and check for these things. Alignment is extremely important; *Te prati prasavah heya sukshmaha*. You have to check, check, and check again.

STEP 4: If there is any pain or discomfort in your right knee, turn your right toes and your right knee slightly out to the right. Always keep your knee and toes pointed in the same direction. Turn them out as little or as much as it takes to alleviate any discomfort in your knee, and as you become more familiar with the pose, you can explore pointing them back toward the front of your mat.

STEP 5: Bend your knee more than in the first two lunges (less than a 90° angle) and keep it tracking forward over your right heel. Soften your hips and sink forward to bring your right sit bone closer to your right heel. Stamp your right heel into the mat and press into the top of your left foot to keep it from dragging forward. Those are your anchors. You need at least two anchors to create a stretch; if you only have one anchor, you're just dragging your tissue in one direction.

STEP 6: Lift your chest and drop your tailbone to lengthen your front body, like you are moving into a backbend. This is the first stage of the lunge. The next step will intensify the stretch so if you're at your threshold, stay here and soften the intensity of your effort. If you're ready to move further, stay here for 15 – 30 seconds before moving on.

STEP 7: On an exhale, press the top of your left foot into the mat and straighten your left leg. Keep your right heel rooted to the mat. Press evenly through the big toe and pinkie toe sides of your left foot and straighten your left knee completely. Straightening your leg may lift your hips an inch or two higher than they were before; soften your right sit bone toward your right heel to lower them. Do not bend your left knee. If straightening your left leg hurts your left knee, bring your left knee back to the mat, curl your left toes under, and then straighten your leg again. Keep sinking your right hip toward your right heel because the lower you keep your hips, the deeper the stretch in your left leg, hip and torso.

STEPS 8 & 9: Roll your shoulders back, drop your tailbone and lift your sternum. Soften your right hip and fully engage your left leg to create a stretch through the entire left side of your body. The last piece of the pose is extending your throat and looking up, but don't force your body to do anything that feels unsafe. If you do choose to look up, lift your head from the extension of your chest, not by simply extending your chin.

STEPS 10 & 11: Look down and bring your left knee to the mat. If you turned your right foot out to protect your knee, point both of them back to center before straightening your right leg. Inhale and lift your hips and exhale to step your right foot back into downward dog. Take a resting breath between sides and then repeat the lunge with your left foot forward.

FIFTH LUNGE

The fifth lunge is similar to the fourth lunge and it has the same contraindications for stiff and flexible people: pain in the front knee and overstretching the labrum. If you skipped the fourth lunge, please review it to address these issues.

From downward dog with your thumbs touching:

1. Inhale and step your right big toe to your outer right wrist.

Lunges

2. Exhale and bend both knees. Bring your left knee to the mat and point your left toes straight back.

3. Look over your left shoulder to align your foot and point your left heel straight up.

4. Shift your right heel slightly to the right and organize your foot and ankle. Press into your right heel, and keep your right knee tracking in the same direction as your right toes.

5. On an inhale, bring both palms to the top of your right thigh, just at the edge of your right knee.

6. Press your right knee forward in the direction of your right toes. Sink your hips and lean back *(6.e.1)*.

7. Place your left hand in the crease between your left thigh and buttock. Stick your thumb into the crease with the other fingers wrapping down around your outer thigh. Hold your thigh firmly, and on an exhale, use the clasp to internally rotate your left leg *(6.e.2)*.

8. Press your right knee forward, drop your tailbone, lift your chest and extend your spine. If it is comfortable on your neck, look up *(6.e.3)*.

9. Exhale, gently release the clasp on your left leg and bring both hands back to the mat to the inside of your right foot.

10. Inhale and lift your hips. Exhale and step back to downward dog.

STEPS 1-4: Point your left toes straight back. Balance the weight between your big toe and pinkie toe so your left heel points straight up. Organize your right foot and ankle, and stamp into your right heel. Keep your right knee tracking forward in the direction of your right toes, unless that action puts pressure on your right knee. If it does hurt your knee, turn your right knee and right toes out to the right. Always keep your knee and toes pointed in the same direction.

STEP 5: Lift your torso and put both hands on your right thigh. Place the heels of both palms on your right knee. If lifting both hands off the mat puts too much pressure on your left kneecap, fold the left side of your mat under to provide

Lunges

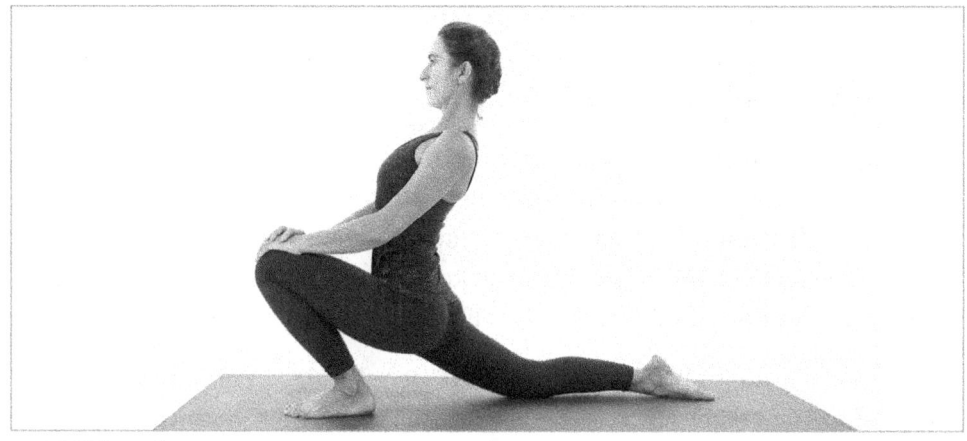

6.e.1 Fifth lunge, first stage

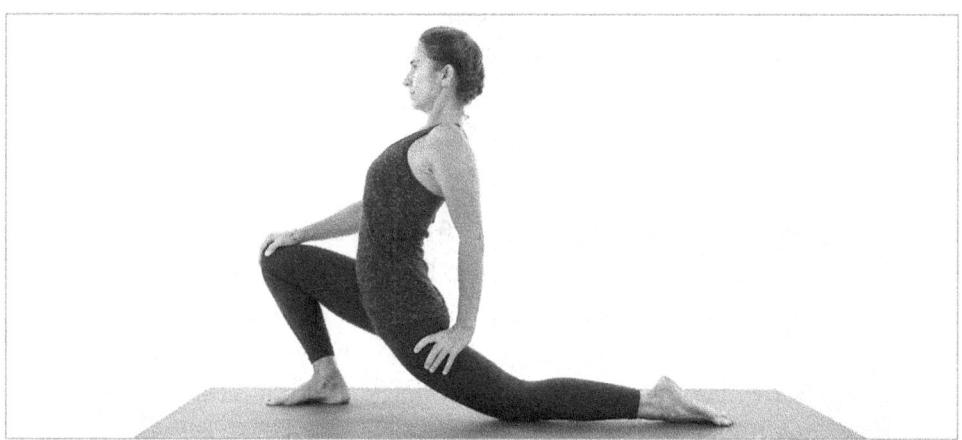

6.e.2 Fifth lunge, second stage

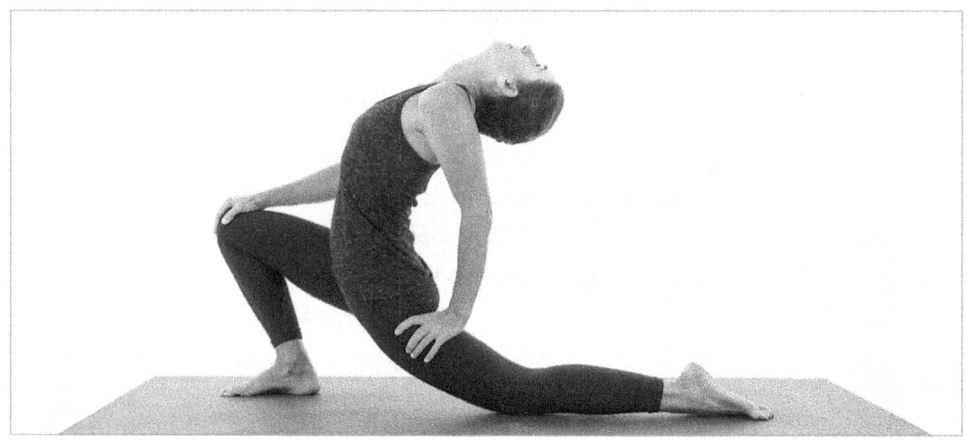

6.e.3 Fifth lunge, final stage

extra padding. The pressure comes from tightness in your psoas and quadriceps, but as those muscles lengthen, it will move out of your kneecap and into the bottom of your quadriceps (more comfortable and anatomically indicated).

STEP 6: Use your hands to guide your knee in the direction of your toes and lean your torso back, away from your right thigh. Drop your tailbone, lift your chest, and increase the space between your sternum and your belly button. Sink your right sit bone toward your right heel, and keep your right heel heavy on the mat. Soften your shoulders and breathe. This is the "first" part of the lunge.

STEP 7: Keep your right hand on the edge of your right knee, and take your left hand to the crease where your left leg meets your left buttock. Stick your left thumb into the crease, as high up onto the back of your thigh as possible, and wrap the rest of your fingers down the side of your left leg. Use this clasp to firmly grab your upper thigh, and on an exhale, roll your thigh forward and down. That action internally rotates your left leg and ideally puts a little more sensation into the front of your left hip. It also tends to lift your right shoulder so soften both shoulders and sink your hips toward the opening.

STEP 8: Use your right hand to press your front leg away from you and use your left hand to internally rotate your back leg. Keep your body tracking forward as if there were walls on either side of your hips; don't let your torso or your right knee splay out to the side. Use *mula bandha* to move your right sit bone closer to your left. Soften your right shoulder, lean back, and if it feels comfortable on your neck, look up.

If you feel any compression in your lower back, please don't lean back. Come forward to relieve the pressure, and simultaneously lift your chest and drop your tailbone. You will be able to explore leaning back as your psoas lengthens, but in the meantime, you must make space for the reality of your anatomy.

STEPS 9 & 10: Release your left hand, look down, and bring both hands to the mat inside of your right foot. If you turned your right foot out to protect your knee, point both of them back to center before straightening your right leg. Inhale and lift your hips and exhale to step your right foot back into downward dog. Take a resting breath between sides and then repeat the lunge with your left foot forward.

SURYA NAMASKAR B

soor·ya nah·mah·scar B | *sun salutations B*

Surya namaskar B is an evolution of *surya namaskar A*. It requires the same foundational work: meticulous alignment, a conscious connection between breath and movement, and a strong *dristi*. It includes two new postures: *uttkatasana* and *virabhadrasana A*. These postures will challenge you to become even more efficient as you work to gracefully incorporate complex movements within the parameters of each breath.

We will begin with a brief introduction to the sequence and follow with a thorough explanation of each breath and its corresponding actions. Many of these postures were explained at length in the earlier section so we'll focus on the new ones. As with *surya namaskar A*, each movement is marked with a Sanskrit number: *ekam* means one, *dwi* means two, *trini* means three, and so forth. Remember: this is a breathing system. Every movement is linked to breath and every breath is married to movement.

UTTKATASANA
oot·kuh·taas·ahn·nuh | powerful pose | *chair pose*

Uttkatasana can be translated into "powerful" pose. It is a relatively simple pose but it is often misunderstood in modern yoga.

Begin in *samastiti*.

1. Ground down through your heels.
2. Inhale as you simultaneously bend both knees and raise your arms overhead.
3. Shift your sit bones back as though you were sitting into a chair, and press evenly into your feet to engage both legs.
4. Look up at your palms to lift your chest and straighten your elbows to lengthen your waist *(7.a)*.

In *surya namaskar B*, these four steps happen within a single inhale. It is a fluid, graceful movement: arms lift, knees bend, and gaze extends upwards. Everything

Surya Namaskar B

NICKI:
When I first went to Mysore, I looked forward in *uttkatasana*—that's what I had been taught in America. Guruji grabbed my ponytail and pulled it back to lift my head, and that simple action completely changed the energy of the pose. Looking up and reaching your arms creates a magnificent lengthening of your entire upper body.

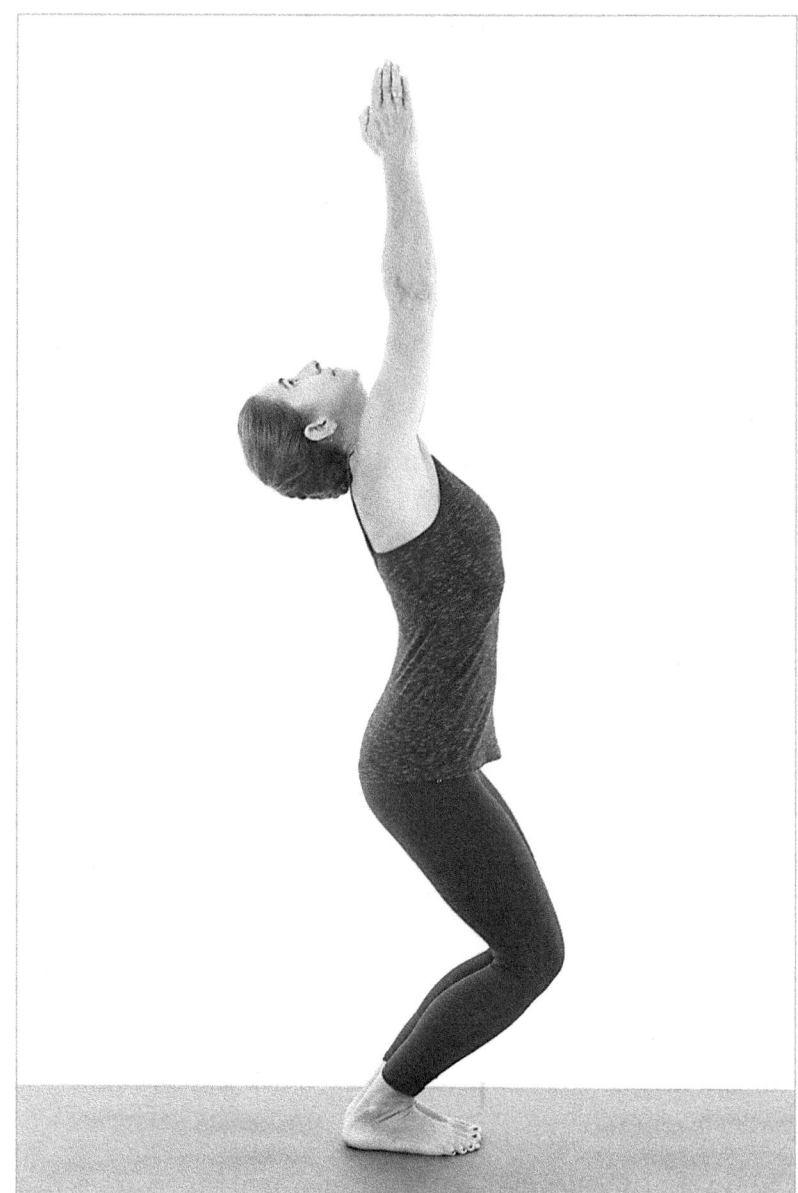

7.a Uttkatasana

below the pelvis goes down and strengthens and everything above the pelvis goes up and lengthens.

It has become popular to bring your fingertips to the floor before moving into *uttkatasana*, but we were taught to simultaneously lift the arms and bend the knees. Bending to touch the floor rounds your back and leans the pose forward, and lifting your torso from that deep forward bend can put pressure on your lower back. The energy of *uttkatasana* is **up**. There is no need to reach down; simultaneously reach your arms overhead and lift your gaze as you bend your knees. Reach your sit bones back as though you were sitting into a chair. Do you tuck your butt under when you sit down? Of course not, so please don't do it here. This is not an abdominally focused squat. It's a fluid, graceful movement that marks the beginning of a beautiful sequence.

Surya Namaskar B

Move your arms and legs in unison to arrive at full *uttkatasana* as you reach the top of your inhale. Stop bending your knees as your palms join overhead, and allow both movements to be fully encapsulated in your breath. When viewed from the side, your heels, sit bones, shoulders, and hands are in a straight line, with your sacrum directly underneath your occiput.

VIRABHADRASANA A
veer·uh·bha·draas·ahn·nuh A | *warrior 1*

Virabhadrasana A is the first warrior pose. It is a fairly complex pose to explore within a single *vinyasa* as it requires strength, flexibility and balance. We generally introduce it as a stationary standing pose before beginning the full sequence of *suyra namaskar B*.

1. Stand in *samastiti* at the top of your mat, facing the short end, and put your hands on your hips. Step your left foot to the back of your mat. The space between your feet should be the length of one of your legs or wider.

2. Bend your right knee until your hip is the height of your knee and your thigh is parallel to the floor.

3. Press through the outer edge of your left foot and lift your inner ankle bone. Straighten your leg completely.

4. Lift both frontal hip bones and drop your tailbone to lengthen your lower back.

5. Reach your arms up and join your palms overhead.

6. Look up at your thumbs and reach through your elbows to lengthen your waist. Drop your tailbone and pull your floating ribs toward your spine to push the opening into your hips. Stay here and breathe *(7.b)*.

7. Exhale and bring your hands to your hips. Inhale and straighten your legs to switch sides.

Surya Namaskar B

NICKI: In surya namaskar B, virabhadrasana A spans a single breath. The actions are much more compressed: the knee bends and the arms lift simultaneously. When we explore the pose as a static posture, it's helpful to set the foundations before you lift your arms and look up.

STEP 1: The space between your feet should be wider than the length of one of your legs and much wider than your stance for straight leg standing poses like *parsvottanasana*. Align your feet heel to heel to stabilize the pose.

STEP 2: Organize your front foot. Bend your knee to 90° so if Nicki were to put a cup of tea on your right thigh it would stay perfectly balanced. There is a tendency to unbend your right knee as you move deeper into the pose. Visualize Nicki's teacup and keep it upright. Maintain stability in your front leg by pressing firmly through your right heel. Keep your right knee tracking in the direction of your right toes.

STEPS 3 & 4: Stiffness in your hips will push your right sit bone out to the right and send your frontal hip bones diving toward the mat. Counteract the stiffness by shifting your right sit bone closer to your left, similar to the action of the 1st and 2nd lunges; engage *mula* and *uddiyana bandha*. Use your hands to find your frontal hip bones and pull them up while simultaneously dropping your tailbone to lengthen your lower back. Increase the space between your right frontal hip bone and your right thigh. Press into the outer edge of your left foot and straighten your left leg completely.

Please note these instructions are suited to introductory practitioners. In a more advanced practice, the action of the pose shifts away from the pelvis and moves toward extension in the upper body. Any anatomical action can be overdone to the point of injury, and overemphasizing the work in the pelvis (lifting the frontal hip bones and dropping the tailbone) when the pelvis is already sufficiently open can endanger the labrum of the extended leg. Remember: always move away from pain in your joints, including your groin and hip socket.

STEPS 5 & 6: Straighten your arms and reach through your elbows to lengthen your waist. Inhale and extend your spine from the foundation of your pelvis, and exhale to bend your right knee back to 90°—it almost always unbends in the effort to align your pelvis. Lift your sternum and soften your ribs to put the action of the pose into your hips and legs; there's definitely a backbend, but the spine should be more upright than bent (no bananas please). Let your head go back and look up at your thumbs.

STEP 7: Exhale and release your hands to your hips. Inhale and straighten your right leg, and then repeat the pose with your left leg forward.

Surya Namaskar B

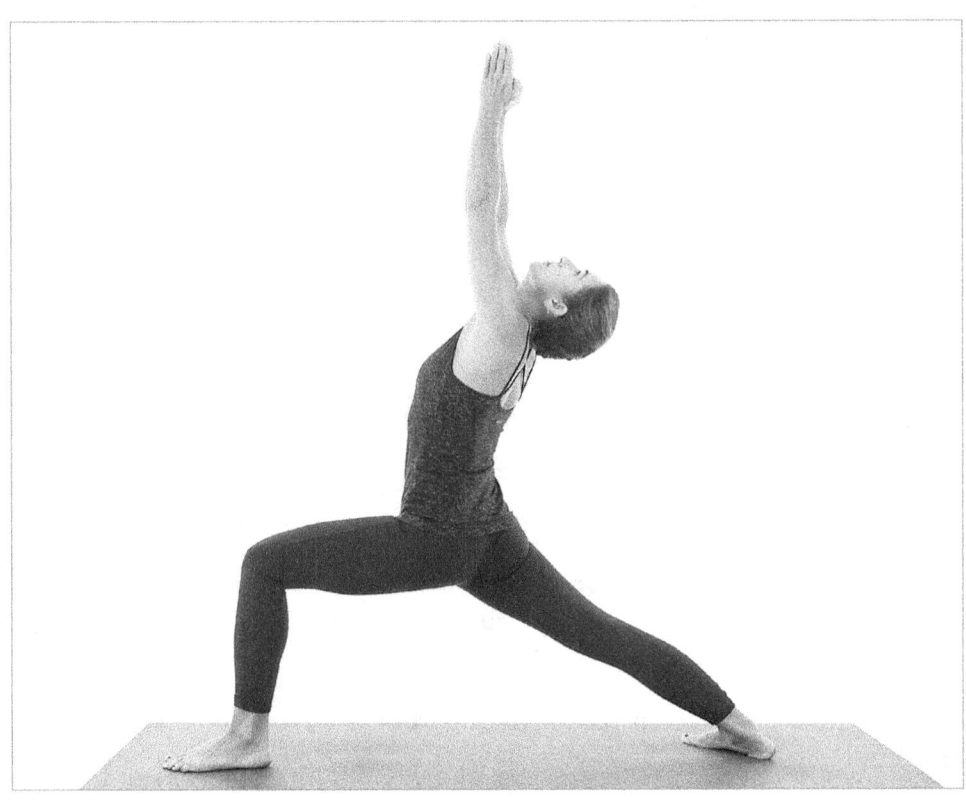

7.b Virabhadrasana A

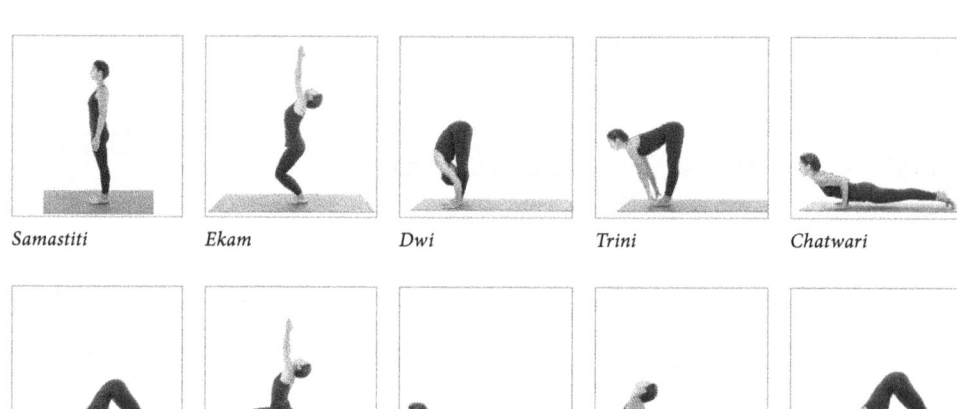

Surya Namaskar B

Samastiti Ekam Dwi Trini Chatwari

Desha Ekadesha Dwidesha Triodesha Chaturdesha

SURYA NAMASKAR B

Begin in *samastiti*.

EKAM: Inhale, lift your arms and bend your knees into *uttkatasana*. Look at your thumbs.

DWI: Exhale, bring your ribs to your thighs and straighten your legs. Lower your hands to the mat and look at your knees.

TRINI: Inhale, lift your head, look forward and extend your spine.

CHATWARI: Exhale, keep your head lifted and step to the back of your mat. Look forward, press your elbows toward your ribs and lower into *chataranga dandasana*.

PANCHA: Inhale, straighten your arms, lift your chest and look up in *urdvha mukha svanasana*.

SHAT: Exhale, lift your hips and reach your heels to the mat. Let your head come back last into *adho mukha svanasana*.

SUPTA: Inhale, look up and step your right foot forward between your hands into *virabhadrasana A*. Bend your right knee to the height of your hip, straighten your left leg, bring your palms together overhead and look up at your hands.

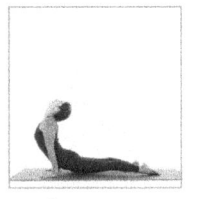
Pancha

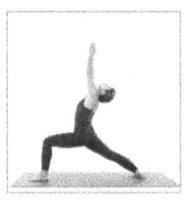
Shat

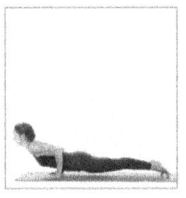
Supta

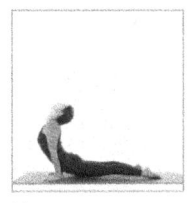
Ashto

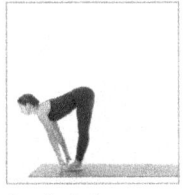
Nawa

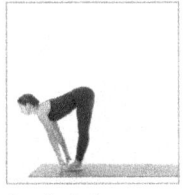
Panchadesha

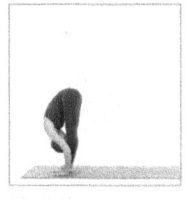
Shodesha

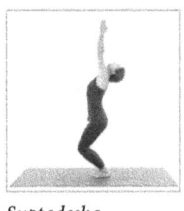
Suptadesha

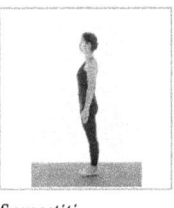
Samastiti

Surya Namaskar B

EDDIE:
When moving from *ekam* to *dwi*, bring your ribs to your thighs before straightening your legs to protect your lower back. If you straighten your legs before there is contact, your hamstrings are able to pull on your spine.

ASHTO: Exhale, bend forward and place your hands on either side of your front foot. Keep looking forward as you step your right foot back and lower into *chataranga dandasana*.

NAWA: Inhale, straighten your arms, lift your chest, and point your toes straight back into *urdhva mukha svanasana*.

DESHA: Exhale and lift your hips into *adho mukha svanasana*.

EKADESHA: Inhale, look up and step your left foot forward between your hands into *virabhadrasana A*. Bend your left knee to the height of your hip, straighten your right leg, bring your palms together overhead and look up at your hands.

DWIDESHA: Exhale, bend forward and place your hands on the mat. Keep looking forward as you step your left foot back into *chataranga dandasana*.

TRIODESHA: Inhale, straighten your arms, lift your chest, and point your toes straight back into *urdhva mukha svanasana*.

CHATURDESHA: Exhale, lift your hips and let your head come back last into *adho mukha svanasana*. Stay in *adho mukha svanasana* for five breaths.

PANSHADESHA: Inhale, look up and step both feet to your hands. Reach your chest forward and your legs back into *trini* position.

SHODESHA: Exhale and soften your spine into a deep forward bend. Gaze at your knees.

SUPTADESHA: Inhale, bend your knees and lift your arms as you sit back into *uttkatasana*. Reach your arms and look at your palms.

Exhale, release your arms and straighten your legs. Return to *samastiti*. As in *surya namaskar A*, the last exhale is not counted.

Surya Namaskar B

EKAM | yay·kum | *one:* Stand in *samastiti*. Press the fingers of each hand firmly together and extend through your inner triads to spread the base of your palm. Begin your inhale and simultaneously lift your arms and bend your knees. Drop your head back and look at your thumbs as your palms join overhead. Straighten your elbows and reach your entire upper body—your chest, shoulders, elbows, and hands—toward the ceiling. Stay strong in your legs and rooted through the center of your heels. At the top of the inhale you are in *uttkatasana*, gazing at your thumbs with your palms touching and your arms fully extended.

DWI | dwhey | *two:* Press through your heels, bring your ribs to your thighs, and bring your arms to the floor. Do not straighten your legs until your ribs touch your thighs. Once they have made contact, straighten your legs and gaze at your knees. Bring your hands to the mat on either side of your legs and lengthen the back of your neck. At the bottom of the exhale you are in a deep forward bend with your hands on the floor, legs straight (unless you need to bend them to protect your back), spine soft and head heavy. The gaze is at your knees.

TRINI | tree·knee | *three:* Inhale, lift your head and look forward to extend your spine. Lift your palms off the mat but leave your fingertips connected. Keep your legs straight and strong and soften your shoulders. At the top of the inhale your legs are reaching back and your torso is reaching forward with a slight backbend in your upper back.

CHATWARI | chut·twar·ee | *four:* Keep your head up and gaze forward. Exhale, bend your knees and step both feet to the back of your mat—still no jumping. Straighten your legs and shift forward onto your tiptoes. Bend your elbows in toward your ribs as you lower forward and down. Reach your chest, throat, and gaze forward to keep your elbows directly over your wrists, and lower your shoulders to the height of your elbows. Keep your inner triads heavy. Find *mula* and *uddiyana bandha* at the bottom of your exhale; be as straight and strong as a four-limbed staff.

PANCHA | pawn·chuh | *five:* Inhale to straighten your arms and roll forward onto the tops of your feet. Point your toes straight back. Externally rotate both arms and roll your shoulders back to open your chest. The eyes of your elbows will naturally roll forward with your arms, but keep your inner triads heavy. Lead with your chest to lift forward and up. Internally rotate your legs, straighten your knees, and drop your tailbone toward your heels to lengthen your lower back. Stretch your throat and look up, if it's okay on your neck. At the top of the inhale you are in full *urdhva mukha svanasan*a (upward-facing dog) with your arms and legs completely straight, shoulders back, chest forward, and gaze upward.

Surya Namaskar B

SHAT | shat | *six:* Exhale, keep your legs straight, lift your hips and roll over your toes. Reach your heels to the mat, lift your sit bones and let your head come back last into *adho mukha svanasana*. Extend your arms and open your armpit chest. At the bottom of the exhale you are in *adho mukha svanasana* with your arms and legs fully extended and your gaze at your navel.

SUPTA | sup·tah | *seven:* Inhale, look up and step your right foot forward between your hands. Bend your right knee until your hip is the height of your knee, and lift your arms overhead into *virabhadrasana A*. Press into the outer edge of your left foot and straighten your left leg. Lift your frontal hip bones and descend your tailbone as you lift your chest and look up. Gaze at your thumbs and straighten your elbows to lengthen your waist. At the top of the inhale you are in *virabhadrasana A*.

ASTO | ash·toe | *eight:* Exhale, look forward and bring your hands to the mat on either side of your right foot. Keep your gaze forward and step your right foot back. Straighten both legs and lower forward and down into *chataranga dandasana*. Keep your inner triads heavy and engage *mula* and *uddiyana bandha*.

NAWA | naah·wah | *nine:* Inhale and straighten your arms into *urdhva mukha svanasana*.

DESHA | dhey·shah | *ten:* Exhale and lift your hips into *adho mukha svanasana*.

EKADESHA | eay·khah·dey·shah | *eleven:* Look up and step your left foot forward between your hands. Bend your left knee until your left hip is the height of your knee, and lift your arms overhead into *virabhadrasana A*. Press into the outer edge of your right foot and straighten your right leg. Lift your frontal hip bones and descend your tailbone as you lift your chest and look up. Straighten your elbows to pull length into your waist. Gaze at your thumbs.

DWIDESHA | dwhey·de·shah | *twelve:* Exhale and look forward. Bring your hands to the mat and lower into *chataranga dandasana*.

TRIODESHA | try·yo·dhey·shah | *thirteen:* Inhale and straighten your arms into *urdhva mukha svanasana*.

Surya Namaskar B

CHATURDESHA | cha·tour·dhey·shah | *fourteen:* Exhale and lift your hips into *adho mukha svanasana*. Stay here for five full breaths.

PANCHADESHA | pawn·chah·dhey·shah | *fifteen:* Finish your fifth exhale and look up at your hands. Inhale and step or walk both feet to the front of your mat. Leave your fingertips on the mat, straighten your arms and legs, and look forward. The top of the inhale finds you in *trini* position: legs strong, arms extended, shoulders soft, chest open and gaze forward.

SHODESHA | show·dhey·shah | *sixteen:* Exhale and bend forward at your hips. Release the weight of your head, soften your spine, and gaze at your knees. At the end of the exhale you are in a deep forward bend with your legs straight, palms on the floor and forehead pressed into your shins.

SUPTADESHA | sup·tuh·dhey·shah | *seventeen:* Inhale, lift your arms and bend your knees to sit back into *uttkatasana*. Lift your chest and gaze at your palms as they join overhead. Press into your heels to engage your legs and straighten your elbows to lengthen your waist. At the top of the inhale you have returned to *ekam* position.

Exhale, straighten your legs and release your palms to your side to return to *samastiti*.

STANDING POSES

Standing poses can be divided into three categories: straight leg standing poses, bent knee standing poses, and balancing poses. Regardless of their categorization, the foundation of every standing pose is your feet, ankles, and knees. We'll start with specific instructions for the front and back leg in the first two categories and then describe the foundational *asana*s for each category. We have divided the poses into categories to make them easier to present, but many of them encompass different physical and energetic actions. Try to think of each pose outside of its primary classification; for example, *parvritta trikonasana* is primarily a standing pose but it's also a twist. All of yoga's *asana*s are alive and dynamic. Systematic categorization endangers their inherent complexity.

Utthita
oot·ti·tah | *intense*

Most the standing poses in this section, with the exception of *vrksasana* and *garudasana*, begin with the word "*utthita.*" *Utt* means intense (as in "*uttanasana*") and it indicates that these poses cultivate a certain degree of intensity. We hope you take it to heart: *Utthita parsvakonasana* is not just "extended lateral angle posture," it is *intensely* extended lateral angle posture. These poses are designed to develop strength and stamina, and you can't do that without challenging yourself. Intensity is part of the package.

STRAIGHT LEG STANDING POSES

Straight leg standing poses are the safest and most basic standing poses. Their simplicity gives them a profound ability to unravel stiffness in your hips and legs. Removing stiffness in your hips releases your lower back and removes pressure from your intervertebral discs, which will keep you walking comfortably on your own two feet for the rest of your life.

The effectiveness of the straight leg standing poses depends on your ability to build a straight line from the floor to your hip. The step-by-step actions for creating this straight line are *(8.a)*:

1. Organize your foot and ankle (as described in the Foundations).

Standing Poses

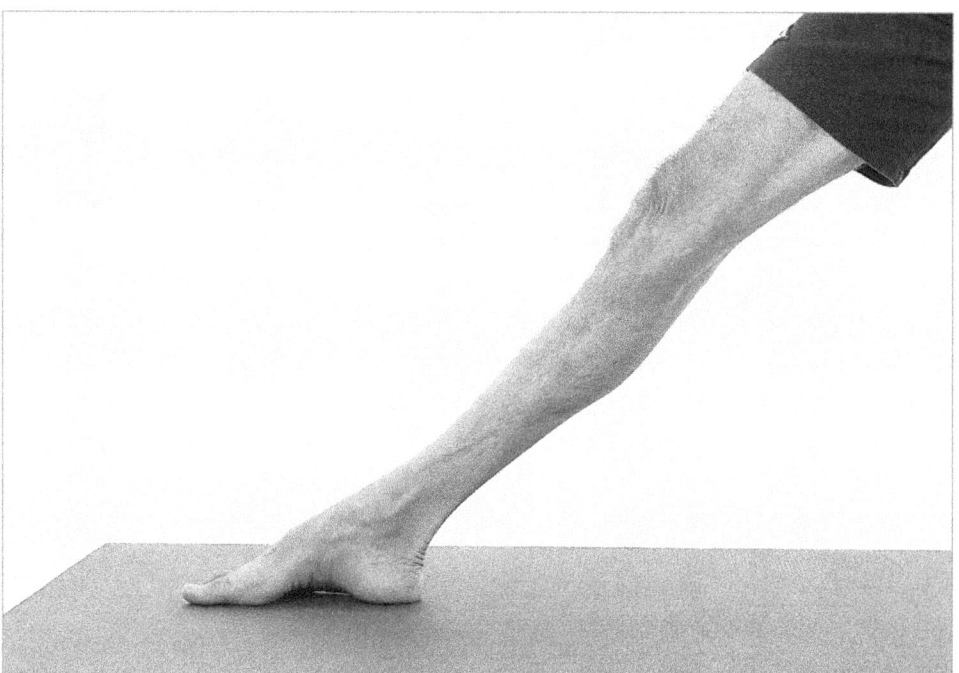

8.a Front leg of a straight leg standing pose

2. Lift your kneecap.

3. Straighten your leg.

4. Externally rotate your leg.

STEP 1: Building a straight line in your leg starts with building a straight line in your foot and ankle, and that work should be very familiar: shift your heel slightly toward the outer edge of your mat, lift your inner arch, press firmly into the knuckle of your big toe bone, and balance your ankle directly over your heel. Straightening your knee transfers stiffness from your hips directly into your outer heel and challenges the weight distribution in your foot. Actively press into the front of your foot to counteract the stiffness, drawing it away from your outer heel and Achilles tendon. The center of your heel should remain heavy, but it should be equal to the pressure in your big toe bone, not greater.

STEP 2: The muscles of your lower and upper leg work in pairs, and these pairs are governed by a nervous system response called the agonist/antagonist relationship. To put it simply: when you engage the muscle on one side of the bone your brain sends a message to release the muscle on the other side of the bone.

The muscle that engages is the agonist and the muscle that releases is the antagonist. In the action of straightening your leg, your quadriceps are the agonist and your hamstrings are the antagonist: engaging your quadriceps tells your hamstrings to release. In the action of bending your knee, the muscles switch sides: the hamstrings become the agonist and the quadriceps are the antagonist.

Yoga utilizes these agonist/antagonist relationships to achieve proper alignment. In the straight leg standing poses, you engage your quadriceps in order to release your hamstrings. Releasing your hamstrings stacks your femur bone (thigh) directly over your lower leg and creates a straight line from your foot to your hip.

The easiest way to engage your quadriceps is to lift the small bone attached to the bottom of the muscle: your kneecap. Lifting your kneecap tightens your quadriceps and straightens your leg. It also protects the structure of your knee by fitting your kneecap into the groove between your lower and upper leg. The kneecap acts as a stabilizing peg between these two moving parts, and it becomes monumentally important in the 4th step.

So look at your kneecap and lift it up. Sounds simple, right? As you will quickly learn, lifting your kneecap is extremely challenging. The patella (kneecap) is a very small bone and you've probably never had a reason to think about it, let alone ask it to do something. The surrounding tissue may be sluggish and unresponsive, and getting it to move often distorts the foundations in your foot and ankle. You have to learn to get it up, and keep it up, while maintaining the very specific organization of your foot and ankle.

Building a relationship with your kneecap is a process of give and take. You have to use *netti netti*, meaning a little of this and a little of that, to explore the relationship between each interconnected part of your leg. Each part must learn to do its job independently and effectively so the cumulative actions of the pose don't get lost in a single joint or muscle. And you have to develop all those new relationships without disturbing your jaw, face, and hands—all the tissue your brain is used to controlling.

The best way to develop a relationship with your kneecap is to look at it and ask it to lift. When it lifts, ask it to stay there. When it drops, ask it to lift again. This process will connect your mind to the tissue of your leg. It develops a strong neurological passageway between your brain and your quadriceps and allows you to fully occupy your own body. That's why you're doing yoga: to be more connected, aware, and present in the entirety of your being. And once that

Standing Poses

EDDIE:
It's just a few simple actions but it can take months to figure them out. You get your kneecap to lift, but then your outer heel takes all the weight. Or you micro-bend your knee to straighten it and then your kneecap drops. It's hard, repetitive work and it might seem tedious at first, but it's really cool. You are developing a stronger relationship with your tissue. You are using your mind to control your body on a cellular level. You are using the precise placement of your body to tune your mind to the frequency of the universe.

neurological passageway is established you can use it to address bigger things, like your hips and spine.

STEP 3: Keep your kneecap lifted and straighten your leg. Press firmly into the front of your foot to shift pressure away from your outer heel. If you are prone to hyperextension, make a slight micro-bend in your knee—even though that makes it harder to lift your kneecap. Straight is straight and bent is bent. Be meticulous.

STEP 4: Externally rotate your leg: spin your thigh toward the outer edge of your mat and point your knee at the little toe side of your foot. External rotation does two things: it protects the medial hamstring tendons that run behind your inner knee and it rotates your femur (thigh bone) in your acetabulum (hip socket) to address stiffness in your hips.

The medial hamstring tendons wrap around the inside of your knee and attach to your tibia (shin bone). When you bend forward in a straight-leg standing pose, stiffness in your groin and hamstrings causes your leg to internally rotate. Internal rotation spins the medial hamstring tendons toward the mat, forcing them to bear the strongest part of the stretch. And if you remember correctly, tendons are not designed to stretch; the stretch belongs in the middle of the muscle, where it is broadest and most resilient. Externally rotating your leg lifts the medial hamstrings and points the center of your hamstrings straight down, pushing the stretch safely into the middle of your hamstring muscle.

External rotation also confronts stiffness in your groin, but to have this external rotation happen at your hip, you must keep the rest of your leg perfectly organized. This is where your kneecap comes in: if it's not lifted, the rotation can happen at your knee instead of your hip, and your knee is not supposed to rotate. Keep your kneecap lifted to ensure your lower leg and upper leg rotate together; otherwise they may torque against each other and trap your knee in the middle. Externally rotating your leg also challenges the alignment in your foot and ankle so press into your big toe bone and keep your ankle directly over the center of your heel.

That is a lot of direction for one leg, and it may seem impossible to maintain all of them at the same time. Your kneecap goes up, but your ankle shifts. Your leg externally rotates, but your big toe bone peels off the mat. You straighten your leg but all your weight falls to the outer edge of your front heel. Trust us, we've been there. We know how frustrating it can be, but we also know how important it is to do this work. You are training your body to listen and training your mind to see. It may feel like a lot of give and take, especially in the beginning, but don't give up. All of this work is definitely possible; otherwise we wouldn't ask you to do it.

BKS Iyengar said students must be able to hold the standing poses for five minutes on each side before practicing *pranayama*. That means engaging your quadriceps—from the top of your knee to the top of your thigh—while keeping your foot and ankle completely balanced and then holding it all in place for five whole minutes. Five minutes may suddenly feel like a very long time. We don't suggest you start with five minute timings, but we want you to be moving in that direction. It will strengthen your physical tissue and refine your nervous system to put you firmly in control of your body.

And that's just the front leg. The back leg is simpler but no less important.

In straight leg standing poses, the general rule is to press into the big toe side of your front foot and the little toe side of your back foot. Always keep your knee and toes pointed in the same direction; once you have set your back foot according to the alignment of the pose, adjust the rotation of your back leg to keep your knee in line with your toes. Press into the outer edge of your foot, lift your inner ankle bone and descend your heel. And if you can, lift your kneecap. It's just as important in the back leg as it is in the front leg, especially to protect your knee from twisting.

All the standing poses will begin from *samastiti* in the center of your mat. Start with one-minute timings on each side and use a stopwatch for accuracy.

PARSVOTTANASANA
pars·voh·tah·naas·ahn·nuh | *flank stretch pose*

We feel *parsvottanasana* is the safest standing pose. Its safety lies in its simplicity: it stretches your legs one at time, and you can see the body part in question (your front leg) for the duration of the pose. But the full expression of the pose is also a deep forward bend, which can be difficult for people with stiff hamstrings and/or lower back pain. If you're one of those people, approach *parsvottanasana* like you approach *uttanasana*: if you can keep the stretch in your legs, explore the forward bend. If doing the forward bend causes discomfort in your lower back, don't do it. Rewind the pose and use blocks, a chair, or the wall to work the action of your pelvis, and slowly make your way into the forward bend without jeopardizing your lumbar discs.

Standing Poses

EDDIE:

These poses have deliberate steps, and you must complete every step before you move to the next one. If the action is difficult to complete, stay there and figure it out—even if it means you don't go into the "full" pose for several weeks. Each additional principle of alignment builds on the previous action, and each new action can affect the previously established foundations. You have to check, check, and check again.

Standing Poses

1. Stand in *samastiti* in the center of your mat, facing the long end, and put your hands on your hips. Inhale and step or jump your feet at least three feet apart.

2. Turn your right toes to the front of the mat and shift your left heel toward the back of the mat. Square your hips and torso over your right leg.

3. Turn your left toes in the same direction as your left knee and press through the outer edge of your foot.

4. Organize your right foot and ankle, and press firmly into your big toe bone.

5. Lift your right kneecap and straighten your leg.

6. Externally rotate your right leg.

7. Move your right sit bone toward your left sit bone in the action of *mula bandha (8.b.1)*.

8. Inhale, lift your chest and press your pubic bone forward. Exhale and come forward over your right leg. Place your hands on the floor or on blocks on either side of your right foot *(8.b.2)*.

9. Organize your right foot, lift your kneecap, spin your thigh toward your pinkie toe, and move your right sit bone toward your left sit bone. Stay here and breathe.

10. Put your hands on your hips, press into your feet, and inhale to standing.

STEPS 1 & 2: The space between your feet should be the length of one of your legs. Adjust them if they're not far enough apart. Turn your right toes out and your left toes in, and square your hips and torso to face over your right leg. Align your feet heel to heel, but if you feel like you're walking on a tightrope, go a bit wider (laterally).

STEP 3: Set your back leg: your knee and toes should always point in the same direction so look at your left (back) knee and turn your toes to follow your knee. Press firmly through the outer edge of your foot. Lift your inner arch and inner ankle bone, and descend your heel and the little toe side of your foot.

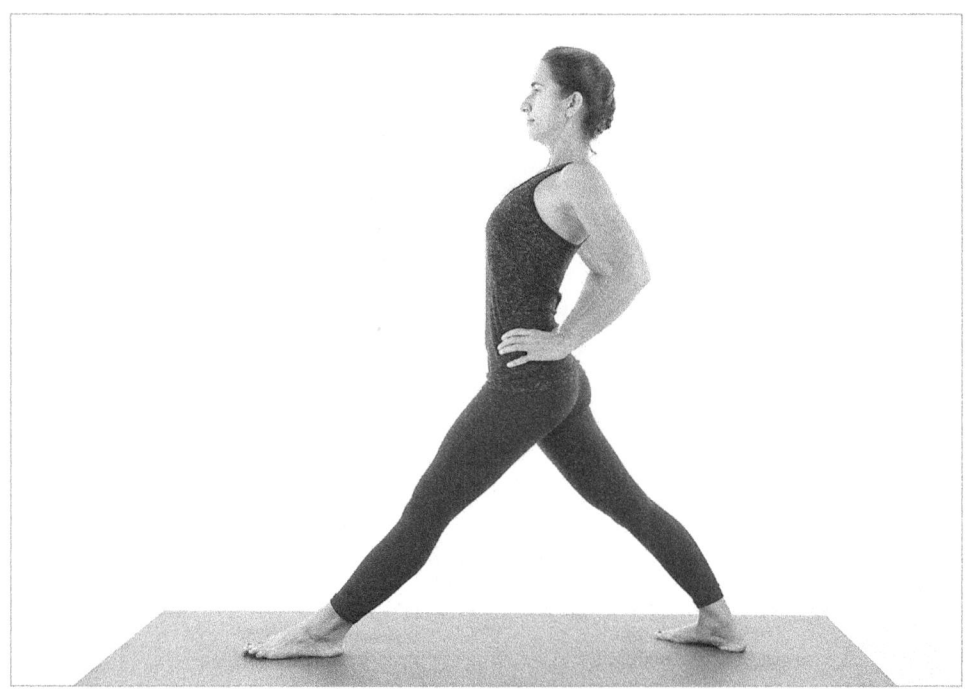

8.b.1 Parsvottanasana setup

Standing Poses

NICKI:
Your foundations are always the most important part of the pose. Yes, your leg needs to rotate but not at the expense of your foot and ankle. You must maintain the foundations as you explore each additional action; otherwise those additional actions are ineffective.

STEP 4: Organize your front leg: shift your heel to the right to make the outer edge of your foot roughly parallel to the long side of your mat, lift your toes and spread them, press deliberately into the big toe bone and the center of your heel, and balance your ankle over your heel. Your foot should begin to resemble your hand in downward dog: the weight rolls forward and down to move pressure away from the outer edges.

STEP 5: Tighten your right thigh and lift your kneecap. Once your kneecap is lifted, straighten your right leg. Be conscious of hyperextension and micro-bend your knee if necessary.

STEP 6: Keep your kneecap lifted and externally rotate your entire right leg. Point your knee at the little toe side of your foot. The external rotation may drag your big toe bone and ankle to the right so press them to the left. It may also push your weight to the outer edge of your right heel so stamp deliberately into the front of your foot.

STEP 7: Keep your gaze on your front leg and bring your awareness to your pelvis. When your hamstrings and hips are tight, parsvottansana pulls your right hip

Standing Poses

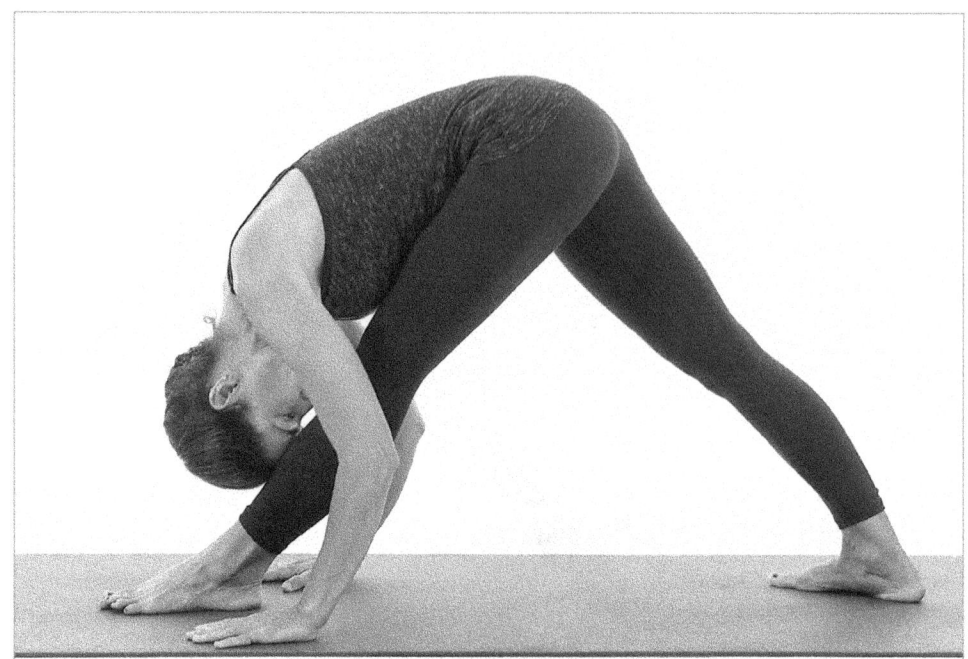

8.b.2 Parsvottanasana with forward bend

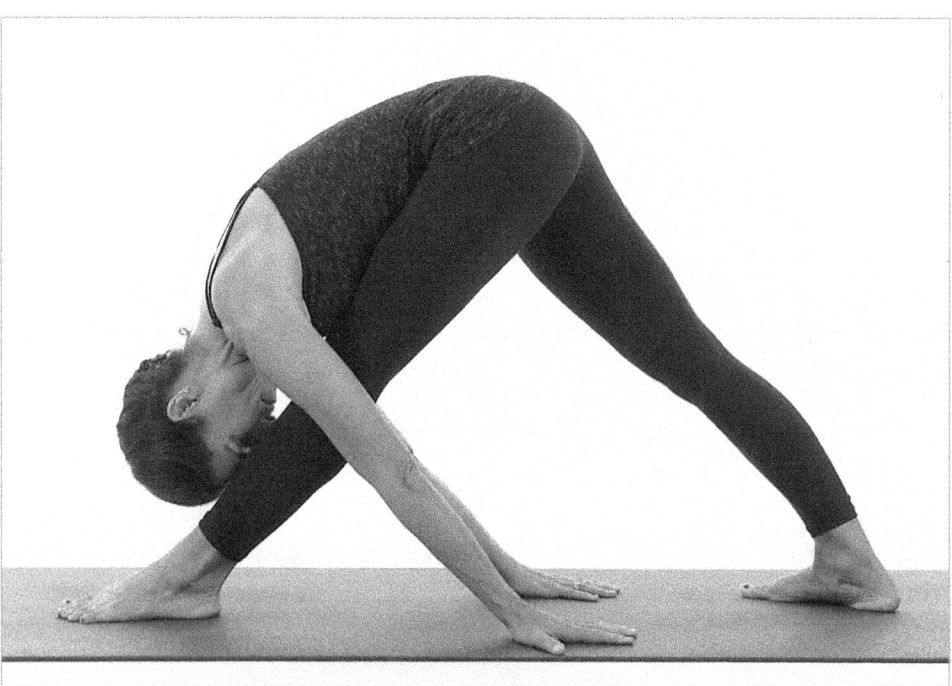

8.b.3 Parsvottanasana with hands fully extended

in the direction of that stiffness: forward and to the right. The flexibility comes from your lower back via recruiting, just like it does in the lunges. The work in *parsvottanasana* is similar to that of the lunges: confront the stiffness by shifting your right hip back and your left hip forward, in the action of *mula bandha*. Move your sit bones toward one another to align your pelvis and create a stable base for the extension of your spine.

We're technically only halfway through the pose, but the first half really encompasses the foundations of the pose and its major anatomical challenges. Adding the forward bend makes everything more difficult so if you're struggling to maintain the foundations thus far, stay here for a while. It's the process that matters, not the external shape.

STEP 8: The traditional hand position for *parsvottanasana* is *viparita namaste*, or reverse prayer, and instructions for *viparita namaste* are included at the end of the pose. We teach *parsvottanasana* with the hands in front because it allows you to focus on your front leg, the main anatomical challenge.

Keep your hands on your hips and, on an inhale, lift your chest and drop your tailbone. Exhale and bend forward over your right leg. Place your hands on either side of your right foot with your wrists directly under your shoulders. Look at your right foot, ankle, and knee and reestablish your foundations: press into the big toe bone and the center of your heel, balance your ankle over your heel, lift your kneecap and externally rotate your leg. If bending forward puts pressure on your lower back, put your hands on blocks or a chair.

STEP 9: The "flank stretch" part of this pose refers to stretching your side body (waist), and to stretch your sides evenly you have to balance your hips. Shift your right hip back and your left hip forward to align your hips, and lengthen the right side of your waist. Watch your foundations and address any imbalances that arise.

With all this focus on your front leg, please don't forget about your back leg. Press into the outer edge of your back foot and lift your inner ankle. Flexible individuals may over-drop the left hip, creating a slant in the sacrum and a corresponding twist in the lower back. It's difficult to detect that subtle misalignment until it becomes a not-so-subtle back problem so be meticulous: press firmly into the outer edge of your left foot and engage your left leg to keep your hips level.

To come out, exhale and bring your hands back to your waist. Inhale and press into both heels to come up, and then repeat the pose with your left leg forward.

Viparita Namaste

veep·pah·rhee·tah nah·muh·stay | *revolved prayer*

Parsvottanasana is traditionally done with hands in *viparita namaste,* or reverse prayer. To practice the pose in *viparita namaste,* place your hands in reverse prayer before you enter the forward bend (Step 8).

1. Internally rotate your arms and bring the tips of your fingers together behind your back with your fingertips pointing up.

2. Roll your shoulders back and press your palms together. Once they are fully connected, move them up toward the middle of your back. Do not move your hands up if your palms are not fully connected.

3. Inhale and reach your elbows back to lift your chest and exhale to bend forward over your front leg. Your hands are no longer available for balance so place your chin or forehead onto your shin.

If *viparita namaste* hurts your wrists or elbows, don't do it. You can create a similar (but less intense) effect by putting your arms behind your back and clasping opposite elbows or stretching both arms toward your back foot *(8.b.3)*.

UTTHITA TRIKONASANA

oot·ti·tah tree·koh·naas·ahn·nuh | intense three angle pose | *triangle pose*

Trikonasana is a lifelong pose. The action of the legs is similar to *parsvottanasana,* but by rotating your hips laterally instead of keeping them straight, it puts you up against the stiffest part of your body. It may be the most overlooked and underappreciated pose in all of yoga, but trust us; this pose definitely deserves your attention, effort, and respect.

1. Stand in *samastiti* in the center of your mat, facing the long end, and put your hands on your hips. Inhale, bend your knees, and step or jump your feet to opposite ends of your mat.

Standing Poses

2. Turn your right toes to the front of the mat and shift your left heel toward the back of the mat.

3. Place a block on its highest setting to the outside of your right shin.

4. Point your left toes in the direction of your left knee and press through the outer edge of your foot.

5. Organize your right foot and ankle.

6. Lift your right kneecap, straighten your leg and spin it to the right.

7. Turn your chest to face the long side of your mat. Inhale and lift and extend your arms to shoulder height.

8. Exhale and keep the right side of your waist long as you bring your right hand down to the block. Place your left hand on your left hip.

9. Look down and address any changes in your foundations. Lean back to bring your chest directly over your right leg.

10. Press your right hand into the block and reach your left arm toward the ceiling. If it feels okay, keep your chin low and look up at your left thumb. Stay here and breathe *(8.c.1 and 8.c.2)*.

11. Exhale and place your left hand back onto your left hip.

12. Press into your feet and inhale to standing.

STEPS 1–3: The distance between your feet should be equal to the length of one of your legs. If you're tall, your feet should be pretty far apart—about four feet wide. Turn your right toes to the right and your left heel to the left, and then align your feet heel to heel. Put a block on its highest setting outside of your right shin, about halfway between your knee and ankle, and place both hands on your hips. You're about to start a detailed conversation with your leg, and unoccupied hands provide an easy outlet for your fidgeting mind.

STEP 4: Most of *trikonasana* is oriented around the front leg, but the back leg is absolutely essential. Adjust your left foot to keep your knee and toes pointed

Standing Poses

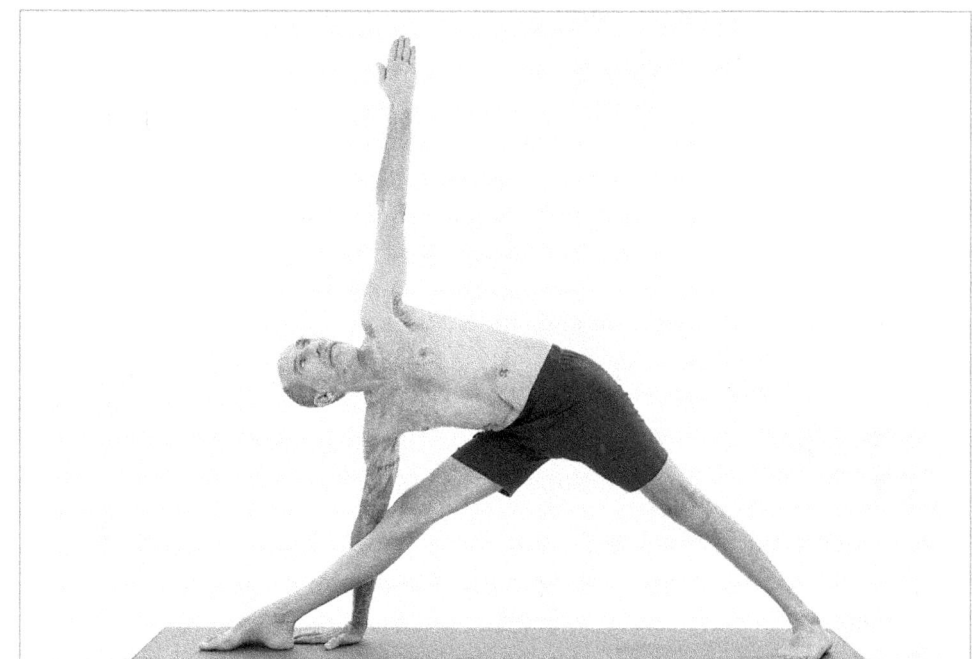

8.c.1 Trikonasana

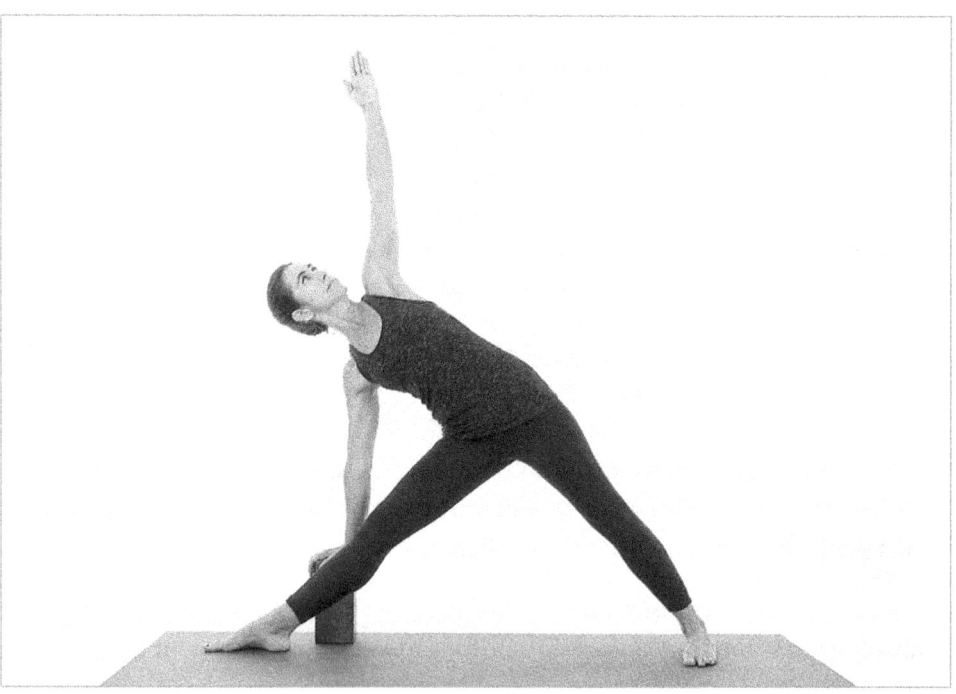

8.c.2 Trikonasana with a block

in the same direction, and then press into the outer edge of your foot. Stamp through your heel, lift your inner arch, lift your kneecap, and soften your hip.

STEPS 5 & 6: Draw a mental line between your heels and see if your hips—specifically the right one—are within that line. If you are like 99.9% of beginners, your hips will be somewhere behind that line—as evidenced by your protruding right buttock. Your right leg cannot externally rotate in relation to your hips so your entire pelvis gets pushed out behind you. *Trikonasana* uses your front leg to plough through this stiffness in your hips, and the primary action is external rotation.

Start by setting the foundations in your right foot and ankle, and then straighten your leg, lift your kneecap, and externally rotate your entire leg. Point your knee at the little toe side of your foot, and be very conscious of how that action can increase pressure in your outer right heel; if your outer right heel turns, micro-bend your knee and press more into your right big toe bone. Spin your thigh to the right and push your ankle to the left to keep it over your heel. Keep your foot, ankle, and knee perfectly organized so the rotation of your leg moves up to your hip, where it belongs.

STEPS 7–8: Turn your chest back to center, and on an inhale, lift your arms to the height of your shoulders. Press the fingers of each hand together and extend the skin on your palms. On an exhale, keep the right side of your waist long and bring your right hand down to the block. Look down and see if that transition affected your foundations and correct any imbalances you find. It should be very clear by now that what's happening in your foot and ankle is indicative of what's happening in your leg and hips. They're connected. Keep your right leg spinning to the right as much as possible (external rotation), but see if it gets pulled to the left (internal rotation) as you go forward; that movement is indicative of the stiffness in your right hip.

If you cannot reestablish your foundations with your hand on the block, place your hand on something higher, like the seat of a chair. If that doesn't help, skip the bend entirely: stay upright and work to solidify your foundations until they're able to follow you into the pose.

STEP 9: Lean back and bring your chest directly over your right leg. Scoop your right buttock under and press your right groin-pit (where your right leg meets your pelvis) toward your front body. Use the external rotation of your right leg to wrap your right hip underneath your left, and extend the inseam of your right

Standing Poses

EDDIE:
This pose is all about your legs. Look at them. In the beginning, your tissues will behave like naughty children; the minute you look away, they stop doing what you want them to do. If you cannot hold your leg accurately without looking at it, then stay here and look at it. You can add the arms and the *dristi* later, but right now, focus on your foundations.

leg toward the front of your mat. Soften your left frontal hip bone to accommodate the movement in your right hip; if your left hip pushes back while the right pushes forward, your sacrum and SI joint can get caught in the middle.

STEP 10: Press your right hand into the block and roll both shoulders away from your ears. Raise your left arm straight up and broaden your chest. If it feels okay on your neck, extend your left arm directly over your face and look up. Keep your chin low, your wrists in line with your shoulders, and your thumb directly over your nose.

STEPS 11 & 12: Exhale and bring your left hand back to your left hip, and look down at your right leg. Inhale, grab the block, and press into both feet to come up. Set the block on the opposite side and repeat the pose with your left leg forward.

In the full expression of the pose, your feet, knees, hips, shoulders and head are on the same vertical plane: your right hip is fully underneath your left and both sides of your waist are evenly extended. When you look at the pose from the front you can see its three namesake triangles: the biggest one is formed by your legs and the floor; a smaller one is formed by your right waist, right leg, and right arm; and the last one is formed by your right arm, right shin, and the floor.

Once you can comfortably maintain all the elements of the pose, experiment with putting your block on a lower setting. Be completely honest about how that action affects the rest of your pose: the weight in your foot, your ankle, kneecap, etc. Don't sacrifice any of those foundations to get your hand to a lower point. Stay connected with the process of the pose, not with the end product.

If you are ready to put your hand on the floor, the Ashtanga lineage instructs you to hold your right big toe. The Iyengar lineage puts the palm flat on the floor with your wrists directly under your shoulders. We're not really attached to what you do with your hand; we're more interested in maintaining the actions that got you there.

PARVRITTA TRIKONASANA
paur·vree·tah tree·koh·naas·ahn·nuh | *revolved triangle pose*

Parvritta trikonasana is revolved triangle pose. It is a twist, a standing pose, and a slight backbend. The legs begin in *parsvottanasana* so we often start with a few rounds of *parsvottanasana* to reinforce those foundations. A strong *parsvottana-*

sana provides a stable foundation for spinal extension, and extension is the key to safe spinal twisting.

1. Stand in *samastiti* in the center of your mat, facing the long end, and put your hands on your hips. Inhale and step or jump your feet at least three feet apart.
2. Turn your right toes to the front of the mat and shift your left heel toward the back of the mat. Square your hips and torso over your right leg.
3. Place a block on the inside of your right foot, at its highest setting, and put your hands on your hips.
4. Turn your left toes to follow your left knee and press through the outer edge of your foot.
5. Organize your right foot and ankle, and press firmly into your right big toe bone.
6. Lift your right kneecap and straighten your leg.
7. Externally rotate your right leg and move your right sit bone toward your left sit bone.
8. Inhale and lift your left arm overhead to lengthen the left side of your waist. Keep your right hand on your right hip.
9. Exhale and bring your left hand to the block.
10. Shift your right hip back and your left hip forward to lengthen your waist.
11. Press into your right big toe bone and your left inner triad, and reach your sternum forward.
12. Lift your face and extend your gaze in the direction of the twist.
13. If you feel stable, reach your right arm up and look at your right thumb. Stay here and breathe *(8.d.1)*.
14. Bring your right hand back to your right hip and exhale. Inhale and press into both feet to return to standing.

Standing Poses

EDDIE:
Twists should always be done in spinal extension—i.e. a backbend. It doesn't have to be an extreme backbend but it should NOT be a forward bend. Twisting in a forward bend is contraindicated for the lumbar spine.

15. Turn your left toes to the front of the mat and shift your right heel toward the back of the mat. Square your hips and torso over your left leg and repeat steps 3-14 with your left leg forward.

Standing Poses

STEPS 1–7: The setup is consistent with *parsvottanasana*. Orient both frontal hip bones toward the front of the mat to face your right leg. Start with a heel-to-heel alignment, but if you feel wobbly, broaden your stance. Place a block on its highest setting inside of your right foot. If you use a higher prop in *parsvottanasana*, like a chair or bench, then use it for this pose as well. The twist will pull strongly on your front foot and ankle so take the time to make sure they're stable. Pay very close attention to the pressure in your big toe bone because it plays a pivotal role in the twisting you're about to do.

STEPS 8 & 9: On an inhale, lift your left arm overhead and extend your spine. Lift your sternum to create a slight backbend in your upper back. Exhale and keep your spine extended as you bend forward at your hips. Put your left hand on

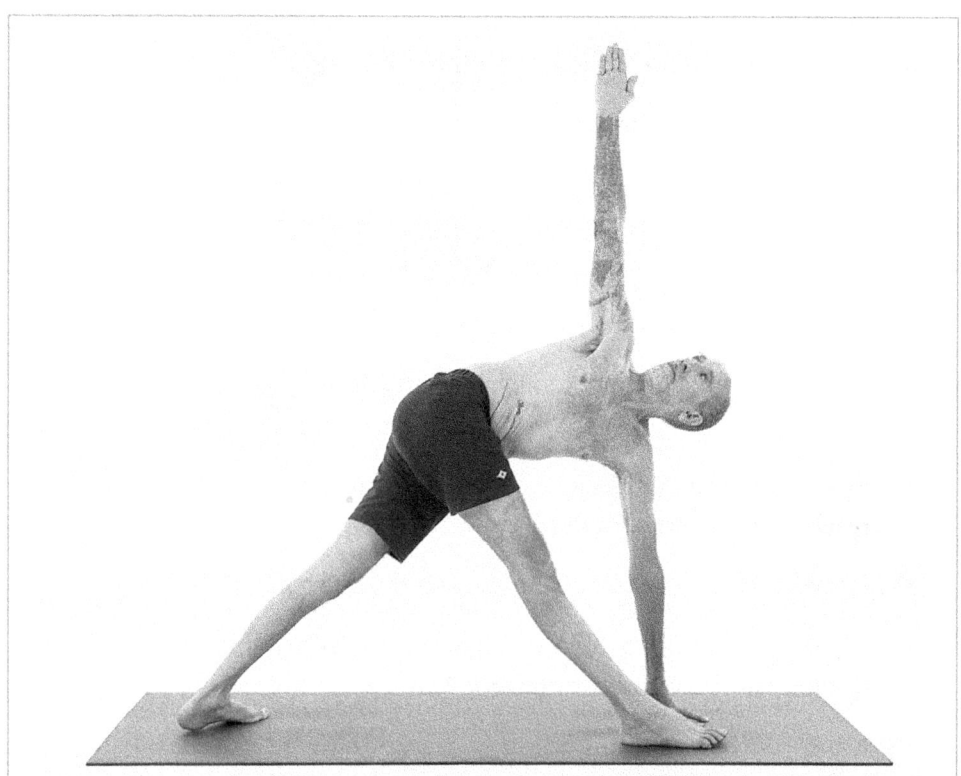

8.d.1 Parvritta trikonasana with hand inside front foot

the block and soften your shoulders away from your ears. Use your right hand to encourage your right hip back. Lengthen the right side of your waist and lift your chest.

STEP 10: Root your right big toe bone to the mat, lift your kneecap, and spin your right leg toward your pinkie toe. If your spine is bending forward to reach the block, get another prop and go higher; twisting in a forward bend is contraindicated. Maintain the extension of your spine. Stamp into the outer edge of your left foot to keep your left hip from dropping below your right, and use *mula bandha* to stabilize your pelvis.

STEP 11: Inhale, extend your spine, lift your chest and twist to the right to deepen the twist. Do not bear down toward your belly or tighten your abdomen; maintain length in your torso to protect your lower back. Roll your shoulders away from your ears and reach your chest forward and up. Once you have established the length (and it's an ongoing process), use each exhale to deepen the twist by pressing into your left hand and your right big toe bone.

STEP 12: If it's comfortable on your neck, look up in the direction of the twist. Eddie calls it "getting snobby;" lift your face, open your throat, and reach your gaze forward and up. Use your breath to continue exploring the twist: use the inhale to build length and the exhale to work the twist.

STEP 13: Roll both shoulders back and press your shoulder blades into the back of your chest; putting them on your back makes them more effective levers for rotating your spine. On an inhale, simultaneously press your left hand into the block and reach your right arm up, over your right shoulder. Look up, keep your chin low and gaze at your right thumb. Reach your arms away from each other to open your chest and extend the twist into your upper back. Roll your left ribs toward your right toe and your right ribs toward the ceiling. Extend your right arm on the same trajectory as your chest; if your right hand is pointed more toward the ceiling than your right shoulder, the ligaments in the front of your shoulder may be at risk.

STEP 14: Look down and bring your right hand back to your right hip. Press into both feet and inhale up to standing; unwind your spine in the direction you went in. Take a breath between sides and repeat the pose with your left leg forward.

If you are able to maintain the fundamental structural alignment of the pose

Standing Poses

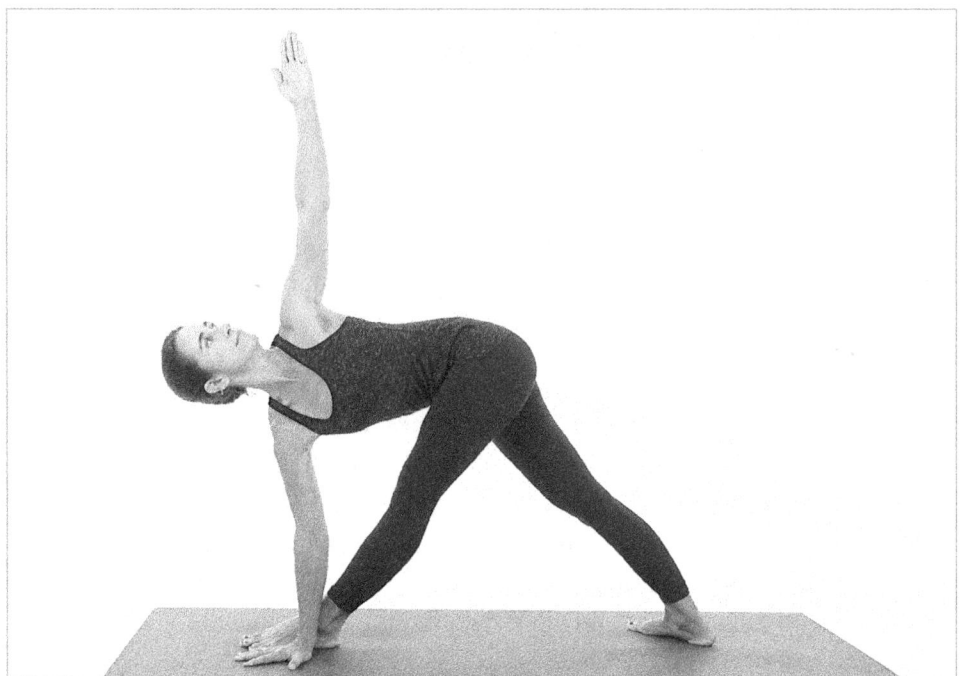

8.d.2 Parvritta trikonasana with hand outside front foot

as described above, flip the block onto its next lowest setting. When the next lowest setting becomes available, put the block back on its high setting and move it to the outside of your right foot. Continue to move lower with the block on the outside of your foot, but pay close attention to your left elbow; if you are prone to hyperextension, it may be easy to hyperextend your elbow around your right leg.

Traditional *parvritta trikonasana* places the left palm flat on the floor outside of your right foot *(8.d.2)*, but it takes a LOT of openness in your hips to get there. We cannot emphasize this enough: the process is always more important than the pose. And your process is your process; it will not, and should not, look like anyone else's process. It belongs to you. Please enjoy it.

PRASARITA PADOTTANASANA
prah·suh·rheet·tah phad·doe·tuh·naas·ahn·nuh | *wide angle foot posture*

Prasarita padottanasana is a straight leg standing pose, but because both feet are pointed in the same direction, the front leg does not externally rotate. Both legs are neutral and pointed in the same direction as your toes. There are four variations of the pose: A, B, C and D. The variations entail different positions for your arms but the work in your legs is the same throughout. We recommend one-minute timings for each variation.

All four variations of *prasarita padottanasana* involve forward bending. If bending forward hurts your lower back, rewind the pose: use blocks or a chair to elevate your hands/head and work the rotation of your pelvis.

*Prasarita padottanasan*a A:

1. Stand in *samastiti* in the center of your mat, facing the long end, and put your hands on your hips. Inhale and step or jump your feet to opposite ends of your mat.
2. Shift your heels away from each other to make the outer edges of your feet roughly parallel to the short ends of your mat.
3. Organize both feet and lift your inner ankle bones.
4. Straighten both legs and lift your kneecaps.
5. Inhale and lift your sternum away from your pubic bone. Reach your elbows back, drop your tailbone and look up.
6. Exhale, bend forward at your hips and bring your hands to the mat.
7. Place your hands shoulder-width apart with your fingertips in line with your toes.
8. Inhale, straighten your arms and look forward.
9. Exhale and bend your elbows to bring the crown of your head to the mat or to a block. Lean forward to put your sit bones directly in line with your heels, and soften your spine *(8.e.1)*.
10. Bring your hands to your hips and exhale. Press into both feet and inhale up to standing.

STEP 1–4: Prasarita means wide. The distance between your feet should be at least the length of one of your legs. Look closely at your feet and make sure they are on the same horizontal plane, i.e. your right heel and toes are directly in line with your left heel and toes. Lift all ten toes and spread them, and then lift your inner ankle bones. Root your big toe bones to the mat, straighten both legs and

Standing Poses

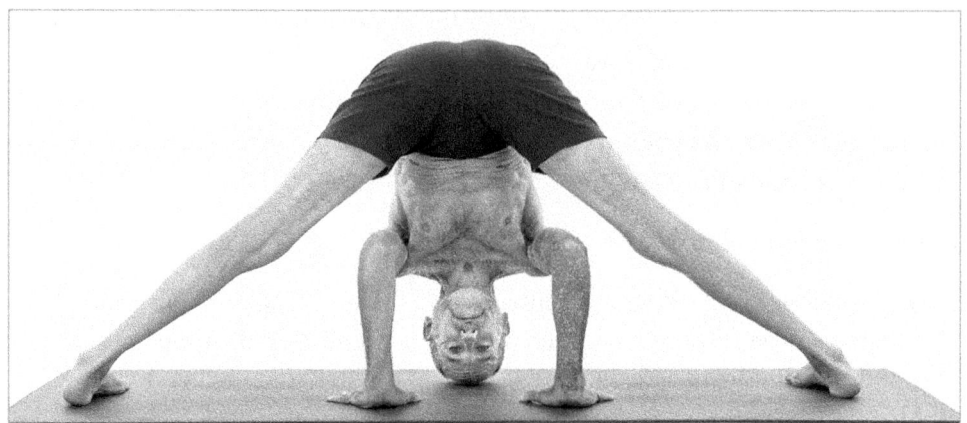

8.e.1 Prasarita padottanasana A

lift your kneecaps.

STEP 5: On an inhale, lift your sternum away from your bellybutton and look up. Press your pelvis forward and keep your perineum pointed down at the mat. Drop your tailbone and extend your front body.

STEPS 6–8: Exhale and hinge forward from your hips to bring your hands to the mat. Place your hands shoulder-width apart with your fingertips in line with your toes. Inhale to straighten your arms and look forward, and exhale as you bend your elbows and bring the crown of your head to the mat. If your head comes all the way down to the mat, walk your hands back until your wrists are under your elbows. If your head does not come all the way down, put a block under it and keep your hands in place.

STEP 9: Press your hands down to lift your shoulders away from your ears, and squeeze your elbows toward each other. Tighten your quadriceps and lift your kneecaps. Press through the outer edge of both feet to lift your inner ankle bones. Lean forward to get your sit bones directly over your heels, just like getting "plumb" in *uttanasana*. *Prasarita padottanasana* is a forward bend so don't open your chest or extend your spine; relax your ribs toward your spine and breathe.

STEP 10: Inhale, straighten your arms and lift your head. Exhale right there. Place your hands on your hips, press into your feet and inhale up to standing. The remaining variations of *prasarita padottanasana* depart from Step 4.

Prasarita padottanasana B: Begin at Step 4 of *prasarita padottanasana A*.

5. Inhale and lift your sternum away from your pubic bone. Reach your elbows back, descend your tailbone and look up.

6. Exhale and hinge forward from your hips to bring the crown of your head to the mat or a block. Keep your hands on your hips.

7. Soften your spine, lift your kneecaps and lean forward.

8. Squeeze your elbows toward each other to broaden your chest, and lift your shoulders away from your ears *(8.e.2)*.

9. Keep your hands on your hips and exhale. Press into both feet and inhale up to standing.

STEPS 5–8: On your exhale, hinge forward at your hips and bring the crown of your head to the mat or a block. Keep your hands on your hips with your elbows bent. You no longer have your hands for balance, but there are still three points of contact with the mat: both feet, and your head. Your feet and legs are doing most of the work, but your head is also part of the equation: shift your weight toward the back of your head and soften your spine. Lift your kneecaps and lean forward into the pose. Squeeze your elbows toward each other to broaden your chest and lift your shoulders away from your ears. Engage *mula* and *uddiyana bandha*, work your legs and breathe freely.

STEP 9: Keep your hands on your hips, press firmly into your feet and inhale up to standing. Exhale and return to Step 4 of *prasarita padottanasana A*.

Prasarita padottanasana C: Begin at Step 4 of *prasarita padottanasana A*.

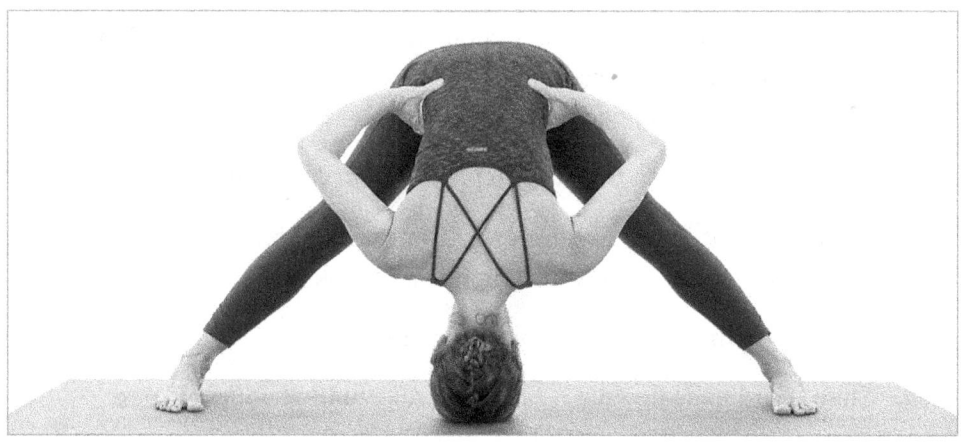

8.e.2 Prasarita padottanasana B

Standing Poses

5. Inhale and extend your arms out to the side at shoulder height.

6. Exhale and interlace your fingers behind your back.

7. Inhale and reach your interlaced hands away from you. Lift your sternum away from your pubic bone, descend your tailbone and look up.

8. Exhale to bend forward and bring your arms overhead. Rest the crown of your head on the mat and reach your interlaced hands toward the mat behind you.

9. Soften your spine, lift your kneecaps and lean forward. Stay here and breathe *(8.e.3)*.

10. Exhale and press into your feet.

11. Inhale and use your interlaced hands to pull up to standing.

STEPS 5–9: Inhale and extend your arms out to the side, and exhale to interlace your fingers behind your back. Inhale and lift your kneecaps, lift your chest, drop your tailbone, and look up. Exhale and bend forward to take your arms overhead. Rest the crown of your head on the floor or a block, and reach your interlaced fingers toward the floor behind your head. Lift your kneecaps and inner ankle bones and bring your hips directly over your heels. Tuck your chin to roll toward the back of your head, and reach your arms away from your chest. Engage your arms and legs, and soften your spine. Stay there and breathe, and keep your eyes open.

STEPS 10 & 11: Press into your feet, and on an inhale, use your arms to pull you up to standing. Exhale to release your arms and bring your hands to your hips. Return to upright *prasarita padottanasana A* (Step 4).

Prasarita padottanasana D: Begin at Step 4 of *prasarita padottanasana A*.

5. Inhale and lift your sternum away from your pubic bone. Reach your elbows back, drop your tailbone and look up.

6. Exhale and hinge forward from your hips.

7. Slide your hands down your legs and take hold of your big toes.

Standing Poses

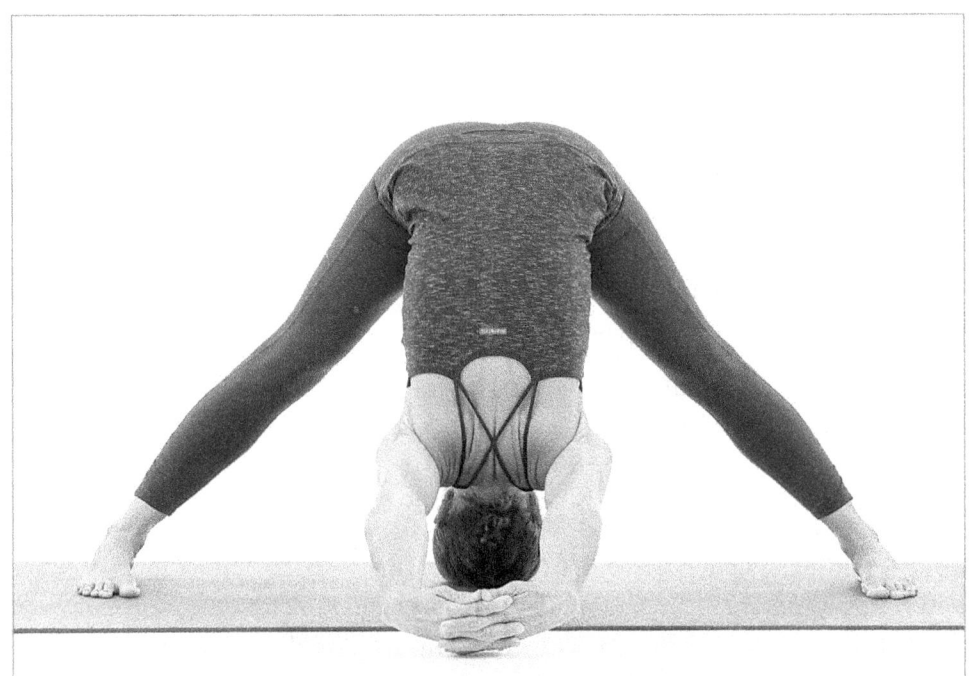

8.e.3 *Prasarita padottanasana C*

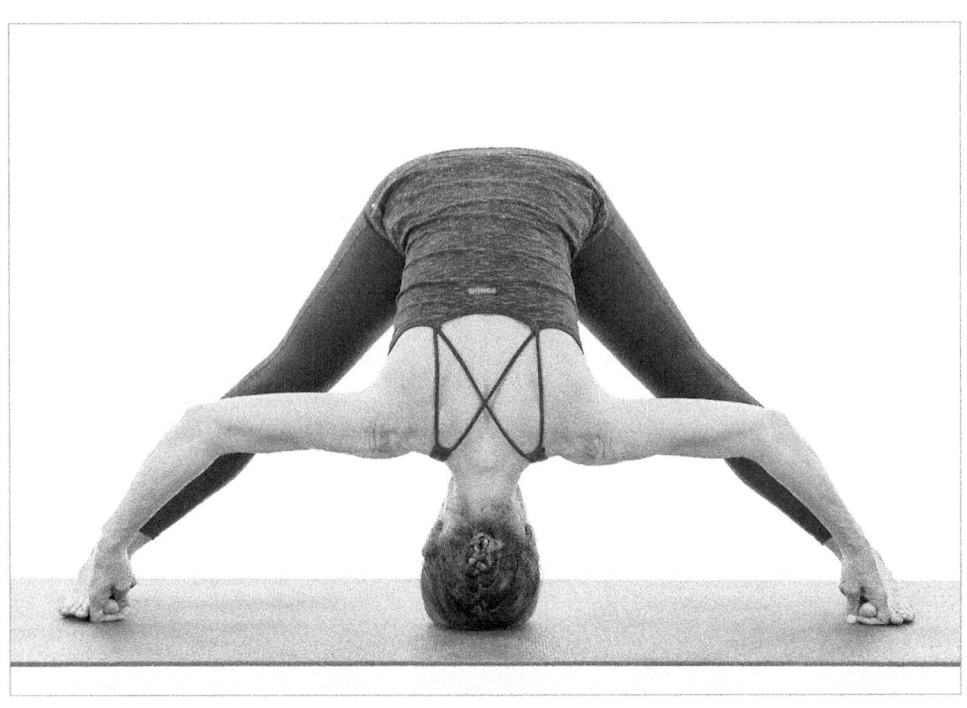

8.e.4 *Prasarita padottanasana D*

8. Inhale, straighten your arms, and look forward.

9. Exhale and bend your elbows to bring the crown of your head to the mat.

10. Lean forward and lift your shoulders away from your ears. Stay here and breathe *(8.e.4)*.

Standing Poses

11. Bring your hands back to your hips and exhale. Press into both feet and inhale up to standing.

STEP 5: On an inhale, lift your sternum away from your bellybutton and look up. Press your pelvis forward and keep your perineum pointed at the mat. Drop your tailbone and extend your front body.

STEPS 6–8: On an exhale, hinge forward from your hips and slide your hands down your legs. Take hold of your big toes with your middle & index fingers and your thumb. Inhale to straighten your arms and look forward, and exhale to bend your elbows and bring the crown of your head to the mat or a block.

STEP 9: Reach your elbows up and away from your knees, without letting go of your big toes, and roll toward the back of your head. Lift your shoulders away from your ears and engage your legs. Stay strong in your legs and pelvis and soft in your spine.

STEP 10: Inhale to straighten your arms and lift your head. Exhale right there. Place your hands on your hips, press into your feet and inhale up to standing. Exhale and return to the upright position of *prasarita padottanasana A*, and then step or jump your feet together into *samastiti*.

BENT KNEE STANDING POSES

Bent knee standing poses are more challenging than straight leg standing poses: bending your knee makes it difficult to align your hips, and stiff hips can jeopardize your front knee as you exit the pose. It may take 30 seconds to set your foundations and get into the pose so start with one-minute timings on each side.

The principles of alignment for the front leg in bent knee standing poses are:

1. Organize your foot and ankle.

2. Bend your knee to the height of your hip (90°).

3. Press into the outer edge of your foot.

4. Keep your knee pointed in the same direction as your toes.

STEP 1: Bent knee standing poses require a wider stance than straight leg standing poses, to accommodate the extra space created by your bent knee. The alignment of your front foot and ankle are similar to the straight leg standing poses, at least in the beginning: shift your heel toward the outer edge of your mat, lift your inner arch, press firmly into the knuckle of your big toe bone, and balance your ankle directly over your heel.

STEP 2: Bend your front knee to the height of your hip to create a 90° angle. The top of your thigh should be parallel with the floor, and if Nicki were to place a cup of tea on your thigh, it should stay balanced for the duration of the pose.

When you bend your front knee, stiffness in your hips drags your knee toward the midline of your body. It pulls your front hip forward (toward your front knee) and pushes your pelvis out behind you. The goal of the bent knee standing poses is similar to that of *trikonasana*: address the stiffness by externally rotating your front leg in relation to your pelvis, and softening your hip. These actions combine to create a straight, uncongested line between your front knee, your pelvis, and your back knee.

STEP 3: Press into the little toe side of your foot to move your knee away from the midline of your body. Keep your right heel heavy, and don't shift so much that your right big toe bone peels off the mat.

STEP 4: The primary contraindication for bent knee standing poses is pain in the front knee, and the best way to protect your knee is to keep it in line with your toes. This is important while you're in the pose, but it is extremely important as you come out of the pose. If your knee and toes are pointed in opposite directions when you straighten your front leg—i.e. your toes are pointed forward but your knee is pulled to the left—your knee will get caught between the opposite actions of your lower and upper leg. It is an extremely dangerous action. Be meticulous with your alignment to protect the entirety of your being.

Finally, it's worth noting the Iyengar system requires the front knee to remain directly above the heel, while the Ashtanga system tends to push the knee forward over the toes. We've done both, and in the end, we're more concerned with lateral movement (as described above) than forward movement.

Standing Poses

The back leg is, again, simple but monumentally important. Most of the bent knee standing poses have the back foot turned in, with the outer edge of your foot roughly parallel to the back of your mat. Your back knee should be pointed in the same direction as your toes. Lift your inner arch and press into the outer edge of your back foot, and use this anchor to pull weight away from your front leg. Lift your inner ankle bone and engage your inner thigh to keep your back hip level with your front hip.

UTTHITA PARSVAKONASANA

oot·ti·tah pars·vah·koh·naas·ahn·nuh | *intensely extended lateral angle pose*

EDDIE: Be graceful with your movements. Getting out of the pose is just as important as getting in, if not more.

1. Stand in *samastiti* in the center of your mat, facing the long end, and put your hands on your hips. Inhale, bend your knees, and step or jump your feet about 4 ft. apart.

2. Turn your right toes to the front of the mat and shift your left heel toward the back of the mat.

3. Place a block inside of your right foot on its highest setting, and then put your hands on your hips.

4. Press through the outer edge of your left foot and lift your inner ankle bone.

5. Organize your right foot and lift your kneecap.

6. Face the long end of your mat and align your sternum over your pelvis.

7. Inhale and extend both arms to shoulder height.

8. Exhale, bend your right knee to 90°, and reach your right arm forward. Place your right hand on the block and keep your left hand on your left hip.

9. Press into the outer edge of both feet, and shift your right knee toward the little toe side of your right foot (away from your elbow).

10. Soften your right hip, drop your tailbone, and lift your frontal hip bones to scoop your buttocks under your hips. Roll your shoul-

ders back and lift your chest.

11. Inhale and extend your left arm overhead, alongside your left ear. Roll your little finger down and your thumb up to externally rotate your arm.

12. Extend the line from the outer edge of your left foot to your left fingertips. Press into your left leg to keep your left hip level with your right hip, and look up at your right thumb. Stay here and breathe *(8.f.1)*.

13. Exhale and bring your left hand to your left hip. Inhale to lift your torso and exhale right there, with your right knee at 90°.

14. Inhale and straighten your legs and exhale to switch sides.

STEPS 1–3: The space between your feet should be wider than the length of one of your legs and much wider than your stance for *parsvottanasana*. Turn your right toes out and your left toes in. Align your feet heel to heel to stabilize the pose. Make the outer edge of your left foot roughly parallel to the back of your mat, similar to the stance for *trikonasana* but wider. Point your left toes in the same direction as your left knee.

STEPS 4 & 5: Place a block inside of your right foot on its highest setting, and bring your hands to your hips. Look at your right foot and organize it: shift your heel slightly to the right, center your ankle over your heel and press firmly into your big toe bone.

STEPS 6–8: Align your chest over your pelvis as you did in *trikonasana*. Inhale and lift your arms to shoulder height, press down through your feet, and engage both legs. Exhale and bend your right knee to 90°. Place your right hand onto the block and your left hand on your left hip. Check that your right hip is the height of your right knee and keep your left leg completely straight.

STEP 9: Examine the relationship between your right foot, knee, and hip. If you are like 99.9% of our students, the stiffness in your hips will prohibit your right leg from externally rotating in relation to your pelvis. Your sit bones will be pulled out behind you and your right knee will be pushed to the left (inward). Counteract the stiffness by moving your knee toward the pinkie toe side of your foot, keeping it in line with your right toes. Bend your right elbow against your

Standing Poses

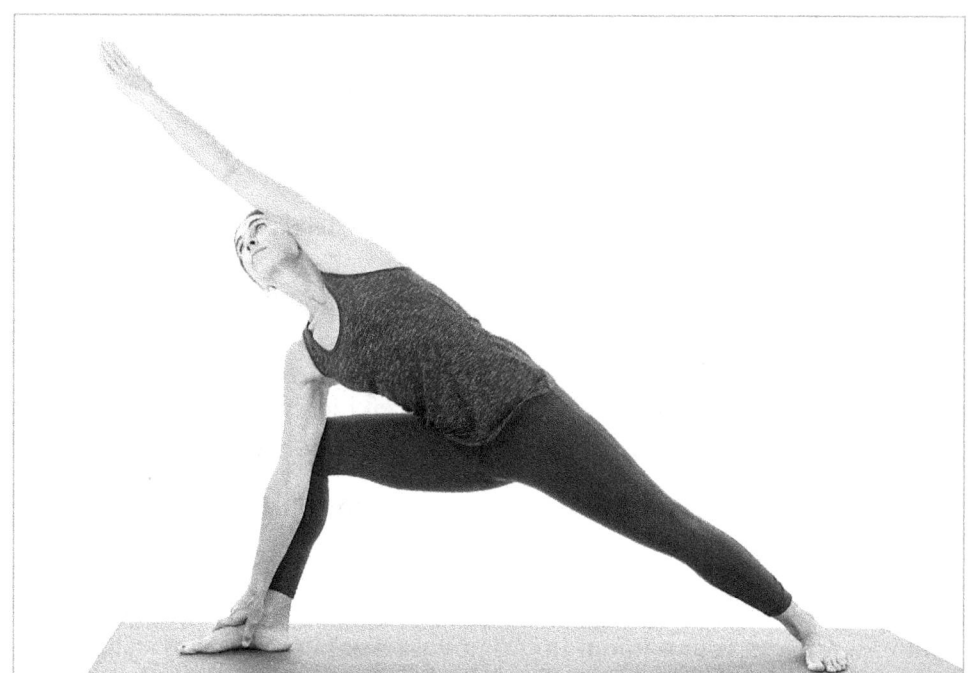

8.f.1 Parsvakonasana with hand inside foot

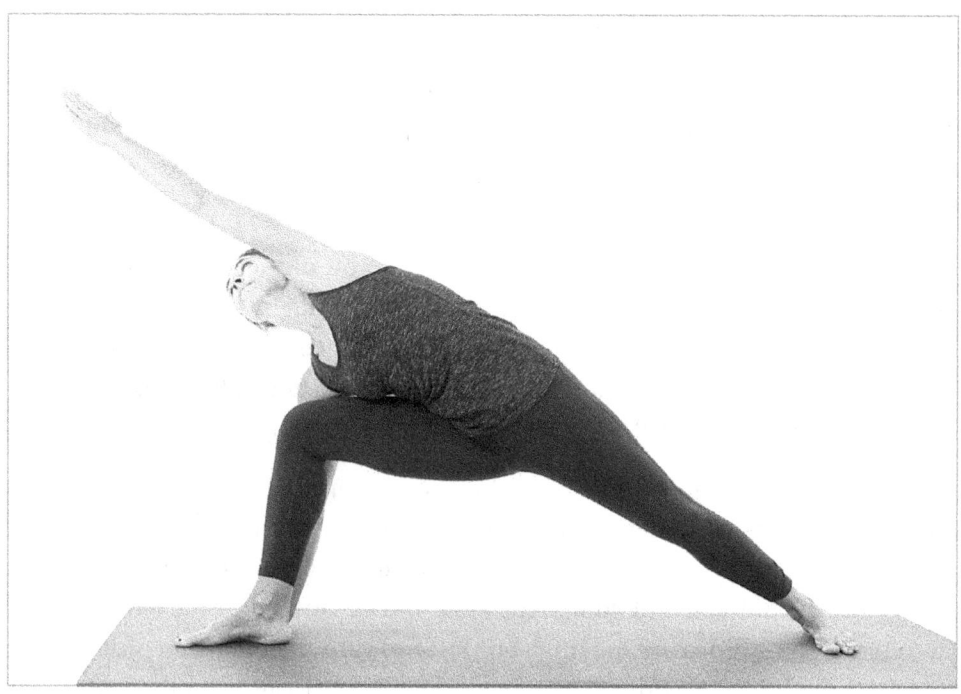

8.f.2 Parsvakonasana with hand outside foot

right inner knee and encourage your thigh to the right, away from the midline of your body.

STEP 10: Reach your inner right thigh toward the front of your mat. Scoop your right buttock forward and under. Keep your right knee bent to 90°. Stamp through the outer edge of your left foot, lift your left inner ankle bone, and engage your left inner thigh to keep your hips level. Roll your shoulders back and lift your sternum away from your pubic bone. If this stage of the pose is sufficiently challenging, stay here and enjoy the sensation in your legs.

STEP 11: Roll your left elbow and shoulder back, and on an inhale, extend your left arm overhead. Press your right hand into the block and reach your left arm alongside your ear. Wrap your left arm in the direction of your little finger to externally rotate it, and reach through the inner triad of your hand. Externally rotating your arm screws your humerus deeper into your shoulder socket and gives it more leverage to lift your spine.

STEP 12: The "intensely extended lateral angle" of *parsvakonasana* is the line that extends from the outer edge of your left foot to the tips of your left fingers, so make this line completely straight and intensely extended. Press firmly into the outer edge of your left foot and engage your left inner thigh to keep your hip from sagging. Straighten your left elbow, and if it is comfortable on your neck, look up toward your left thumb. Keep your chin low, soften your jaw and breathe.

STEPS 13 & 14: Look down and put your left hand on your waist. Inhale and press into your feet to bring your torso over your pelvis. Keep your right knee bent to 90° and exhale in that position. Enjoy that invigorating sensation in your right quadricep; it's a reminder you are alive and working. Look down to ensure your knee is pointed in the same direction as your toes, and then inhale to straighten your right leg. Take a breath between sides and repeat with your left leg forward.

In the traditional expression of *parsvakonasana* your front hand is flat on the floor outside of your front foot *(8.f.2)*—but that's one heck of a journey. Start with a block inside of your front foot on its highest setting (as instructed above) and gradually move it lower. Using the block gives you more leverage into your hips and allows you to use your elbow to encourage the lateral movement of your front knee: bend it to give your thigh a little nudge in the right direction or lift your knee away from your elbow to achieve the same result.

Standing Poses

EDDIE:
Parsvakonasana uses your bent knee as a lever to attack the stiffness in your hips.

Standing Poses

Putting the block on the outside of your foot is a bit harder. Start with the block on its highest setting on the outside of your front foot. You no longer have your elbow to encourage your knee back, but now you can focus on reaching your knee toward your elbow.

When you're ready to put your front hand lower (without altering the fundamental structural alignment of the pose, of course), hold the inside of your ankle and use your thumb to lift your inner arch. But please don't sacrifice your foundations to get there; your personal evolution is much more important than "completing" the pose.

VIRABHADRASANA A
veer·uh·bha·draas·ahn·nuhA | *warrior 1*

See Chapter 7 (*surya namaskar B)* for a full exploration of *virabhadrasana A*.

VIRABHADRASANA B
veer·uh·bha·draas·ahn·nuh B | *warrior 2*

Start in *samastiti* in the center of your mat, facing the long edge.

1. Stand in *samastiti* in the center of your mat, facing the long end, and put your hands on your hips. Inhale, bend your knees, and step or jump your feet about 4 ft. apart.

2. Turn your right toes to the front of the mat and shift your left heel toward the back of the mat.

3. Press through the outer edge of your left foot and lift your inner ankle bone.

4. Organize your right foot and lift your right kneecap.

5. Align your sternum over your pelvis and look over your right leg.

6. Inhale and extend both arms to shoulder height. Press your fingers together and face your palms down.

7. Exhale and bend your right knee to 90°. Keep your torso centered over your hips and extend both arms.

8. Press into the outer edge of both feet and shift your right knee

toward the little toe side of your foot.

9. Soften your right hip, drop your tailbone, and lift your frontal hip bones to scoop your buttocks under.

10. Reach back through your left arm and turn your head to look forward over your right fingertips.

11. Lift your chest, reach your arms, and charge your legs. Stay here and breathe *(8.g)*.

12. Inhale to straighten your right leg, and exhale to release your hands and switch sides.

Standing Poses

NICKI:
Stay in the pose and breathe. You are stronger than you think you are.

STEPS 1–3: The space between your feet should be wider than the length of one of your legs, similar to the stance for *parsvakonasana*. Turn your right toes out and your left toes in, and align your feet heel to heel. Make the outer edge of your left foot roughly parallel to the back of your mat; similar to the stance for *trikonasana* but wider. Point your left toes in the same direction as your left knee.

STEPS 4 & 5: Look at your right foot and organize it: shift your heel slightly to the

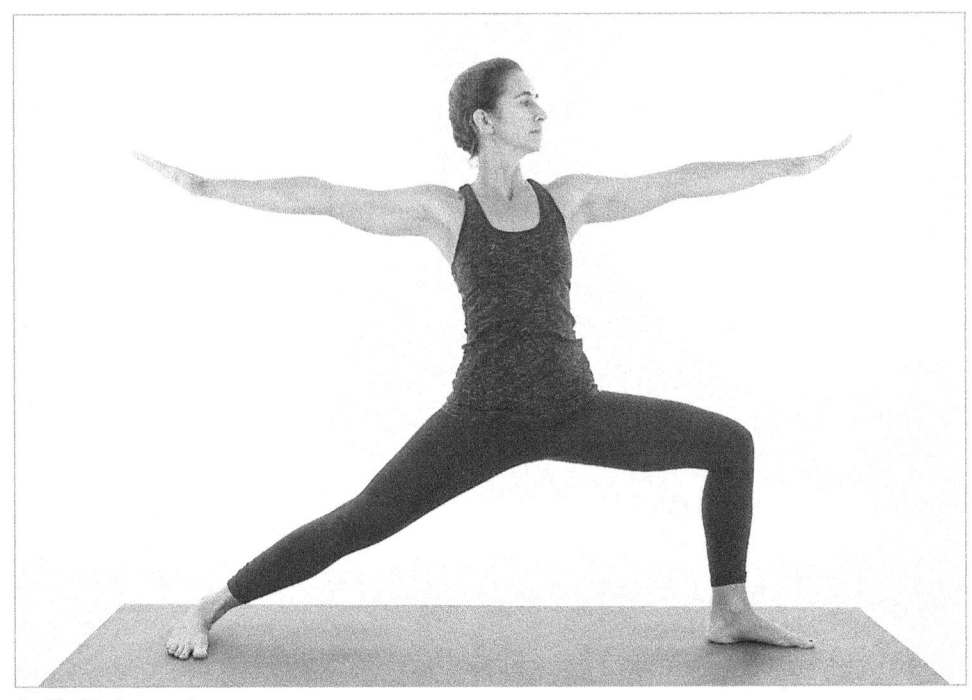

8.g Virabhadrasana B

right; center your ankle over your heel and press firmly into your big toe bone. Align your chest over your pelvis as you did in *trikonasana* and look over your right leg.

STEP 6: Inhale and extend your arms out to your side. Lift your hands a tiny bit higher than your shoulders to energize the pose. Turn your palms up to externally rotate your shoulders (away from your ears), and then turn your palms down for the duration of the pose. Press your fingers together and reach through the inner triads of both hands.

STEP 7: Exhale and bend your right knee to 90°. Your right knee should be over your ankle—or a bit past if you're a real Astangi—and your right hip should be the height of your right knee. Keep your back leg completely straight. Reach your right knee forward and your left leg back.

STEPS 8 & 9: *Virabhadrasana B* is similar to *parsvakonasana* in that it uses the front knee as a lever to attack stiffness in your hips. The goal is to have a straight line through your feet, knees, and hips. Press through the outer edge of both feet, and move your right knee toward the pinkie toe side of your foot to keep it in line with your toes. Stamp through the outer edge of your left foot, lift your inner ankle bone, and engage your inner thigh to keep your left hip in line with your right. Lift your frontal hip bones and drop your tailbone to scoop your right buttocks forward and under. Roll your shoulders back and lift your sternum away from your pubic bone.

STEPS 10 & 11: Look over your left hand and lean back, as though someone were pulling your left arm in the direction of your left leg, to create space between your right thigh and your right frontal hip bone. Maintain that space and look back over your right hand. Reach your arms away from each other to broaden your chest. Charge your legs and savor that invigorating burn in your right quadriceps. Lift your sternum away from your pubic bone and extend your gaze beyond your right fingertips.

STEP 12: Inhale to straighten your right leg and exhale back to release your arms. Take a breath between sides, and then repeat the pose with your left leg forward.

BALANCING POSES

Balancing poses draw on the same physical and energetic actions as the rest of

Standing Poses

the standing poses. The standing leg is paramount, and the work is consistent with everything you have learned thus far: press into the knuckle of your big toe bone and the center of your heel, lift your inner arch, and set your ankle directly over your heel. Lift your kneecap and engage your standing leg as much as possible.

VRKSASANA

vrick·shas·ahn·nuh | *tree posture*

Standing Poses

Vrksa means tree. Start in *samastiti* with your hands on your hips.

1. Ground down through your left foot and lift your left kneecap.

2. Bend your right knee and place the sole of your right foot onto your left inner thigh. Take hold of your ankle and bring your right heel as close to your pubic bone as possible.

3. Allow your right knee to come forward. Use your hands to find your frontal hip bones and bring your pelvis to neutral.

4. Explore moving your right knee back, but don't let it affect the alignment of your hips. Be sensitive to any discomfort in your right knee.

5. Press your right foot into your left thigh and press your left thigh into your right foot.

6. Bring your hands to *anjali mudra* and set your gaze at eye level, at least 10 ft. in front of you.

7. Press into your left foot and straighten your arms overhead. Keep your palms together, and if you are stable, look up at your thumbs. Stay here and breathe *(8.h)*.

8. Exhale and release your hands and right foot into *samastiti*.

STEP 2: Use your right hand to place your right heel as high as possible onto your inner left thigh. Allow your right knee to come forward to accommodate the placement of your foot. If it's difficult to keep your right foot stationary, move it further down your left inner thigh but do not put it against your left knee. The knee is not designed to be pushed sideways.

STEPS 3 & 4: This pose is more about your pelvis than your knees. Use your index fingers to find your frontal hip bones and bring your pelvis to neutral. You can explore moving your right knee back but as soon as it starts to pull on your right hip, stop moving it. Stay at that point, even if your right knee is still forward of your hips, and work on developing strength in your left leg and softness in your right hip.

STEPS 6 & 7: Set your *dristi* on a stationary point somewhere in front of you. If this variation of the pose is sufficiently engaging, stay here and enjoy your experience. If you would like to move further, ground down through your left leg and inhale as you raise your arms overhead. Lift your gaze to follow your hands and press your palms together overhead. Drop your head back, straighten your elbows, and reach your arms to extend your waist.

Exhale and bring your hands back to your hips. Bring your right knee forward and release your right foot to return to *samastiti*. Take a full breath between sides, and then repeat these directions on the opposite side.

GARUDASANA
gha·roo·daas·ahn·nuh | *eagle posture*

Garuda means eagle. *Garudasana* is a strong standing balancing pose with intricate action in both the arms and legs. Start by practicing the arms and legs separately, and once you're comfortable with both, bring them together into the full pose.

Garudasana arms:

1. Stretch your arms out in front of you and turn your palms up.

2. Press all your fingers together to make your hands sharp, and extend through your inner triads.

3. Cross your right arm over your left. Bend your elbows and turn your palms to face each other.

4. Move your forearms toward each other and place your left fingers onto your right palm. Your left fingertips should be in line with the bottom of your right fingers.

5. Turn your hands to bring your thumbs in line with your nose, and

Standing Poses

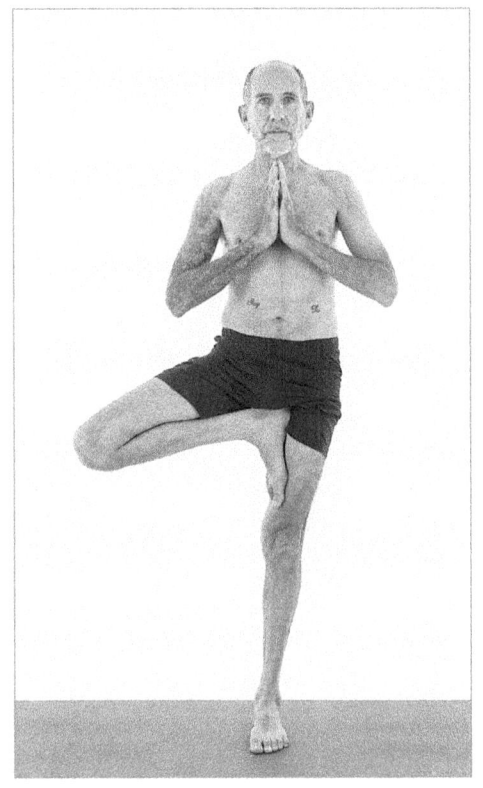
8.h Vrksasana

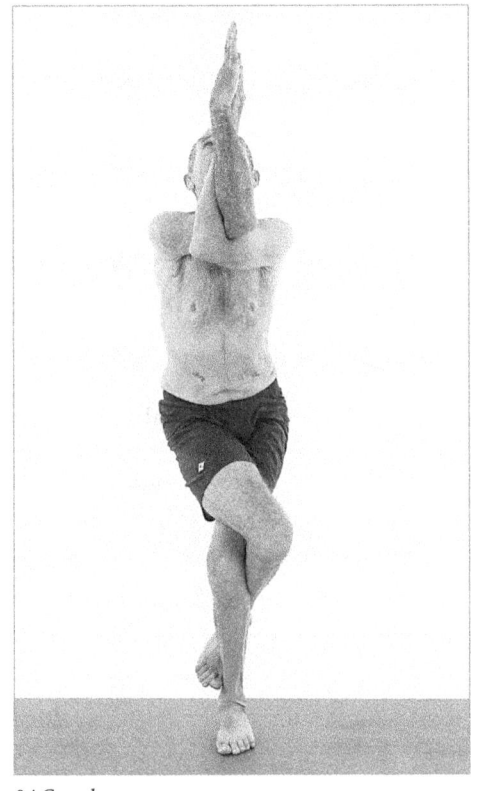
8.i Garudasana

Standing Poses

straighten your wrists.

6. Lift your elbows up, press your shoulders down, and move your hands away from your face.

7. Look up at your fingertips, soften your jaw and breathe.

Garudasana legs, from *samastiti*:

1. Bend both knees and cross your right leg over your left.

2. Hook your right toes behind your left shin; use your hands if necessary.

3. Lean back to bring your torso over your hips and lift your chest.

Full *garudasana*, from *samastiti*:

1. Bend your knees and cross your right leg over your left. Hook

your right toes behind your left shin.

2. Extend your arms out in front of you and turn your palms up.

3. Cross your right arm over your left into *garudasana* arms.

4. Lean back and lift your chest. Find your balance and be still.

5. Soften your shoulders, lift your elbows, and press your palms away from your face.

6. Gaze at or beyond your thumbs *(8.i)*.

7. Exhale, and then inhale to unwind and return to *samastiti*.

Standing Poses

ARMS: Stiffness between your shoulder blades may make it difficult to wrap your forearms around each other, and your palms & fingertips may not meet on the first try. Use your fingers to create some sort of a clasp (many people use the pinkie and thumb) without injuring your wrists, and try to soften your shoulders into the pose. Once your hands are able to connect, there is a tendency for the thumbs to spin toward the shoulder of the top arm (i.e. toward your right shoulder). Counteract the stiffness by spinning your palms until your thumbs face your nose and then move your palms away from your face and up.

LEGS: Tight hips will make this pose somewhat challenging. In the beginning, Eddie would reach his right leg out like a ballet dancer and quickly throw it to the left, using the momentum to get his right foot wrapped behind his left calf. There's no right or wrong way, and your movements will become more fluid as your hips open. Once you're in the pose, finding balance is different for everyone: some find stability by straightening the left leg; others find stability by bending the left knee more. Try both actions to see what works for you and be sensitive to any discomfort in your knees.

ARDHA CHANDRASANA
aur·dah chawn·drah·suh·nah | *half-moon pose*

Ardha chandrasana is a standing balancing pose that begins in *trikonasana*.

1. Set a block on its highest setting about 1' in front of your right foot, toward the little toe side of your foot.

2. Get into full *trikonasana* with the right foot forward and both

kneecaps lifted.

3. Put your left hand on your waist and look down.

4. Inhale. Bend your right leg and lift your left leg off the mat. Shift forward and straighten your right leg as you place your right hand on the block. Flex and lift your left foot to the height of your hip.

5. Press your right hand into the block to lift your left shoulder up. Open your chest to the left and scoop your right buttocks under to lean back, just like *trikonasana*.

6. Extend your left arm overhead. If you feel stable, keep your chin low and look to the left, and then look up at your left thumb. Stay here and breathe *(8.j)*.

7. Look down and place your left hand on your left hip. Bend your right knee and reach your left leg to the back of the mat, back into *trikonasana*. Release the block and straighten your right leg as soon as the left foot is down.

Standing Poses

STEPS 1–3: In *trikonasana*, spin your right leg to the right and scoop your buttocks under. Look down, and then look at the block to orient your next movement.

STEP 4: The next few movements happen simultaneously. Bend your right knee to step your left foot off the mat, and as your left leg lifts, give it a little push to shift your hips forward over your right leg. Reach your right arm forward and place your hand on the block so your wrist is underneath your shoulder. If you have a very long torso you may need to move the block forward a scooch to accommodate the extra length. Lift your left foot to the height of your left hip and flex your foot with your toes pointed forward (i.e. to the left, in the same direction as your left knee).

STEP 5: Press into your right hand to bring the pose forward, away from the weight of your left leg. Engage both kneecaps and lift your left leg higher as it tends to get very heavy. Roll both shoulders back, and lift your left shoulder to open your chest to the left. Scoop your right buttocks under and lean back—toward your back body, not your left leg. It is similar to the action of *trikonasana*: externally rotate the right leg to reach the right inner thigh forward and move

Standing Poses

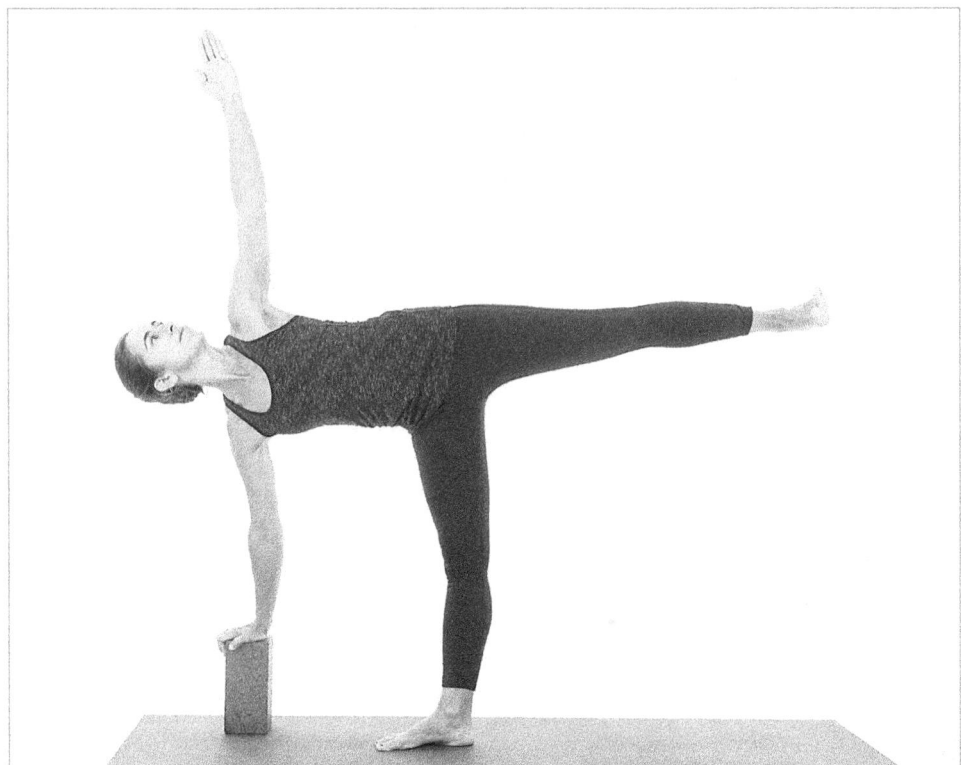

9.j Ardha chandrasana with a block

the sit bones toward each other in the action of *mula bandha*.

STEP 6: If you are comfortable here, lift your left arm straight up over your left shoulder. Press your right hand into the block and reach your left hand toward the ceiling. Keep your fingers together and stretch your palm. Keep your chin low and look to the left, and if you feel stable, look up at your left hand.

STEP 7: Bend your right knee (a lot!) and reach your left leg way back to achieve the proper alignment in *trikonasana*. Straighten your right knee as soon as your left foot reaches the back of the mat, and try to land as gently as possible. Stay here for a few breaths, and on an inhale, return to standing. Move the block to the opposite side, again about 1' in front of your foot and toward the little toe side, and then switch sides.

If you no longer need the block, place your hand on the floor with your thumb in line with your little toe. Your hand should be at least one inch in front of your foot—if you have a very long torso you may need to place it further forward.

BACKBENDS

Backbends are the shining light of yoga *asana*s. They embody health, youth, and spinal integration. They create shared movement among the 24 vertebrae of your spine, a kinetic symphony unlike any other anatomical action. But if the action of backbends is not shared—that is, the movement intended for 24 bones is pushed into just a few bony segments—they can do more harm than good.

The most important anatomical concept for backbends is balance. A sustainable backbend is one that spreads the "bend" evenly among all the segments of your spine instead of hinging into anatomically vulnerable areas. Healthy backbends are round and expansive; harmful backbends angular and compressed.

EDDIE: When I studied with BKS Iyengar, he said backbends in motion are the most physiologically beneficial poses in yoga.

BACKBENDS AND BACK PAIN

Backbends are a fantastic tool for addressing back pain. Eddie used them regularly for many years and they continue to be his go-to poses, along with inversions, when his back pain resurfaces. But backbends have a set place in yoga's hierarchy; they come after the foundational work that includes *adho mukha svanasana*, standing poses, and lunges. These poses open your legs, hips and shoulders to ensure that backbends do not aggravate any existing spinal imbalances. Backbends also have their own internal hierarchy that starts with very simple supine backbends, like *setu bandha sarvangasana*, and it's important to spend time with these simple backbends before moving on to more complicated *asana*s.

In our experience, back pain is usually caused by uneven pressure on lumbar discs. The pressure comes from a long-term shortening of the front body, which is a direct result of spending life in a seated position. Sitting creates stiffness in the front of your pelvis, shortens your psoas, and moves your shoulders toward your front body. Sitting is the new smoking—a silent societal scourge. It puts pressure on the front of your intervertebral discs and causes them to bulge toward the back of your spine. Doing a forward bend can increase the pressure on the front of these already bulging discs but doing a backbend (properly!) can reverse the pressure; it expands the front of your spine and encourages your discs to regain their natural balance.

Quick disclaimer: this book is not intended to diagnose or treat your back pain. Only you can do that, with internal sensitivity and (possibly) diagnostic imaging. But we firmly believe backbends are an integral part of addressing generalized back pain, and we hope yoga guides you to the same relief Eddie was able to find many years ago.

KING ARTHUR

Backbends

King Arthur is one of the keys to removing pain in backbends. It lengthens your front body, from your toes to your sternum, and it does so without jeopardizing your knees. It does not have a Sanskrit name because it's not a traditional pose; Eddie found it in a yoga book produced by a running magazine over 30 years ago, and it quickly became his secret weapon against chronic stiffness.

EDDIE:
I felt pain in my lower back for years, especially when I did backbends. The front of my body was stiff and my legs were not working. When I came out of a backbend, I would feel it in my lower back more than I felt it in my legs—and that's not good. King Arthur and the standing poses removed the congestion from my front body and paved the way for backbends to open my spine. Without the foundational work, there was pain. With the foundational work, there was progress.

Your knee has several delicate ligaments that crisscross the joint from top to bottom. When your knee is bent, the ligaments in the front face of the knee—from the bottom of your thigh to the top of your shin—are most at risk. King Arthur presses this front face of your knee against the mat and uses your body weight to hold it down, which pushes the stretch into the tissue above your knee. It protects the front of your knee and all its vulnerable ligaments by moving the stretch straight into your stubborn quadriceps.

If this pose causes discomfort in the top of your foot, put a mat or blanket on the wall for extra padding. This pose is contraindicated if you have had surgery to repair your ACL (anterior cruciate ligament). If you have had other kinds of knee surgery, explore this pose in the presence of an experienced instructor. Start with 30-second timings and use a stopwatch for accuracy—you may be amazed at the difference between sides.

1. Fold your mat four times and put the straight edge flat against a wall.

2. Start on hands and knees with your toes toward the wall.

3. Walk back to the wall and bend your right knee. Place the top of your right foot against the wall with your toes pointed straight up.

4. Put your right knee into the space where the wall meets the floor, with your shin vertical against the wall and the front face of your knee pressed against the floor.

5. Shift your hips to bring your right buttock inside of your right foot, similar to *virasana*. Point your right heel away from your right hip to externally rotate your right leg.

6. Place your left foot on the floor and walk it forward until it is under your left knee. Use your left leg to lift upright. Place your right hand on your right heel and your left hand on your left knee.

7. Press into your left leg and move your right hip toward the wall. Use your hands to balance your frontal hip bones and drop your tailbone. Bring your right knee, right frontal hip bone, and right shoulder into a straight vertical line.

8. Lean back into the wall. Press your right hip back and your left hip forward. Extend your left knee toward the center of the room to create space in your left groin. Soften your shoulders, soften your jaw and breathe (*9.a.1 and 9.a.2*).

9. Come forward onto your hands and gently unbend your right knee.

STEPS 1–4: King Arthur isolates the stiffness in your front body to protect the delicate tissue of your knee. The face of your knee should be flat on the floor so your quadriceps can only pull from the top of your knee to the top of your shoulder. If you do feel discomfort in your knee you have a couple options: 1) move your knee further away from the wall; 2) use a thicker mat to cushion the front of your knee; 3) and lift your hips, ever so slightly, to put less downward pressure on your knee. Be cautious with that last option; the downward pressure is intended to protect your knee from stretching. Try just a little lift to adjust the skin on your leg and then put the pressure back down to protect your knee.

STEP 5: If you were able to get your right buttock on the wall it should sit inside of your right foot, not on top of your right foot. Your right knee and right shoulder should be in a straight vertical line with your right heel slightly outside of that line. It is similar to the action of *virasana*: the heel points away from the hip and the leg externally rotates to open the front of the pelvis.

STEP 6: It may be difficult to get upright if your front body is very stiff. Use your hands to pull yourself up your left leg, and if you really can't get up, put a chair in front of you for leverage. Once you're up, move your body away from the chair and toward the wall.

STEP 7: Sneaky, persistent stiffness will do everything it can to twist you away from the pose: it will push you away from the wall, raise your left hip up and to the left, and drop your right hip forward and in. Confront your stiffness by spinning your body toward its epicenter: put your fingers on your frontal hip bones and use them to lift your right hip and drop your left—i.e. make them level. Press your right buttock toward the wall and reach your left knee away from the wall. Make a straight line from the center of your right knee to the center of your right shoulder.

STEP 8: Drop your tailbone and encourage your lower back toward the wall. Lean back and breathe. Soften your shoulders and bring your sternum directly over your pubic bone. Channel every ounce of your awareness into softening and releasing the stiffness in your right quadriceps muscle.

STEP 9: Lean forward and put your hands on the floor. Gently release your right knee from the wall and switch sides.

Backbends

EDDIE:
This pose may try to chase you away, but you need to RUN toward it. Turn and face the shadow. Age is just the shadow of congestion chasing you out of your body. That shadow will haunt your life unless you turn and face it. If you turn and face it, you will find the fountain of youth.

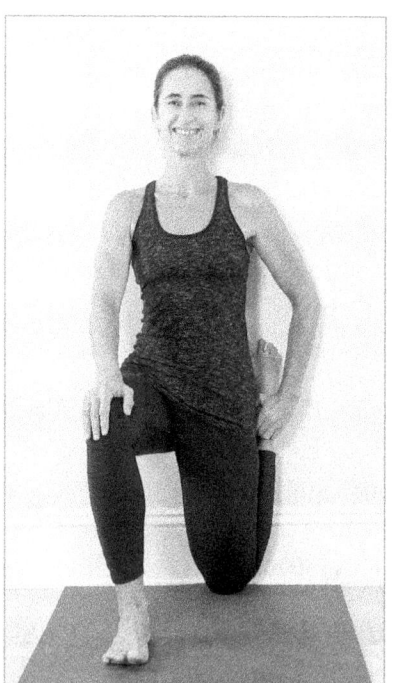

9.a.1 Nicki in King Arthur

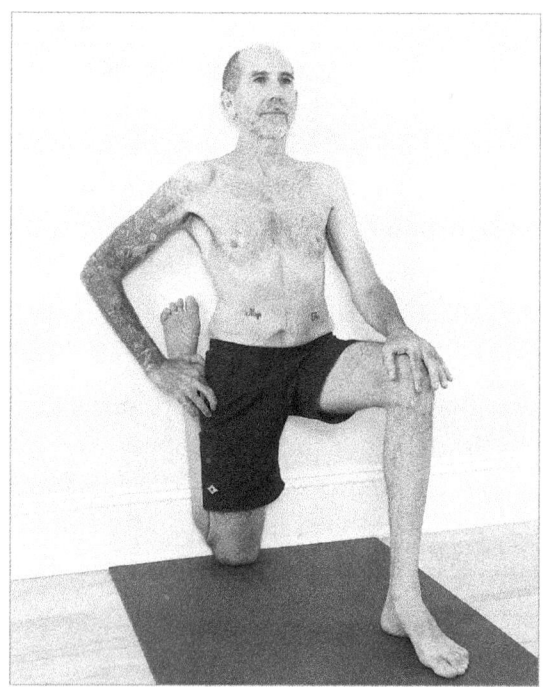

9.a.2 Eddie in King Arthur

King Arthur can evolve to the point that your entire back body rests comfortably on the wall, and to take it further, you can take your foot off the wall and begin to push it forward. But for most of us, that is a very, very long way away—and that's fine. Be patient and enjoy your experience because it's **yours**.

USTRASANA
oo·stras·ahn·nuh | *camel pose*

Backbends

If standing on your knees is uncomfortable, fold your mat over to provide more padding. We usually introduce this pose with the heels up because it makes them easier to reach, but once you're comfortable in the pose, put the tops of your feet flat on the floor.

1. Stand on your knees at the front of your mat. Spread your knees and feet hips-width apart. Point your toes straight back and your heels straight up.
2. Bring your hands to your hips and press the bottom of your sacrum forward. Lift both frontal hip bones.
3. Inhale and lift your sternum, press your pelvis forward, and curl your toes under.
4. Exhale and reach your arms back to put your hands on your heels.
5. Push your feet down to lift your chest, and if it's comfortable on your neck, look up and back (*9.b*).
6. Exhale and release your hands to your sacrum.
7. Inhale and press into both feet to lift straight up.

STEP 1: Look over both shoulders to ensure your heels are pointed straight up. Press evenly through the big toe and little toe sides of both feet.

STEP 2: Your sacrum is a triangular-shaped bone at the base of your spine. The bottom of the triangle is just above the top of your buttocks. Place your thumbs onto the bottom of your sacrum and press it forward. This action pushes your pubic bone forward to open the front of your pelvis and create space in your lower back.

Backbends

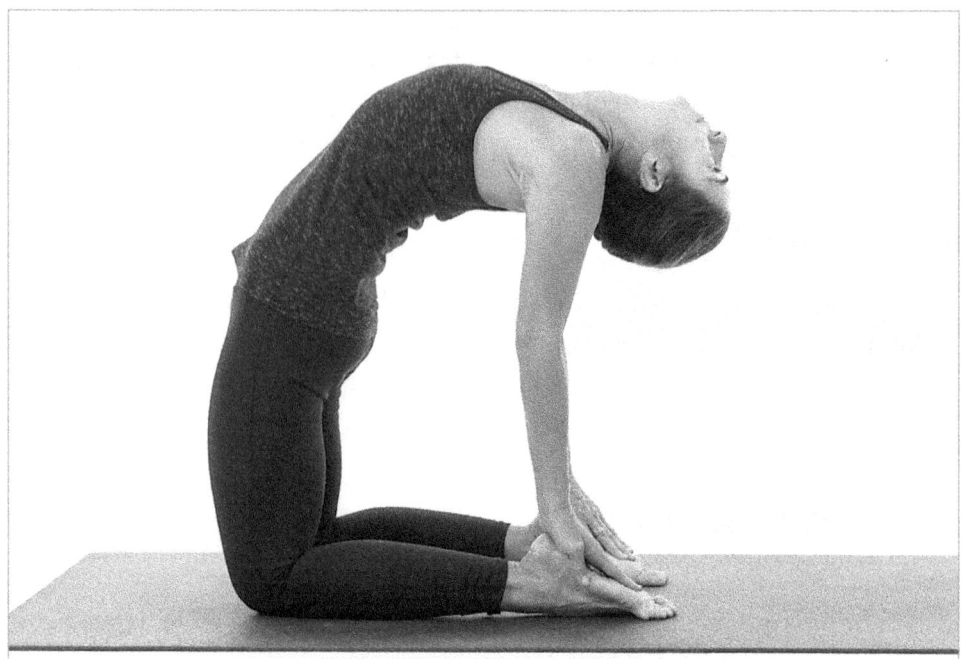

9.b Ustrasana

STEP 3: Curling your toes under makes it easier to find your feet in the backbend. Traditionally, the pose is done with the tops of the feet flat on the floor. If finding your heels is easy the first time, do the next one with your feet down and press evenly through both sides of your feet.

STEP 4: You may need to lean your hips back to reach your heels, but once you have them, reach your pubic bone forward to bring your pelvis directly above your knees. Lift your chest up and back. Get your shoulders over your heels by lifting and extending your spine, not by shifting your hips backward.

STEP 5: Roll your shoulders away from your ears and push your feet down to lift your chest up. If it's okay on your neck, release your head and look back. If that bothers your neck, look straight up or forward.

STEPS 6: Release your hands to your sacrum, and on an inhale, press both feet down to come straight up. Don't twist as you come out of the pose; lead straight up with your chest and let your head come up last.

STANDING BACK ARCH

Standing back arch is not a traditional pose but it will help train your legs to support your torso in backbends.

Start in *samastiti*:

1. Separate your feet hips-width apart and put your hands on your hips.
2. Bend your knees and press into your heels. Keep your knees tracking in the direction of your toes.
3. Exhale. Keep your knees bent and press the bottom of your sacrum forward to lift your pubic bone.
4. Inhale, lift your sternum and look up.
5. Keep your knees bent, lift your pelvis, press through your heels and lean back. Stay here and breathe (*9.c*).
6. On an inhale, press into your heels and straighten your legs. Let your head come up last.

STEPS 1 & 2: Bend your knees enough to hide your toes; if you can still see your toes when you look down, bend your knees more. Keep your knees tracking straight forward in the direction of your toes; don't let them collapse toward each other or spread wider than your hips. If you cannot keep your heels down with your knees bent, put something under them (a narrow slant board is best). You need to be able to press your heels down to lift your spine up.

STEP 3: Place your thumbs on the bottom of your sacrum and press it forward to open the front of your pelvis. Lift your frontal hip bones and drop your tailbone to lengthen your lower back. Ground down through your heels to anchor your pose and keep from leaning forward.

STEPS 4 & 5: Inhale and lift your chest away from your pubic bone. Bend your knees, lean back, and press through your heels to lift your sternum. Squeeze your elbows toward each other to broaden your chest and open the front of your throat. Lift your sternum and look up and back—unless that hurts your neck or makes you unstable.

Backbends

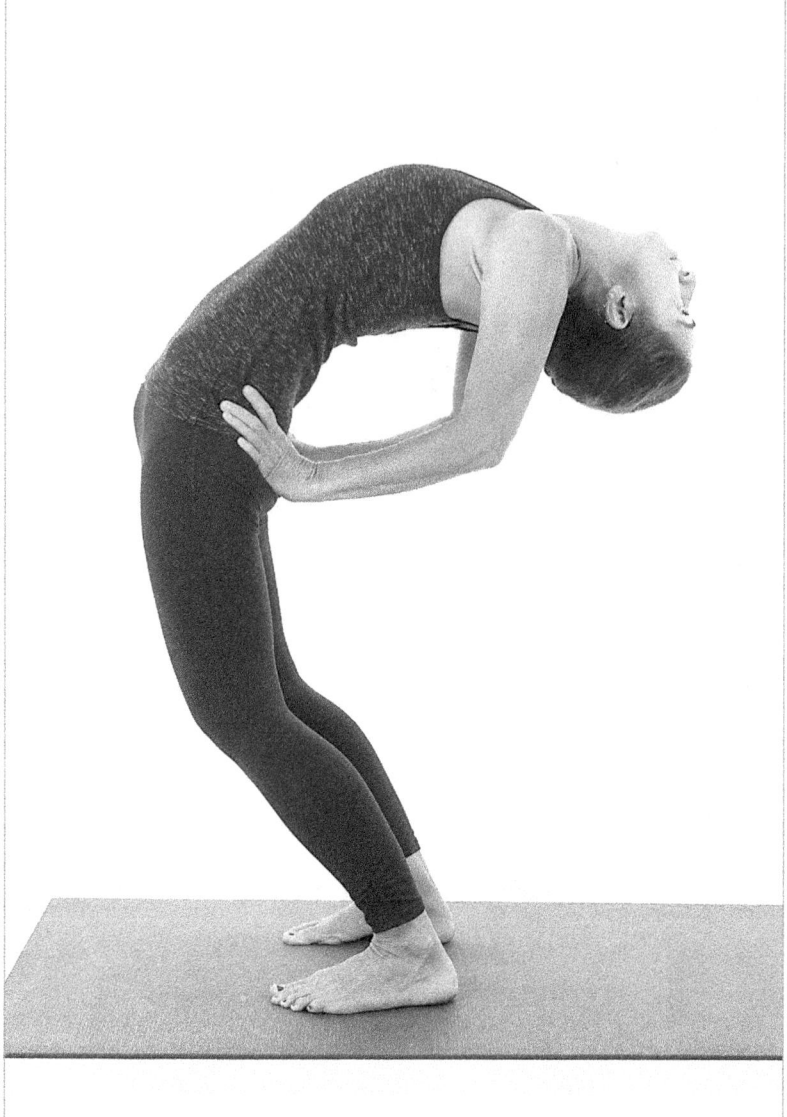

9.c Standing back arch

STEP 6: Maintain the backbend as you exit the pose. On an inhale, press into your heels and lift your chest as you straighten your legs. Let your head come up last. Return to samastiti.

URDHVA DHANURASANA
urhd·vha dawn·yur·aas·ahn·nuh | *upward facing bow pose*

Urdhva dhanurasana is an advanced backbend. Previous backbends have used your legs to leverage your spine; this pose uses the full extension of your legs and your arms. It is a much stronger pose. If it hurts your wrists, use a slant board to protect them while you open your shoulders.

1. Lie on your back with your feet flat on the floor. Bend your knees and bring your feet toward your hips.

2. Reach your arms overhead. Bend your elbows and place your hands on the mat. Hide your fingertips under your shoulders.

3. Exhale and squeeze your elbows toward each other to broaden your shoulders.

4. Inhale and lift halfway up, onto the top of your head. Stay here and adjust your setup: squeeze your elbows and knees toward each other and roll onto the top of your head (*9.d.1*).

5. Exhale in the setup, and then inhale to straighten your arms and legs into *urdhva dhanurasana*.

6. Press evenly into your hands and feet to open your spine. Stay here and breathe (*9.d.2*).

7. Inhale, come up onto your tiptoes and bring your chin toward your chest.

8. Exhale, lift your head and bring your shoulders to the mat, and then lower the rest of your body.

STEPS 1–3: Use your hands to pull your feet toward your hips. Reach your arms overhead and put your palms on the mat. Stiffness in your shoulders will pull your elbows away from each other so press them toward each other in front of your face.

STEP 4: You may be used to going straight up into *urdhva dhanurasana* but we use a very specific two-step process to set the foundations of the pose. Press into your hands and feet to lift halfway up onto the top of your head. Don't go into

Backbends

EDDIE:
Do not stay in your bright areas; push yourself toward your shadows.

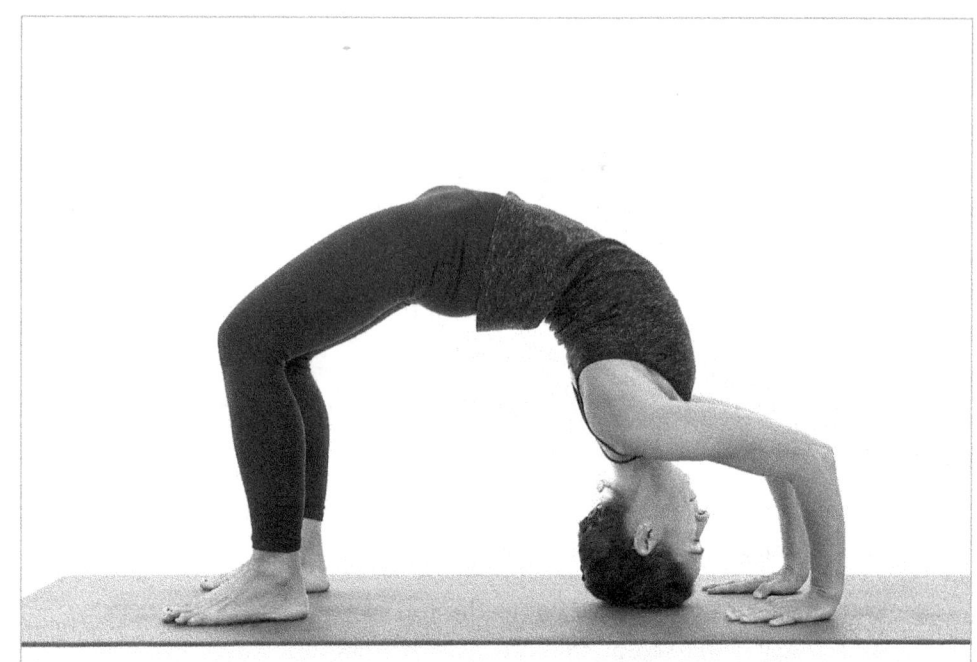

9.d.1 Setup for urdhva dhanurasana

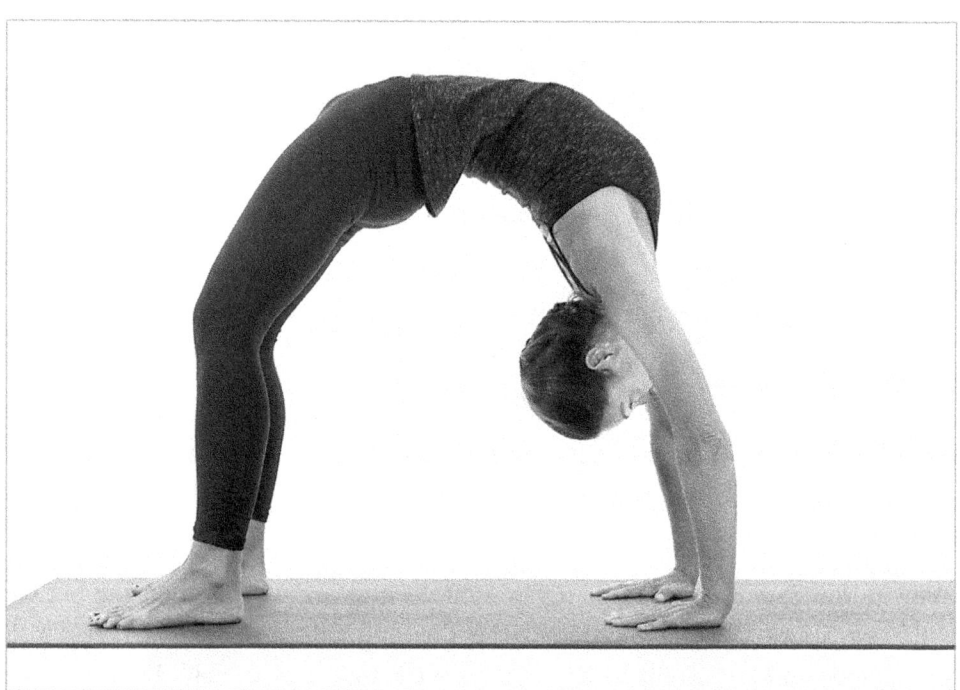

9.d.2 Urdha dhanurasana

the full pose; keep your elbows and knees bent to roughly 90°. Press the back of your head into the mat as you roll up and move your chin toward your throat to lengthen the back of your neck. Look at your hands and walk them away from your shoulders until you can see your wrists. Squeeze your elbows together to put them directly over your wrists. Press into the inner triads of your hands. Lift your shoulders and press into the back of your head to lift your sternum. Squeeze your knees together. Lift your pubic bone and press your pelvis up like you are in *setu bandha sarvangasana*.

STEPS 5 & 6: Inhale and simultaneously straighten both arms and legs. Gaze at the floor between your hands. If your chest is stiff the pose will push you toward your legs; if your pelvis is stiff the pose will push you toward your shoulders. Figure out which one applies to you and use your arms and legs to develop balance. Press into your inner triads and straighten your elbows to lift your chest. Squeeze your legs together and press into your heels to lift your pelvis. Straighten your arms and legs to create an even arc in your spine where your pubic bone and your floating ribs are perfectly level.

STEPS 7 & 8: Inhale and tuck your chin to your chest to get your head out of the way. Exhale and gracefully lower your shoulders to the mat first, followed by the length of your spine and then your pelvis and head.

LOWER BACK RELEASE

Use this pose to decompress your sacrum and lower back at the end of your backbending practice.

1. Lie on your back and bend your knees toward your chest.

2. Reach your arms around the back of your thighs and hold on to your legs. Use each hand to grab the opposite elbow or hold on to opposite forearms.

3. Flex your feet and reach your heels away from you, up and toward the center of the room, as though you wanted to straighten your legs but your arms wouldn't let you.

4. Keep your neck long and soft. Stay here and breathe.

TWISTS

Twists have two very simple rules: 1) they should always be done in extension, and 2) the pelvis should move freely in the direction of the twist. These rules are grounded in spinal anatomy. The shape of your thoracic spine (chest/ribcage) is best suited to twisting, followed by the cervical spine (neck). The lumbar spine (lower back) cannot twist so twists should move up your spine instead of down; they should start in your pelvis and lift up toward your neck.

Unfortunately, many students tighten their abdomen and bear down as they move into a twist. Contracting your abdomen is actually counterproductive: it pulls your chest toward your pubic bone, and bearing down forces the twist into your lower back—right where it's not supposed to go.

The safest way to twist is to inhale and lift and then exhale and twist. The inhale lifts your spine and moves the twist toward your chest where it belongs. Keep your spine extended as you exhale and twist. The movement is up, not down. Lead with your sternum, soften your belly, and allow your pelvis to move in the direction of the twist. Lifting your chest and releasing your pelvis allows your bones to work together and puts the movement of the twist where it belongs.

BHARADVAJASANA
bah·har·aud·vaa·jahs·ahn·nuh | *Baharadvaja's pose*

Bharadvaja was a great Indian sage who is said to have composed several Vedic chants, and this fantastic twist is named in his honor. It sets the pelvis at an angle and uses that angle to rotate the spine, and is thus a perfect example of *asana* following anatomy: the twist originates in the pelvis and lifts through the entire spine; not the other way around.

1. Start on hands and knees. Look back and shift both feet to the right so your left foot is behind your right knee.

2. Point your right foot straight back and put the top of your left foot across your right arch. Flex your left foot to press your toes against the outer edge of your right foot.

3. Walk your hips straight back to put your right hip on your left

heel and your left hip on the mat. Let your thighs spread as you sit back so your right knee is further forward than your left.

4. Place your left hand on the floor outside of your left hip and put your right hand on your left knee. Lean to the left, in the direction of your pelvis.

5. Inhale and lift your chest, exhale and twist to the left. Keep your right hip heavy and expand the line from your pubic bone to your sternum *(10.a.1)*. If you want more, move your left hand back to increase the twist and wrap your right hand under your left knee *(10.a.2)*.

6. Exhale and keep your chest lifted as you return to center. Switch sides.

Twists

SET UP: Start with your knees hip-width apart. Your right hip will be higher than your left hip so most of your weight should be on your left. If this pose puts any pressure on your knees, put something soft and stable between your heels and your sit bones.

STEP 4: Don't try to sit up straight in this pose. Lean to the left, in the direction of your pelvis. Your right hip is higher than your left so your right shoulder should also be higher than your left.

STEP 5: Inhale to lift your chest and keep it lifted as you exhale and twist. The thoracic spine twists more than the lumbar so lead with your sternum. Roll both shoulders back and lift the right side of your body as you twist to the left. If it's comfortable on your neck, lift your head and gaze in the direction of the twist. Allow your gaze to follow the line set by your chest, but keep the action of the twist centered in your thoracic spine. If you want more, move your left hand back and continue to spin the right side of your body to the left. Stay for one or two minutes. Exhale to unwind and return to center.

This is the first of *bharadvajasana*'s three variations. The second variation puts the left foot on the bottom and the right foot on top. The left toes point to the right like they're in the third *vajrasana*, and the right foot rests across the left arch with toes pointed straight back. Everything else is the same. The third variation is the most advanced—it brings the left foot into *padmasana* on top of the right thigh—and is not appropriate for introductory students.

Twists

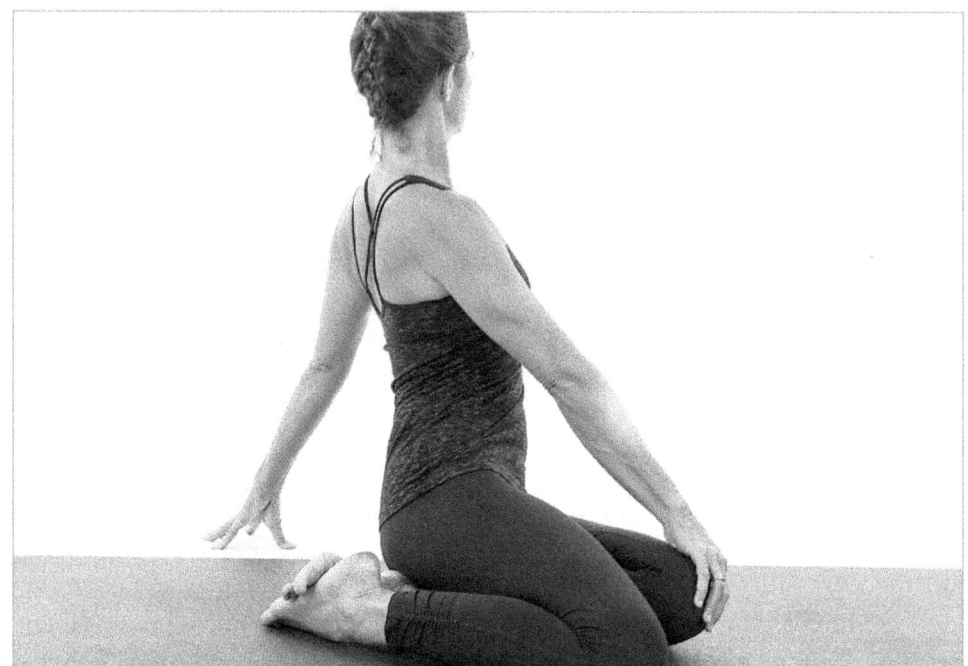

10.a.1 Bharadvajasana

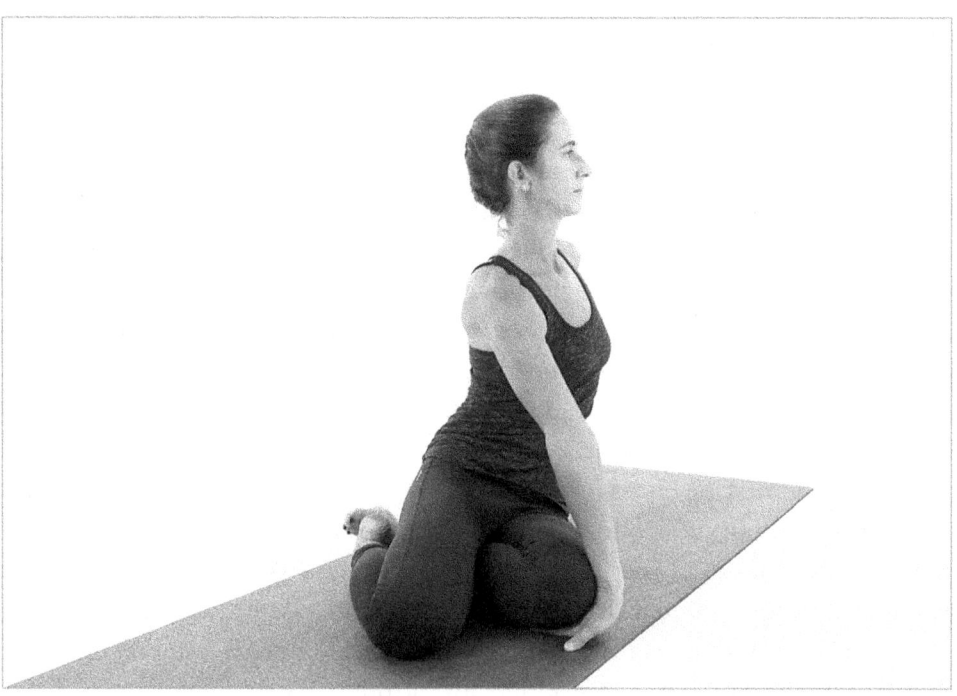

10.a.2 Bharadvajasana with second hand variation

ARDHA JATHARA PARIVARTANASANA
aur·dah juh·tha·ruh paur·ree·vah·ta·naas·ahn·nuh | *half revolved belly pose*

Ardha means half, *jathara* is your belly and *pariva* means to rotate. *Ardha jathara parivartanasana* is a dynamic supine pose that rotates your legs around your belly. It combines twisting with core strength, but in yoga, your core is not your abdomen; your core is your spine. The name of the pose instructs us to rotate around the belly, not from the belly. When done properly, *ardha jathara parivartanasana* is a fantastic way to strengthen and integrate your spine after backbends and inversions.

Twists

1. Lie on your back. Spread your arms at shoulder height and turn your palms up.

2. Bend your knees into your chest, squeeze your knees together, and flex your feet.

3. Inhale and reach your arms away from each other.

4. Exhale and lower your knees to the right. Use your right foot to lift your left and keep both feet higher than your knees. Look at your left hand and reach to the left *(10.b)*.

5. Inhale, press into the back of your hands and lift your head and knees to center.

6. Exhale and lower your knees to the left. Use your left foot to lift your right, and keep both feet higher than your knees. Look at your right hand and reach to the right.

7. Inhale, press into the back of your hands and lift your knees and head to center.

8. Repeat steps 4-7 for three to five rounds. Exhale on your left and return to center. Straighten your legs and rest.

STEPS 3–5: Stretch your hands away from each other to broaden your chest. Keep your knees bent as they lower to move the twist up your spine, away from your lower back. Your heels should stay close to your butt. If your outer right knee can touch the floor it should land just below your right elbow, but your feet should not touch the floor. Flex your feet and use your bottom foot to push your

Twists

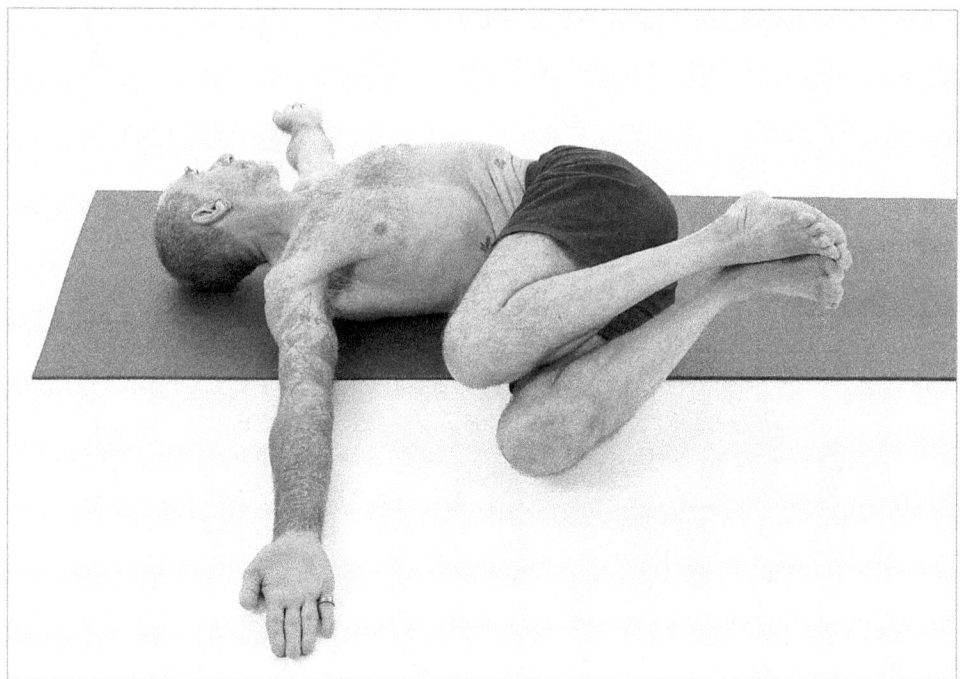

10.b Ardha jathara parivartanasana

top foot higher; your knees go down and your feet go up. Look at your left hand and reach your left arm away from the twist. Roll your left shoulder blade toward the mat and open the left side of your chest. Inhale, press your hands down to return to center, and then repeat on the opposite side.

JATHARA PARIVARTANASANA
juh·tha·ruh paur·ree·vah·ta·naas·ahn·nuh | *revolved belly pose*

Ardha jathara parivartanasana uses half of your leg and *jathara parivartanasana* uses the whole leg.

1. Lie on your back. Spread your arms at shoulder height and turn your palms up.

2. Straighten your legs overhead, squeeze them together and point your toes *(10.c.1)*.

3. Inhale and reach your arms away from each other.

4. Exhale and keep both legs completely straight as you lower your feet to hover over your right hand. Use your right leg to lift your left leg. Look at your left hand and reach to the left.

5. Inhale, press into the backs of your hands and lift your head and feet to center.

6. Exhale and lower your feet to hover over your left hand. Use your left leg to lift your right leg. Look at your right hand and reach to the right *(10.c.2)*.

7. Inhale, press into the backs of your hands and lift your knees and head to center.

8. Repeat steps 4-7 for three to five rounds. Exhale on your left and return to center. Bend your knees and rest.

The action of the pose is similar to its *ardha* variation: keep your feet high to move the twist up your spine, away from your lower back. Bring your feet over

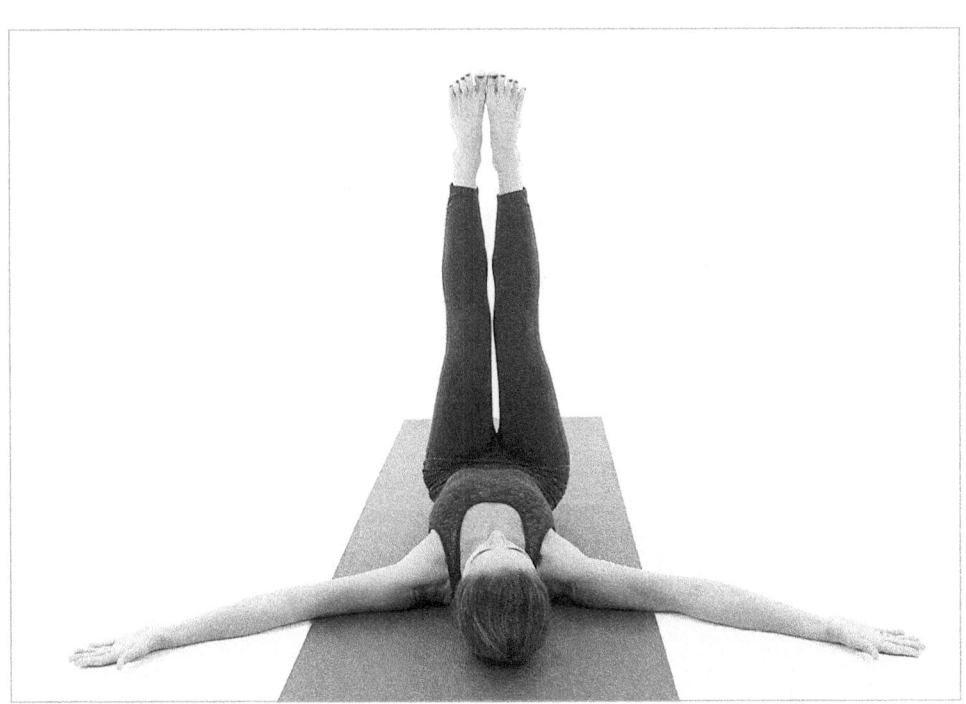

10.c.1 Jathara Parivartanasana setup

Twists

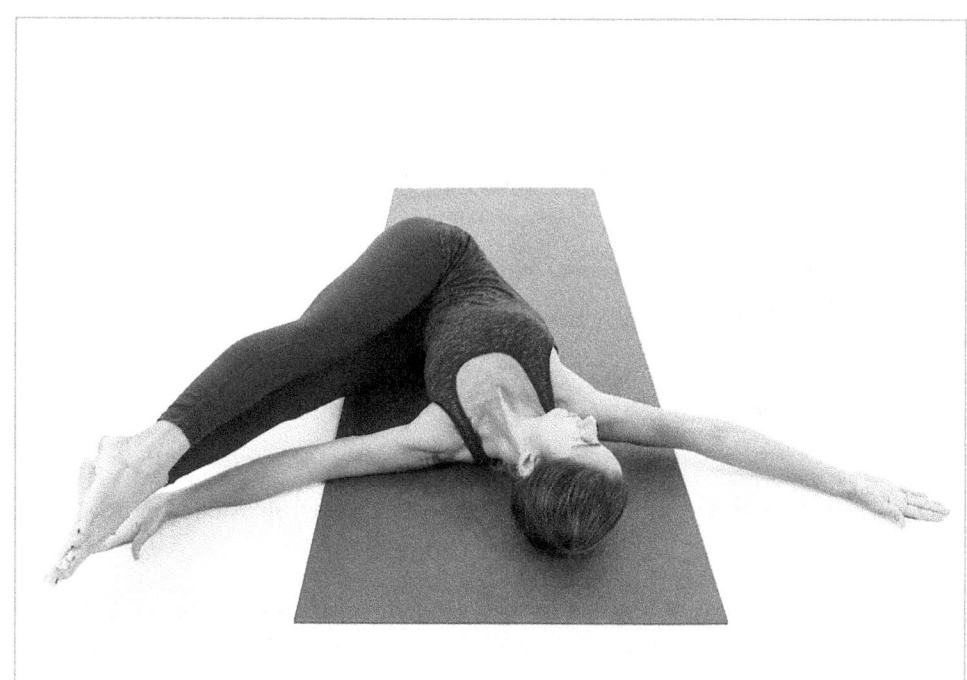

10.c.2 Jathara parivartanasana to the left

your face to start, and then lower both legs to hover over your right hand. Placing your feet lower than your hands pushes the twist toward your lumbar spine, so keep them up. Use your bottom leg to lift your top leg and point your toes. Look to the left and roll your left shoulder toward the floor to open your chest. Inhale, press into your hands to return to center, and then repeat on the left.

INVERSIONS

Inversions are at the top of *asana*'s hierarchy. Other *asana*s work with the axial skeleton—arms, legs, shoulders and hips—but inversions work directly with your spine. They continue the process of moving from the outside in, and from the gross to the subtle. Inversions bring you from your superficial muscles and bones into the deep tissue of your spine and internal organs.

Inversions have a direct effect on your endocrine system, the system that tells everything in your body what to do. The glands of the endocrine system regulate growth, development, metabolism, reproduction, sleep, and emotions—the list goes on. Headstand and shoulderstand are capable of balancing this entire system: headstand balances the pineal and pituitary glands and shoulderstand balances the thyroid gland. These two poses have the power to stabilize your entire physiology. They're the pot of gold at the end of *asana*'s rainbow but as you well know, there is no pay without work. It can take years of standing poses to hold these inversions properly and years of practice to hold them for long enough to be physiologically significant.

It takes seven minutes of stillness for an inversion to be physiologically significant and optimally beneficial. Seven minutes may sound like an eternity, but don't let that dissuade you. Benefits are present in shorter timings as well. Inversions put your heart over your head to provide oxygen to your brain. They drain stagnant blood out of your limbs and take pressure off the veins in your legs. They encourage efficiency in your entire circulatory system. You can feel these positive effects after just a few minutes upside down, and hopefully that feeling will encourage you to stay longer. Start with short timings and build them with daily practice. We usually work up to a 20 minute shoulderstand and a five to seven minute headstand in our teacher trainings.

Inversions have an internal hierarchy: headstand is the king and shoulderstand is the queen, and all the others live below them. Shoulderstand and handstand are the most appropriate for introductory students, and that's what we'll cover in this book, along with *viparita karani*.

SETU BANDHA SARVANGASANA
seh·too baun·dah saar·vun·gaas·ahn·nuh | *bridge pose*

Inversions

Setu bandha sarvangasana is a variation of *sarvangasana*, or shoulderstand. It develops the anatomical foundations of shoulderstand without bearing the full weight of the pose and provides an incredible amount of leverage into your shoulders, chest, pelvis, and legs. *Setu bandha* puts your shoulders on your back, where they belong, so they can support your spine in the journey to *sarvangasana*.

The primary contraindication for *setu bandha* is pain in your knees. If this pose causes an uncomfortable sensation in your knees, or if your knees are visibly spreading wider than your hips, please turn your feet to follow your knees. Always point your toes in the same direction as your knees, and vice versa. If you feel pain in your neck, place one to three neatly folded blankets under your shoulders to set them higher than the back of your head.

1. Lie on your back. Bend your knees and bring your feet toward your hips.

2. Set your feet flat on the floor and parallel to each other, unless that causes pain in your knees. If there is pain in your knees, turn your feet out and allow your knees to follow.

3. Place your hands on your thighs with your fingertips pointed at your knees. Exhale and extend your lower back toward your heels.

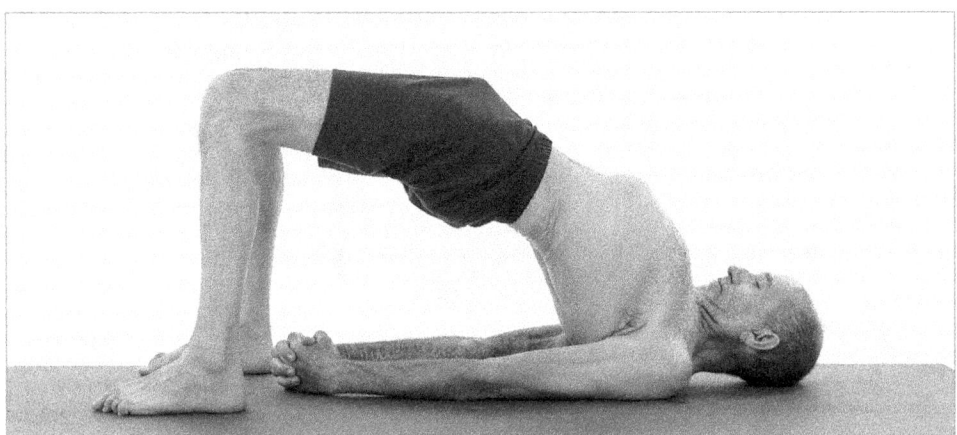

11.a.1 Setu bandha sarvangasana with first arm variation

4. Inhale, press your thighs forward and lift your hips.

5. Take your hands off your thighs and interlace your fingers behind your back. Shift your body to the left to roll your right shoulder under your chest and then to the right to roll your left shoulder under.

First arm variation (*11.a.1*):

6. Press your arms down to lift your chest and press your feet down to lift your pelvis. Reach your pubic bone up and lengthen your lower back.

7. Lift your toes and press into your feet to roll onto the tops of your shoulders. Squeeze your knees toward each other, unless that hurts them. Engage your legs to lift your pubic bone.

8. Stay in the pose until your quadriceps are burning.

9. Inhale and come up onto your tiptoes.

10. Exhale, release the clasp, and gently lower to the mat.

Supported arm variation (*11.a.2*):

6. Release your hands and bend your elbows.

7. Lift your hips higher (come onto your tiptoes if necessary) and walk your elbows toward each other to broaden your shoulders. Shift to the left and place your right hand under your right hip. Shift to the right and place your left hand under your left hip.

8. Lift your toes and press into your feet to roll onto the tops of your shoulders. Squeeze your knees toward each other, unless that hurts them. Engage your legs to lift the weight of your hips away from your hands.

9. Inhale and come up onto your tiptoes.

10. Exhale, release your arms, and gently lower to the mat.

STEPS 1–4: Place your feet so your heels will be directly under your knees when you lift your hips. If your knees are tightly bent—i.e. your feet are closer to your

Inversions

EDDIE:
Come out of the pose when your legs are burning. If you need to come out of the pose because your back hurts, your legs aren't working hard enough. Go back to King Arthur to remove the congestion in your legs, and then use your legs to lift your pelvis away from your lower back.

Inversions

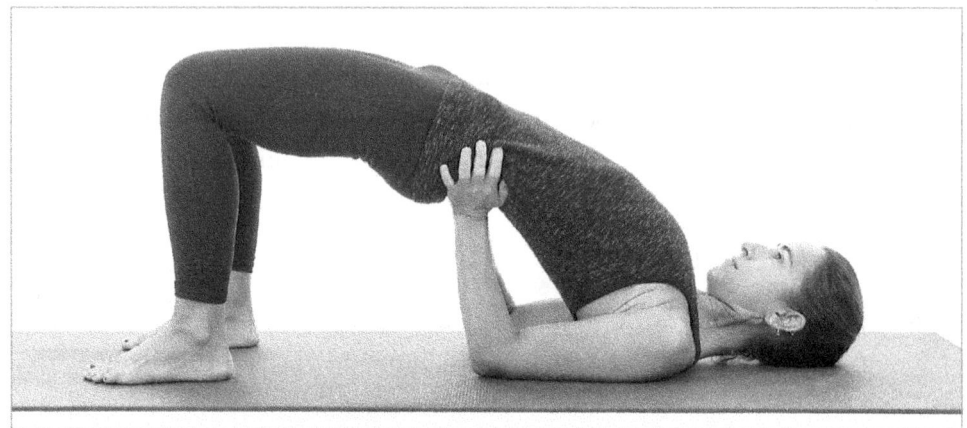

11.a.2 Setu bandha sarvangasana with second (supported) arm variation

hips than your knees—you will have less leverage to lift your pelvis. As you lift, press your thighs toward your knees to create space in the front of your pelvis and lift your tailbone to maintain a corresponding space in your lower back.

STEP 5: *Setu bandha* will put your shoulders on your back, but in the beginning, your weight may rest more on your shoulder blades than the tops of your shoulders. Your armpit chest may be sucked toward your front body, leaving your neck and upper back pressed into the mat, and that's not comfortable. Counteract that stiffness by reaching your arms away from your chest and rolling your shoulders back to sit underneath your sternum. This will move your weight to the tops of your shoulders, away from your neck, and allow your chest to lift away from your upper arms. This action is the anatomical foundation of shoulderstand, and it's important to learn it here without the weight of your legs stacked above you.

STEP 6: The first arm variation provides the most leverage into your chest and shoulders: reaching your clasped hands toward your feet opens your armpit chest.

STEPS 7 & 8: *Setu bandha* is about your legs and pelvis, and the work in your legs is consistent in both variations. Press your feet down to roll onto the tops of your shoulders, and press your outer arms down to lift your sternum. Engage your quadriceps to lift your thigh bones and open the front of your pelvis. Lift your tailbone and pubic bone toward the ceiling. Squeeze your knees toward each other to engage the inseam of both legs—the line that extends from your pubic bone to your inner foot.

Lift your toes to make your feet work harder. Press into the front of your feet and through the center of your heels. If you want more, lift the fronts of your feet off the mat and press into your heels; press them down and lift your pubic bone up. The pose should be ascending; the longer you're there, the higher you get. If you are no longer ascending, come down and rest.

STEPS 9–10: Come out of the pose in the same way you came in. Inhale and lift up onto your tiptoes, and exhale to release your hands and roll your back toward the mat. Bring your hips down last to protect your lower back. Straighten your legs and soften your entire body. Scan your body for pain, and if you find it, use your awareness to diagnose it. If it's in your knees, you need to turn your toes out; if it's in your back, you need to use your legs more. If your quadriceps are burning and your body is free of pain, the *asana* is effective.

SALAMBA SARVANGASANA
saa·lum·bah saar·vun·gaas·ahn·nuh | *supported shoulderstand*

Sarvangasana is the mother of all poses. She is a beautiful, nurturing, inviting and challenging pose that will carry you gracefully through all the stages of your life.

Shoulderstand is a very physiologically effective pose. It balances the thyroid gland that sits at the base of your throat and opens your ribcage for unimpeded respiration. There are 15+ variations that build on the basic pose, and each variation is designed to address a specific organ. That's where it gets really cool. When Eddie studied with BKS Iyengar he called it soaking and squeezing the organs: the shoulderstand variations compress certain areas of your body to squeeze old blood out of your organs and then open those areas to bathe them in fresh blood. It massages your internal organs to keep them soft, supple, and functional.

In a more tangible sense, shoulderstand lengthens your neck and removes congestion in your chest and shoulders. It puts your shoulders on your back body where they belong, and frees the upper ribs to expand your lungs. It also begins the process of strengthening your spine to support its own weight—a process that will eventually lead you to headstand.

Shoulderstand is an inversion and a slight backbend: your legs reach away from your shoulders to create a lever that opens your chest: when your legs go back your chest lifts; when your legs come forward your chest collapses. Most of us come to yoga with stiff shoulders, weak legs, and a closed chest; and when that anatomy is placed on the floor in shoulderstand, the legs fall forward and dump their weight into the cervical spine (neck). That's where shoulderstand gets its dodgy reputation, but it's completely unfounded. If your feet are over your face you're not actually doing shoulderstand; you're doing neckstand, and that's not a real pose.

We teach shoulderstand with props—blankets under your shoulders and upper arms—to provide enough leverage to open your chest and stay in the pose comfortably. The blankets lift your shoulders higher than your head to protect your neck, and encourage your shoulders and upper arms toward your back body to support your torso. They provide leverage to lift your feet away from your face, which opens your armpit chest and the front of your pelvis. They also provide a level of comfort that allows you to stay longer than 30 seconds, and that's the shoulderstand we want you to experience.

Shoulderstand can be introduced shortly after the standing poses. Use props and pay close attention to your alignment because without proper alignment it quickly becomes neckstand (as described above). If there is pain in your neck, reevaluate your pose and get whatever props you need to put the work into your arms and legs. Start with one to three minutes in shoulderstand—not counting the time it takes to set up—and build from there.

1. Open four blankets into wide rectangles and stack them at the end of your mat. Align the folded end of each blanket to face the short end of your mat, and smooth out any wrinkles in the blankets. The stack should be three to four inches tall.

2. Fold the bottom half of your mat over the blankets. Align the bottom edge of the mat with the folded edge of the blankets.

3. Lie on the mat with your head toward the top edge of the blankets. Scoot toward the end of the stack until your head is off and the top of your shoulders are about two inches from the edge.

4. Lift up and interlace your fingers behind your back. On an exhale, roll both legs over your torso, curl your toes under and place them on the floor over your head. This is *halasana* (plough pose). Your shoulders are on the blankets but head and neck are off.

5. Use your clasped hands to roll your shoulders under your chest, one by one, like you did in *setu bandha sarvangasana*. Release the clasp, put your hands on your back as close to your ribs as possible and squeeze your elbows toward each other. Internally rotate your legs and straighten both knees.

   A. *Halasana* is a forward bend and can be dangerous for people with lumbar disc injuries. If there is pain in your lower back, keep your knees bent and do not linger.

6. Inhale and lift your legs, one by one, into shoulderstand. Bring them together, straighten both knees and spin your thighs toward each other. Reach up through your big toe bones.

7. Bring your feet over your elbows and lift your tailbone toward your heels. Walk your hands down your back (toward the top of your ribs) and squeeze your elbows toward each other to open your chest. Lift your chest. Stay here two to three minutes. There should not be any pressure in your neck *(11.b.1)*.

   DO NOT TURN YOUR HEAD at any point.

8. On an exhale, release your feet overhead into *halasana*. Release your arms onto the mat and slowly roll your legs back over your body to lie flat.

9. Scoot off the blankets in the direction of your head, until your shoulders are on the floor but your chest remains elevated. Bend your elbows and release your arms out to the side.

SET UP: The setup should be specific to your needs. If your chest, neck, and shoulders are very stiff, start with more blankets. We've had people start on six or seven; it doesn't matter how many you use because you are more important than the "rules" of the pose.

STEP 4: *Halasana* is a variation of shoulderstand. You will pause in *halasana* on your way into shoulderstand and on your way out, and we'll often visit *halasana* to re-set our shoulders during a long shoulderstand. *Halasana* is a forward bend so please be sensitive to your lower back. If there is any pain in your lower back, keep your knees bent and do not stay longer than necessary.

Inversions

Inversions

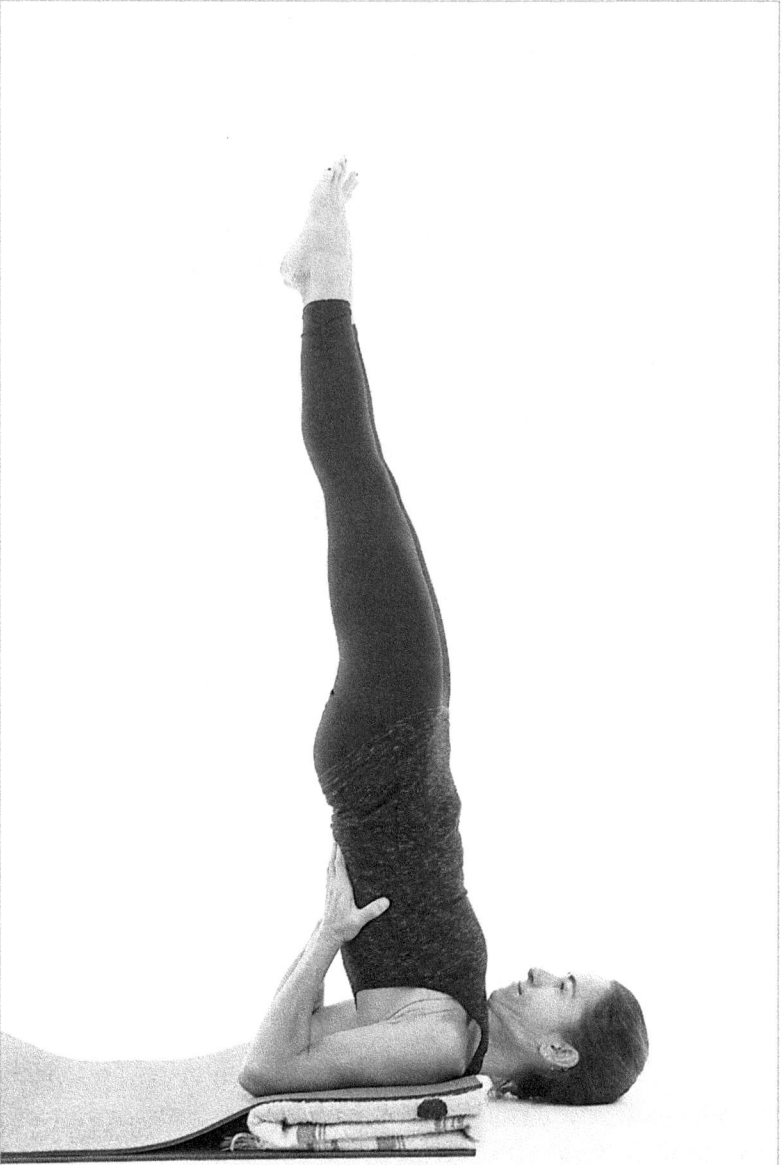

11.b.1 Salamba sarvangasana with folded blankets

STEP 5: Interlacing your hands behind your back broadens your chest and moves your shoulders toward your back body. When your hands release their clasp to support the torso, squeezing your elbows toward each other has a similar effect. If your elbows begin to slide apart, use a belt just above the elbows to keep them together. Put the belt around one arm during the set up and loop it through your other arm while in *halasana*.

STEPS 6–8: You need the strong legs of *uttanasana* to carry you into shoulderstand. Lucky for you, your legs are actually visible in this pose. Straighten both knees, lift your kneecaps, spin your thighs together (internal rotation), and then take your feet back toward your elbows. Reach through your heels and your big toe bones. Lift your tailbone toward your heels to lengthen your lower back, and to keep the pose from tipping over. Walk your hands down your back in the direction of your chest and use them to push your chest open. Stay here until your quadriceps start to burn, and then stay a wee bit longer.

STEP 9: To come out, exhale back to *halasana*. Release your hands and slowly roll your legs back to a supine position. Shift your head and shoulders off the blankets and rest.

We've said that props should always move you in the direction of yoga and these blankets are no exception: they move your anatomy in the direction of *salamba sarvangasana*. But there's a fair chance you'll use the blankets in shoulderstand longer than many other props, and that's fine. Eddie used the blankets for 10 years before he did shoulderstand on the floor, and he's an intensely intense practitioner. The props cultivate a soft, stable pose, and that stillness allows you to reap shoulderstand's many physiological benefits. You can't get to your internal organs if you're shaky or fidgeting so use props to build your anatomy in the shape of yoga.

Shoulderstand should be practiced for at least six months before headstand is introduced. If you currently have a headstand practice but omit shoulderstand, please give shoulderstand the respect it deserves. If they are practiced together, shoulderstand should be held for twice as long as headstand; if you do headstand for five minutes, shoulderstand should get at least ten.

Modifications

Shoulderstand can be done against a wall for additional support. Bring your setup close to a wall with your head pointed toward the center of the room. Lift into the pose and then bend your knees to put the soles of your feet flat on the wall. Use the wall as leverage to get your shoulders under your ribcage, lift your tailbone, and open your chest. We also teach a wonderful therapeutic applica-

Inversions

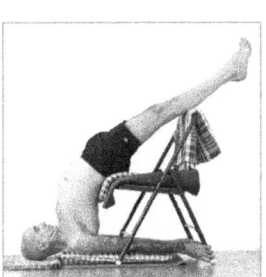

11.b.2 Chair shoulderstand

tion called chair shoulderstand, where the pose is supported by a metal folding chair *(11.b.2)*.

ADHO MUKHA VRKSASANA
aud·ho·moo·kah vrik·shas·ahn·nuh | downward facing tree pose | *handstand*

Inversions

Handstand is an extension of downward dog; hence the similarity in Sanskrit names—downward dog is *adho mukha svanasana* and handstand is *adho mukha vrksasana*. Cultivate a two-minute downward dog and one-minute standing poses before approaching handstand, and do it against a wall for stability. Balance comes from proper alignment, not the other way around.

Handstand continues the process of opening the armpit chest and training the legs to support their own weight. The armpit chest is where many of your lymph nodes reside, which are a vital part of your immune system. It's one of your bodily seats of health, along with your groin, and opening these areas bathes the lymphatic system in fresh blood. Circulation keeps them fluid and devoid of the stagnation that breeds disease. It's especially important for women: the armpit chest is adjacent to the breast tissue and the groin is adjacent to the reproductive organs.

We typically do handstands in sets of three or four, with 30 second to one-minute timings. If you can get up and stay up, move closer to the wall for the next one. Moving closer to the wall gives you less room to jump forward as you go up; it requires more opening in the armpit chest and brings you closer to the alignment of the pose.

1. Start in downward dog with your fingertips 6-8" from the wall.

2. Look at your hands and organize them. They should be shoulder width apart with middle fingers pointed straight forward, fingers evenly spaced, and weight firmly grounded in the inner triads.

3. Exhale, walk your feet in and bend one knee. Look at your hands.

4. Inhale and kick up into handstand.

5. Spin your legs together and stretch your heels up the wall. Lift your tailbone toward your heels and bring your ribs toward your spine. Look down at your hands. Press your inner triads into the

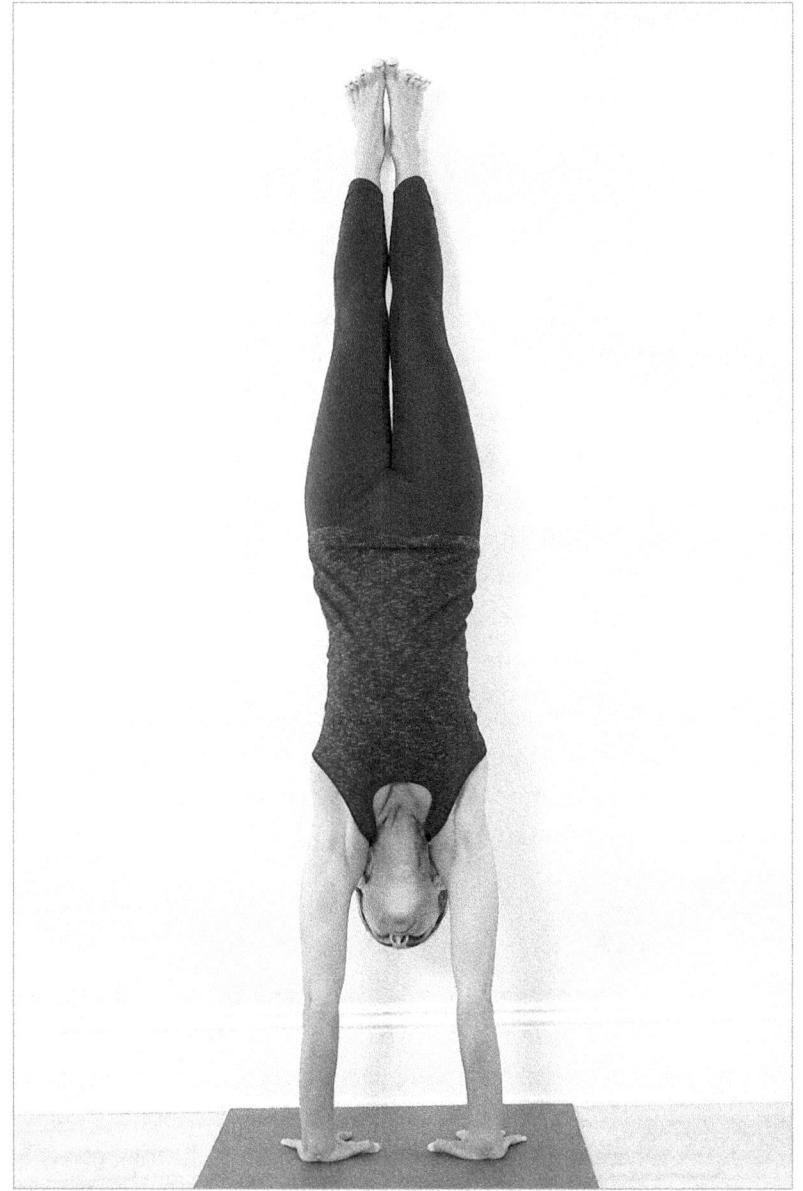

Inversions

11.c Vrksasana

floor and stretch your legs up to the ceiling. Keep your feet on the wall *(11.c)*.

6. Exhale and come out the way you came in: gracefully, one leg at a time. Rest in *uttanasana*.

SET UP: The setup is downward dog. Gather any specific props you use for that pose—belt for your elbows, slant board for your wrists, etc.—and bring them into handstand. If you're not familiar with downward dog, don't do handstand. Start with the foundations.

STEP 4: Kick into the pose with one leg right after the other. The bent leg pushes away from the floor and straightens the instant it leaves the ground. The straight leg arrives first but the push-off leg should be right behind it. Do not hesitate, and don't let your knees bend on the way up. Straighten your legs and pull them together immediately.

STEP 5: Handstand is all about your legs. Use them to pull your torso away from the weight in your shoulders. Do not sag into your ribs or lower back. This is downward facing tree pose, not downward facing banana pose. Lift your tailbone and your lower floating ribs to lengthen your spine in the direction of your heels. Straighten your arms and go up. Resist the urge to peel your heels off the wall, even if you feel quite stable. Keep your heels on the wall and focus on alignment, and your balance will grow from that alignment.

STEP 6: If you cannot exit gracefully you probably stayed too long. Lower one leg and then the next and stand in *uttanasana* between handstands. Study your legs in *uttanasana* and bring them with you into the next handstand. When you have completed your final handstand for the practice, or if you need a break between sets, rest in *balasana*.

SWINGS

We've said there are no shortcuts in yoga but there is one fantastic exception: pelvic swings. You don't have to open your spine or strengthen your legs, just drop in and let go. Hanging in the swing decompresses your spine and feeds the endocrine system in the same way as headstand, but with none of the effort. To be fair, it doesn't have the exact physiological effects as headstand—headstand puts more pressure on the cranium to stimulate the pituitary gland and thus produces more serotonin—but the swing creates a similar effect with a fraction of the work. You can also stay much longer in the swing than in a freestanding headstand so it's easier to reach the threshold for physiological benefits.

VIPARITA KARANI
vee·pah·ree·tah kar·aah·knee | inverted action pose | *legs up the wall*

Viparita karani is a restorative pose that provides the benefits of inversions with minimal effort. Anyone can do it, and everyone should do it. It is one of the friendliest poses in all of yoga. It puts your heart over your head, drains blood out of your legs, and relieves pressure on your veins. It's fantastic for varicose veins and is generally rejuvenating for the legs and feet. Once you are comfortable, spending a few minutes in the pose can relieve pressure in your entire being.

Viparita karani is safe for women on their menstrual cycle because it does not invert the uterus. It requires a bolster and a wall. The bolster provides maximum comfort but *viparita karani* can be done without it: just put your butt against the wall and roll onto your back.

1. Place the bolster against the wall, long ways, and then pull it three to four inches away from the wall.

    A. You can also place a block against the wall, long ways with the narrow side up, and then put the bolster in front of it. The block will keep the bolster from moving toward the wall as you get into the pose.

2. Get on hands and knees next to the bolster, with the soles of your feet on the wall. Bend your knees and put your butt against the wall.

3. Bend your elbows to put your outer hip onto the bolster, and then roll onto your back on top of the bolster. Keep your butt against the wall and straighten your legs.

4. Align your body in the middle of the bolster, with your feet over your hips and your shoulders in line with your pelvis. Release your arms to the side and stay for 5-20 minutes *(11.d.1)*.

5. Bend your knees into *baddha konasana* against the wall *(11.d.2)*. Stay there for a few moments, and then bend your knees into your chest and roll to your side to come off the bolster.

Inversions

11.d.1 Viparita karani

11.d.2 Exiting viparita karani with baddha konasana

Inversions

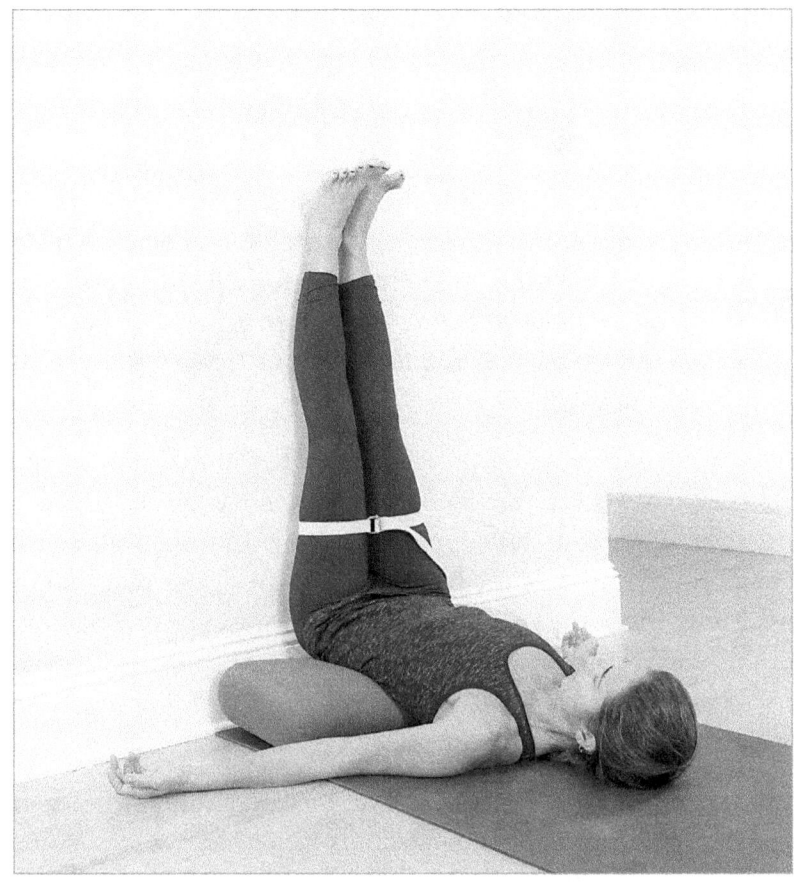

11.d.3 Viparita karani with a belt

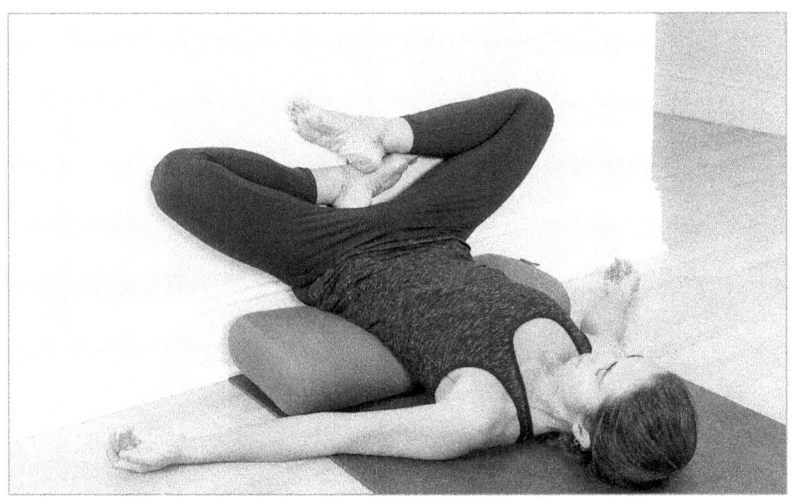

11.d.4 Exiting viparita karani with simple crossed legs

Inversions

SET UP: We often introduce *viparita karani* with the block to set the distance from the wall: the block touches the wall and the bolster touches the block. If you like the block, keep it; if not, get it out of there. This pose is about your maximum comfort so please use whatever props you need to get there.

STEP 3: Start with your butt against the wall and try to keep it there as you roll onto your back. Ideally your sit bones touch the wall when you straighten your legs, but if your hamstrings are tight, don't force it. This pose is not about stretching your legs; it's about softening your entire being, so get as close to the wall as possible and then relax. If you feel like your legs are going to fall apart, use a belt to hold your thighs together *(11.d.3)*.

STEP 4: Getting into the pose may feel a bit awkward at first, and you may need a few adjustments to get comfortable. The bolster should be under your sacrum, not under your heart; if it shifted, press your feet into the wall and lift your hips to adjust it. The curve of the bolster should drop your butt into the space between the bolster and the wall, which encourages your sit bones to make contact with the wall. The bolster also supports your reproductive organs, and if you're a woman, it keeps your uterus from spilling toward your heart. Your head and shoulders should be firmly on the floor.

Introductory students may lose sensation in their feet after just a few minutes, and if that's uncomfortable, bend your knees into *baddha konasana* or simple crossed legs *(11.d.4)*. You can go back and forth to develop your circulatory capacity; Nicki's legs used to fall asleep after about five minutes in this pose, now it takes closer to 45. Ironically, as you become relaxed, your legs get heavy and may actually slide down the wall. If that's your experience, use the belt as described above.

SEATED HIP OPENERS

Seated hip openers represent the *tha* side of *Hatha* yoga. *Ha* is the sun and *tha* is the moon, and together they bring balance to your being. Most of the poses in this book are *ha* poses and modern yoga generally gravitates toward their bright, athletic energy; but you can't just *ha ha ha* all the time. Doing only *ha* poses creates an extreme energetic polarization, and while extremes can be very interesting they are rarely sustainable. Sustainability lies in the middle path: the ability to cultivate both sun and moon on a micro and macro scale. You can include these poses at the end of a more rigorous *asana* sequence to balance the energy of your practice or link them together into a fully restorative practice to balance the energy of your life.

Some of these seated postures involve a forward bend; you put your legs into position and bend forward to rotate your pelvis against that position. If you are very stiff in your hips and legs, explore the forward bend with caution and intelligence—the same way you explore standing forward bends like *uttanasana*. If you feel the stretch in your legs and hips, it's probably in the right spot. If you feel the stretch in your lower back, rewind the pose: take your torso up instead of forward and use props to support your extension.

Aside from pain in your lower back, the primary contraindication for seated hip openers is pain in your knees. Knees are less anatomically stable than hips; there is less bone and more moving parts. When you rotate your pelvis in a seated forward bend, stiffness in your hips may pull on your knees instead. Watch your poses carefully to ensure the rotation intended for your pelvis doesn't spin your knees.

Finally, it's worth reiterating that seated forward bends are the most dangerous poses for the lumbar discs (lower back). If you are very stiff or have known lumbar disc injuries, please do not attempt any seated forward bends until you have spent a few months opening your hips with lunges and standing poses. The seated poses may look "easy" because they're on the floor, but they are far more advanced than they appear.

EDDIE:
Restorative yoga teaches you to be still. Be quiet. Do nothing; just watch. Release the frenetic energy that lives inside you, and become comfortable enough to fall in love with the beautiful being you are.

EDDIE:
If you are open enough to comfortably bend forward, then bend forward and be soft. If you are very stiff, it may be more effective to lift your chest and work the rotation of your pelvis. Those are two different actions for two different people. Modern yoga is getting them confused: flexible people are being taught to open their chest in forward bends, and stiff people are being taught to bend their knees in forward bends. Please take the time to figure out where you are in that spectrum and follow the lines of yoga to do what is right for your anatomy.

VIRASANA
veer·aas·ahn·nuh | *hero's pose*

This pose is contraindicated if you have had surgery to repair your ACL (anterior cruciate ligament). If you have had other kinds of knee surgery, please learn this pose in the presence of an experienced instructor.

Seated Hip Openers

1. Start on your hands and knees.
2. Look between your legs and set your feet slightly wider than your hips. Place the tops of your feet on the floor and point your toes straight back.
3. Place a block between your feet and sit on it. Bring your thighs parallel in front of you with your feet on either side of your hips.
4. Walk your torso back until your head and shoulders are directly over your hips. Rest your hands on your thighs. The front edge of the block should be just in front of your sit bones.
5. Press evenly through the big toe and pinkie toe sides of each foot to point your heels straight up.
6. Balance your sit bones evenly on the block and bring your pelvis to neutral. Align your sternum over your pubic bone, soften your shoulders, and breathe. Stay three to five minutes *(12.a)*.
7. Exhale and lean forward to bring your hands to the mat. Curl your toes under and straighten your legs into *uttanasana*.

STEPS 1–4: *Virasana* externally rotates your femur bones (thighs) within your hip sockets. In a perfect world your thighs would spin away from each other but stiffness in your hips may cause them to spin inward and down, as though your inner leg is being sucked toward the mat. This creates an anatomical predicament: your lower leg is externally rotated while your upper leg is internally rotated, and your knees are caught in the middle. Your knees are not supposed to twist, so let's address this with some simple anatomical geometry.

The front faces of your knees form two little squares and the orientation of those squares can help reveal the rotation of your thighs. If the squares are standing upright (i.e. the tops of your knees are level), then your femur bones are

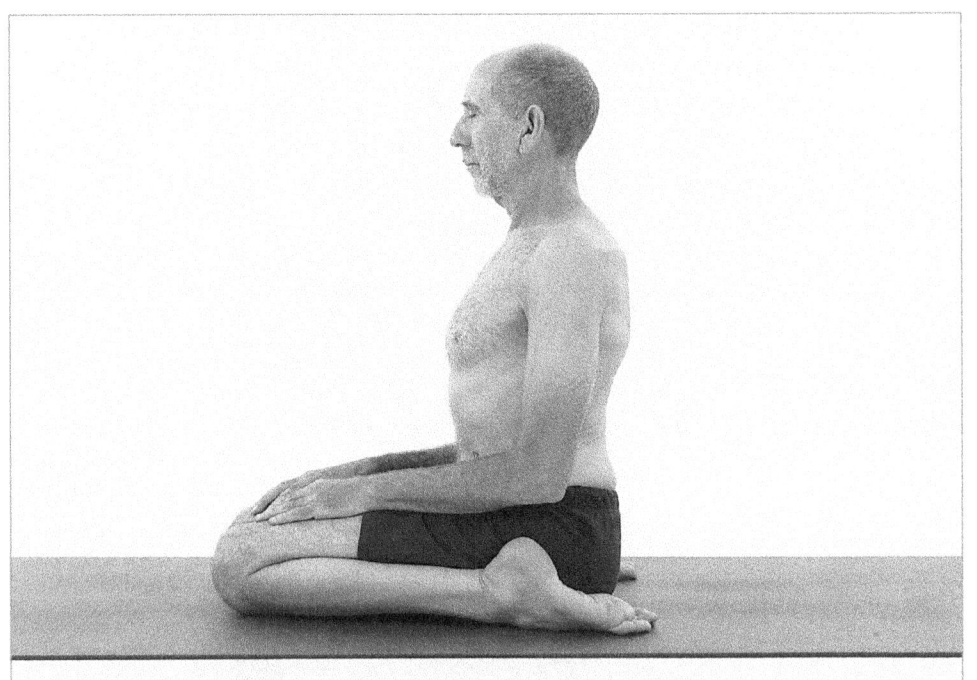

12.a Virasana

Seated Hip Openers

EDDIE:
Uttanasana and *virasana* are complementary poses. In *uttanasana* you use your mind to penetrate your quadriceps; the message goes from the mind to the muscle. In *virasana* the message goes the other way: the pose lengthens the muscle in a passive way that signals a corresponding release in the mind.

rotating in your hips instead of your knees—and that's great. If the squares are tilted down toward the space between your thighs (i.e. the plane across the top of your knees is more of a "v" than a straight line), your femur bones are internally rotating and your knees are at risk. If that's the case, even if it's only a slight rotation, put another block or half-block under your hips to elevate your pose. Watch the change in your knees as you take the pose higher. Elevation reduces the spin between the hips and the thighs; it takes the stretch out of your knees and puts it into your hips where it belongs. And please don't be self-conscious about the props: get as high as necessary to protect your knees. The higher you go the closer you get.

STEP 5: Your heels should point straight up outside of your hips but stiffness may cause them to sickle toward your hips instead. If that's the case, press evenly through the big toe and pinkie toe sides of both feet to move your heels away from your hips. If this causes any pain or discomfort in your knees, even slight discomfort, get more props and bring your sit bones higher until the pain goes away.

STEP 6: Use your hands to find your frontal hip bones and bring your pelvis to neutral. Visualize your pelvis as a bowl of water, filled to the brim, and try not to spill a single drop. Align your sternum directly over your pubic bone. Rest your hands on your thighs, close your eyes, and lower your head. Keep your chest lifted and your spine tall. Your shoulders should be directly over your hips and your sit bones resting evenly on the block. Stay here and breathe.

STEP 7: When your knees ask you to straighten, exhale and come forward into *uttanasana*.

SUPTA VIRASANA
soup·tah veer·aas·ahn·nuh | *reclined hero's pose*

Supta means reclined (think supine) so this is the reclined version of *virasana*. It has the same contraindications as *virasana* but it adds a backbend: from *virasana*, you walk your hands back to rest your torso on a bolster or folded blankets. This soft, supported backbend can do magnificent things for your anatomy. It opens the front of your pelvis by elongating the line from your knees to your shoulders. It increases the space between your pubic bone and your sternum in a gentle, passive way. It opens the sides of your chest and moves your shoulders toward your back body, where they belong. It's also fantastic for digestion and is a soothing, nurturing tonic for all the organs in your abdomen and pelvis.

But if the front of your pelvis is stiff, as is the case for most of humanity (chairs!), the backbend in *supta virasana* may cause compression in your lower back: stiff legs will pull your frontal hip bones down and push the bend into your lumbar spine instead of sharing it with the rest of your body. The best long-term solution is to lengthen the front of your pelvis with King Arthur and the lunges, but in the short term, you can use props to navigate your discomfort. Place more blankets or bolsters under your torso to pull the backbend out of your lumbar spine, and reach your sternum away from your pubic bone to decompress your lower back.

Before you enter the pose, collect the blocks, blankets, and bolsters you require to protect your anatomy and cultivate stillness. Set the block(s) or half block to support your sit bones (you should be familiar enough with *virasana* to know what you need), and then place the bolster(s) or blankets behind the block to support the length of your spine. Keep a couple folded blankets nearby: one to go under your head and one to provide more support if necessary.

1. Begin in *virasana*. Place the blankets/bolsters behind your hips, close enough to support your entire body when you lie back.

2. Inhale and lift your chest. Exhale and walk your hands back to rest your torso onto the blankets/bolster.

3. Place a folded blanket under your head to create a gentle slope from your forehead to your chin.

Seated Hip Openers

4. Press your hands into your heels to lift your sternum away from your pubic bone. If there is no compression in your lower back, bend your elbows and release your arms to the side, palms up.

5. Be still and relax. If you cannot be still, use props to address your discomfort and then return to the pose. Stay 5-10 minutes *(12.b.1)*.

6. Place your hands onto your heels. Inhale and press your elbows into the floor to come up. Lead with your sternum to maintain the backbend as you lift, and let your head come up last.

7. Exhale and lean forward to bring your hands to your mat. Curl your toes under and straighten your legs into *uttanasana*.

STEPS 1 & 2: Take the time to set *virasana* meticulously. Be sensitive to any discomfort in your knees and lower back. On an inhale, lift your chest and extend your spine. Keep your front body lifted as you exhale and lower onto the bolster. Use your hands to support your descent but do not twist; go straight back onto the bolster.

If you don't feel supported, come up and add more props. There shouldn't be any space between you and the props beneath you. Make any necessary adjustments to stay in the pose without fidgeting.

STEP 3: Use a folded blanket to raise your forehead slightly higher than your chin. This gentle downward slope creates a corresponding expansion in your occiput, which sits at the base of your skull. Expanding your occiput stimulates the parasympathetic nervous system, the internal catalyst of rest, relaxation, and nourishment. If your chin is higher than your forehead you are subconsciously stimulating the sympathetic nervous system—the highly tensioned "fight or flight" response—and that energy will prohibit you from letting go.

Seated Hip Openers

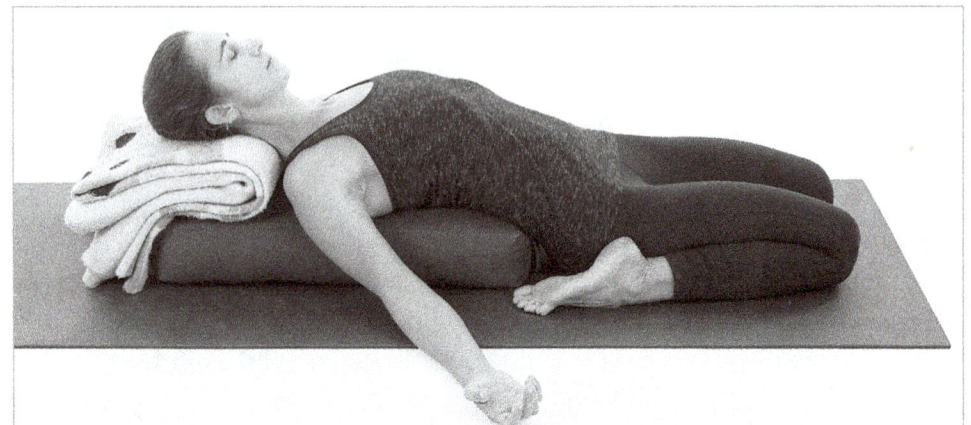

12.b.1 Supta virasana with props

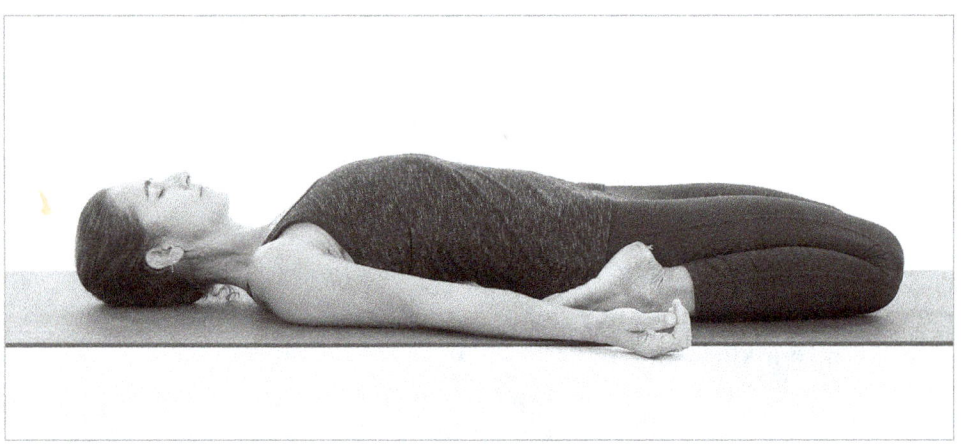

12.b.2 Supta virasana without props

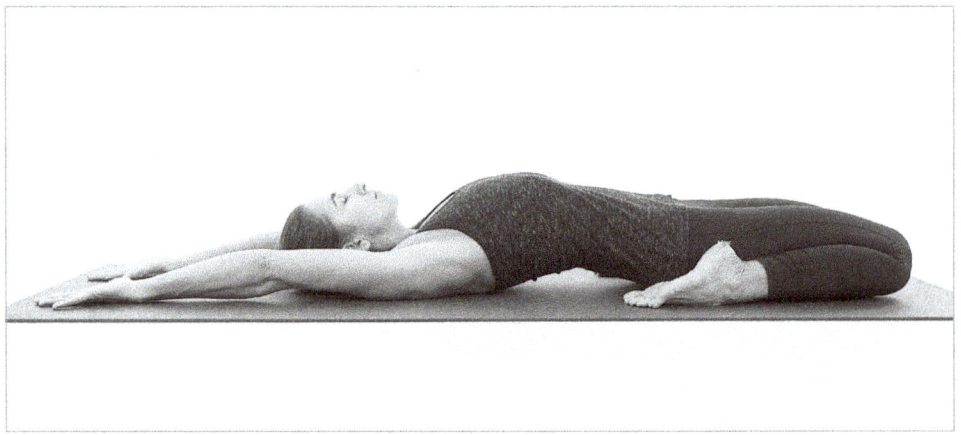

12.b.3 Traditional supta virasana with arms overhead

STEPS 4 & 5: If you have discomfort in your lower back that cannot be alleviated with props, press your hands into your heels and lift your sternum toward your chin. This action will move the backbend toward your chest instead of dumping it into your lumbar spine. If your lower back is comfortable, release your arms out to your sides, turn your palms up and soften your elbows. Allow your shoulders to move away from your spine and down the rounded side of the bolster(s) so gravity can pull them toward your back body. Breathe freely and sink.

STEPS 6 & 7: Come out of the pose as gracefully as you went into it. Put your hands on your heels for leverage, and on an inhale, lift from your sternum into *virasana*. Use your hands to support your ascent but do not twist—go straight up and maintain the backbend as much as possible. Bring your head up last and exhale forward into *uttanasana*.

Traditional variations are done on the floor without props *(12.b.2 and 12.b.3)* but it may take a long time to get there; Nicki has been doing serious yoga for decades and she still prefers supported variations. Traditional variations can be fun to explore as your body opens, but when you're looking for complete stillness and relaxation please use as many props as it takes to get there.

UPAVISTHA KONASANA
oo·pah·veesh·ta koh·nahs·ahn·nuh | *seated angle pose*

There is a strong relationship between *upavistha konasana* and *baddha konasana*. If one of them is open the other one will probably be closed, and together they hold the key to opening your hips. You should spend more time in the one that is closed.

Keep a bolster or blanket nearby to support your torso, if necessary.

1. Sit on the floor with your legs in front of you.
2. Spread your legs to 90° and point your toes straight up.
3. Walk your hands behind your hips and press into the center of your sit bones *(12.c.1)*.
4. Straighten both legs and press your inner knees down to the mat.
5. Inhale and lift your chest *(12.c.2)*. Exhale and walk your hands forward into the space between your legs.

Seated Hip Openers

Seated Hip Openers

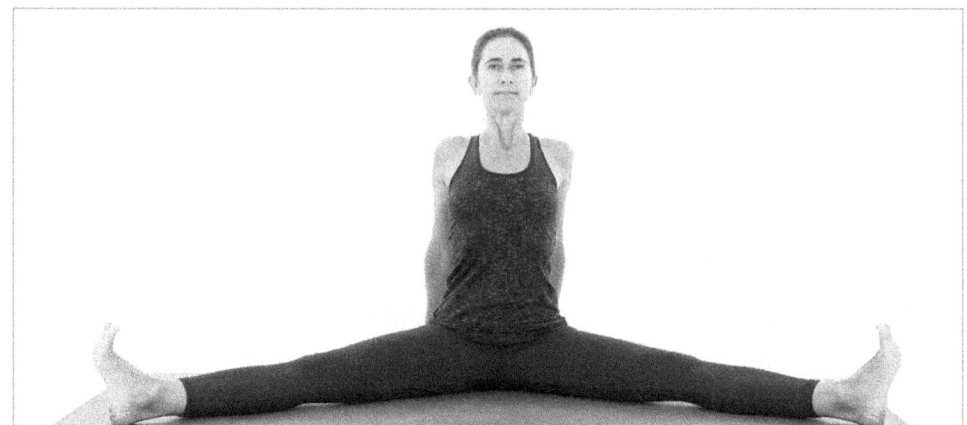

12.c.1 Upavistha konasana with spinal extension to encourage rotation in the pelvis

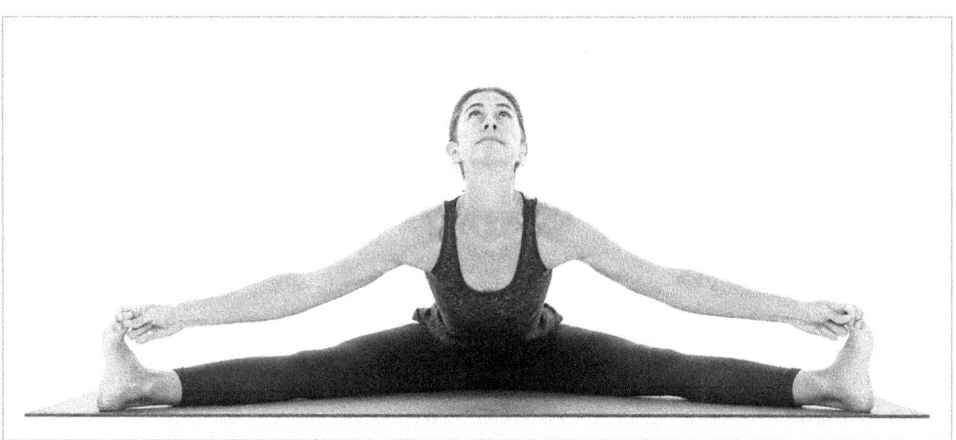

12.c.2 Upavistha konasana preparing for the forward bend

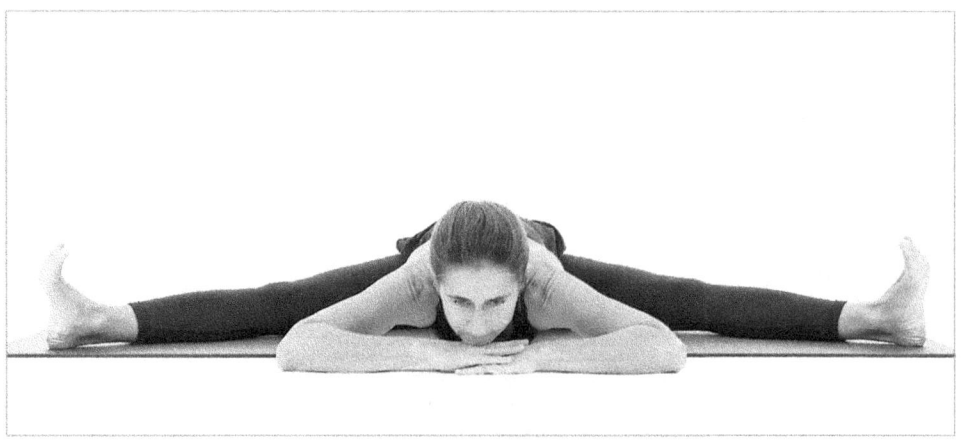

12.c.3 Upavistha konasana with forward bend

6. Press the entire inseam of your legs into the mat. Soften your torso and breathe. Stay three to five minutes *(12.c.3)*.

7. Use your hands to press up to seated and bring your legs together.

STEPS 1 & 2: Set your legs at a 90° angle in *upavistha konasana*; going wider than 90° will narrow your pelvis. Once your legs are set point your toes straight up and press the back of your heels into the mat.

STEP 3: Use your hands behind your hips as leverage to lift your chest and press into the center of your sit bones. Stiffness in your hips may pull your sit bones toward your legs so you're sitting more on the back of your pelvis than the front, and that's not good. Bending forward from that position can push your lumbar discs to the place they are most at risk. If you feel like you are sitting on the back of your sit bones—i.e. toward your sacrum—elevate your hips with blankets or a bolster until you can press your sit bones down evenly. If this stage of the pose pulls very strongly on your legs and pelvis, consider staying here instead of bending forward.

STEP 4: Press the inseam of your legs into the mat. Bring your inner knees down faster than your outer knees; BKS Iyengar wanted the entire inseam of the leg ironed to the floor. If you have very large calf muscles, you may need to pull your calves backward and to the side to remove the space under your knee. Your toes might roll forward a tiny bit to get your inner knee down, but keep the backs of your heels pressed firmly into the mat.

STEPS 5 & 6: Inhale and lift your chest. Exhale and walk your hands forward to lower your torso between your legs. Press your inner knees down and keep your toes pointed up as your pelvis rotates forward. If you cannot rest comfortably on the floor, put something in front of you to support your torso and head. If bending forward strains your lower back, please stay upright and work on releasing tension in your hips and legs.

STEP 7: Use your hands to press up to a seated position. Let your head come up last and use your hands to bring your legs together.

Seated Hip Openers

BADDHA KONASANA
bah·dah koh·nahs·ahn·nuh | *bound angle pose*

Baddha konasana means "bound" angle pose. It binds your feet together to open the front of your pelvis. The primary contraindication is pain in your knees, which can be addressed by elevating your hips to bring your pelvis to neutral.

Seated Hip Openers

1. Sit on the floor with your legs in front of you.
2. Bend your knees and bring the soles of your feet together.
3. Walk your hands behind your hips and lift your chest. Sit on the center of your sit bones and stick your butt out behind you.
4. Press into your hands to lift your sit bones off the mat. Scoot your groin toward your heels and then put your sit bones back on the mat. Lift your chest and stick your butt out to find the center of your sit bones *(12.d.1)*.
5. Continue this progression until the backs of your heels are touching your pubic bone without pulling on your chest or lower back.

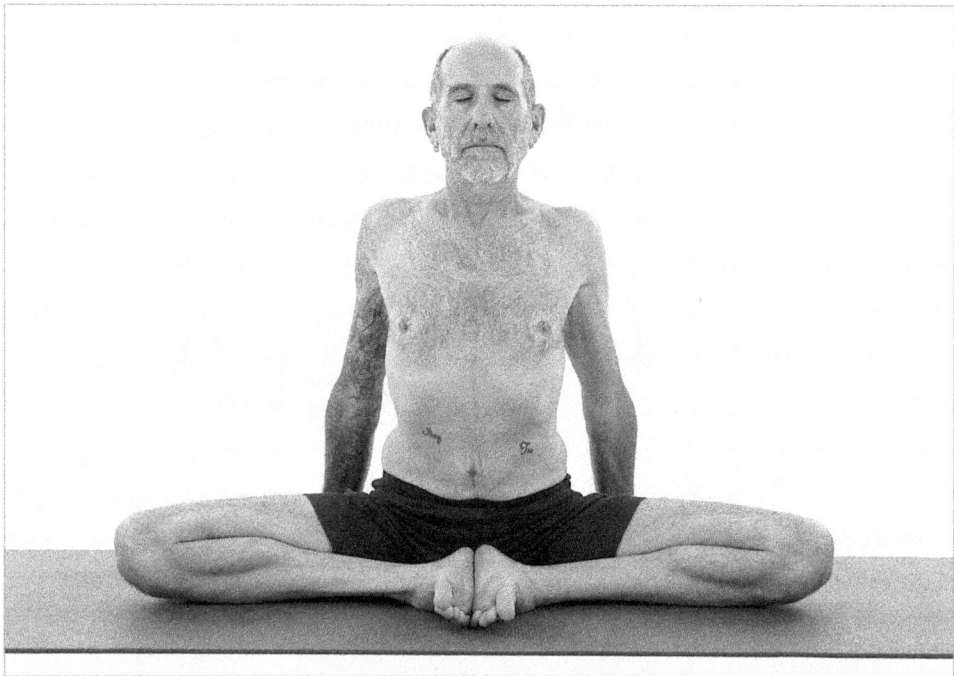

12.d.1 Baddha konasana with upright spine to facilitate rotation in the pelvis

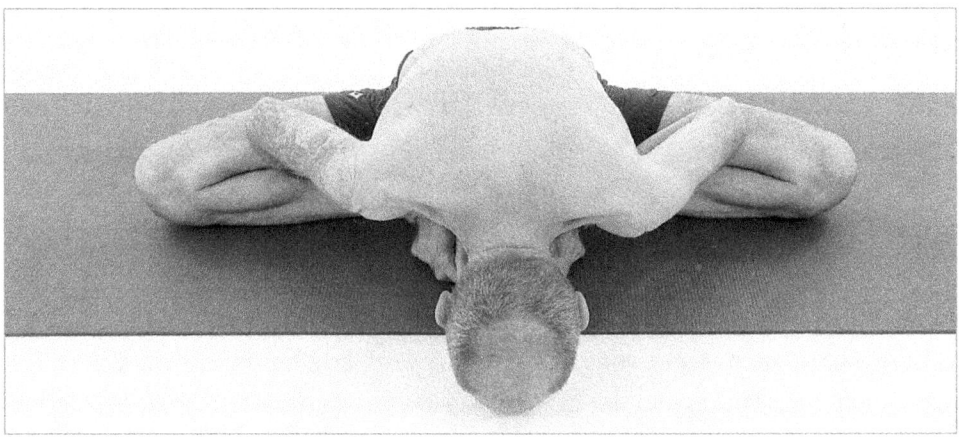

12.d.2 Baddha konasana with forward bend

Seated Hip Openers

EDDIE:
The action of *baddha konasana* is in your pelvis, not in your torso; your belly should reach your feet before your chest reaches the floor. Soften your spine and wait for the invitation to move deeper.

6. Inhale, lift your chest and press into the center of your sit bones.

7. Exhale and walk your hands forward to release your torso over your feet.

8. Press your heels together and encourage your belly toward your feet. Soften your spine. Stay three to five minutes *(12.d.2)*.

9. Inhale and use your hands to push up to seated. Let your head come up last, and then straighten your legs.

STEPS 1 & 2: Bring the soles of your feet together. Align your heels, arches, and big toe bones. Try to make each foot a mirror image of the other, and if one does not perfectly reflect the other, look closely to figure out how they differ. Those tiny incongruencies are part of the treasure map that leads to your hips. Press your heels together and reach your toes away from each other to engage both feet.

STEP 3: Place your hands outside of your pelvis. Use them to lift your chest and sit squarely onto the center of your sit bones. This is similar to the work of *upavistha konasana*; you want to sit in the center, not the front or back. If your butt is sucked under you're not in the center, you're on the back. Rotate your pelvis forward, or use props to lift your sit bones and keep your spine extended.

STEP 4: This pose is often taught by pulling the heels into the pelvis; we prefer to move the pelvis to the heels. Press into your hands, lift your sit bones, and

Seated Hip Openers

scoot your pelvis toward your feet. Release your hips to the mat and stay there for a moment. See if that action shifted weight toward the back of your sit bones, as though the bowl of your pelvis were spilling out behind you. If so, press into your hands and rotate your pubic bone closer to the mat. Stick your butt out behind you and find the center of your sit bones. If you cannot find center, put more props under your sit bones to gain leverage into your pelvis. You may need to stay here for a while to safely move further into the pose, and that's fine. Honor your journey.

STEP 5: Continue to scoot your sit bones forward, and be conscious of how that action pulls on your spine: the closer you get to your heels the more your spine will hunch forward as the stiffness in your pelvis pulls on your chest and lower back. Rotate your pelvis forward to keep your chest lifted, and always find the center of your sit bones before moving further forward. The goal is to shift your pelvis forward until the backs of your heels are touching your pubic bone but that progression may take several months. Be patient and remain sensitive to your knees. Please resist the urge to force your knees down—your knees are not the lever of the pose. The lever of the pose is your pelvis: your pelvis rotates forward and down as your thighs roll back (external rotation). Once you can bring your pubic bone to your heels without props, your knees will be all the way down and your pubic bone will be slightly lower than your heels.

STEPS 6–8: Keep your chest lifted, and on an exhale, walk your hands forward to lower your torso. Press your heels together and roll your pubic bone toward the mat. The weight of the pose will fall more toward your outer foot (pinkie toe side), and your inner foot may separate like the pages of a book. Soften your spine and use props or your hands to support your head and chest. The action of *baddha konasana* is in your pelvis, not in your torso; your belly should reach your feet before your chest reaches the floor. Soften your spine and wait for the invitation to move deeper.

STEP 9: Use your hands to press up to a seated position. Let your head come up last. Use your hands to bring your knees together and straighten your legs in front of you.

SUPTA BADDHA KONASANA
soup·tah bah·dah koh·nahs·ahn·nuh | *reclined bound angle pose*

The reclined variation of *baddha konasana* is often used in restorative classes and is particularly beneficial for women suffering from menstrual cramps. It is softer than *supta virasana* and generally quite comfortable for all body types as it limits the psoas' ability to pull on the lower back. The primary contraindication is pain your knees, which can be addressed by placing folded blankets under them to provide support.

Start with one bolster and keep a couple folded blankets nearby, one to go under your head and one to provide more support if the bolster is not high enough.

Seated Hip Openers

1. Sit on the floor with your legs in front of you. Place the bolster behind your hips, close enough to support your entire body when you lie back.

2. Bend your knees and bring the soles of your feet together. Pull your heels into your groin.

3. Inhale and lift your chest. Exhale and walk your hands back to rest on the bolster.

4. Place a folded blanket under your head to create a gentle slope from your forehead to your chin.

5. Release your arms to the side, palms up, and breathe. Stay three to five minutes *(12.e)*.

6. Before exiting the pose, straighten your legs and stay for one to two minutes. Bend your knees and roll to one side to come off the bolster. Rest on your side and then return to seated. Let your head come up last.

STEPS 1 & 2: Upright *baddha konasana* rotates the pelvis forward in relation to the legs to challenge the stiffness in your hips. The *supta* variation allows the pelvis to rotate in the direction of the bolster, which usually makes it easier to keep your heels close to your groin. If your heels do begin to slide, use a belt to keep them in place. Make the belt into a very wide loop and bring it over your head to rest in your lap. Set the back of the loop at the very top of your hips (right below the flare of the pelvic brim), and then put the front of the loop around the outside of your bound feet. Tighten the belt to bring your heels into your groin

Seated Hip Openers

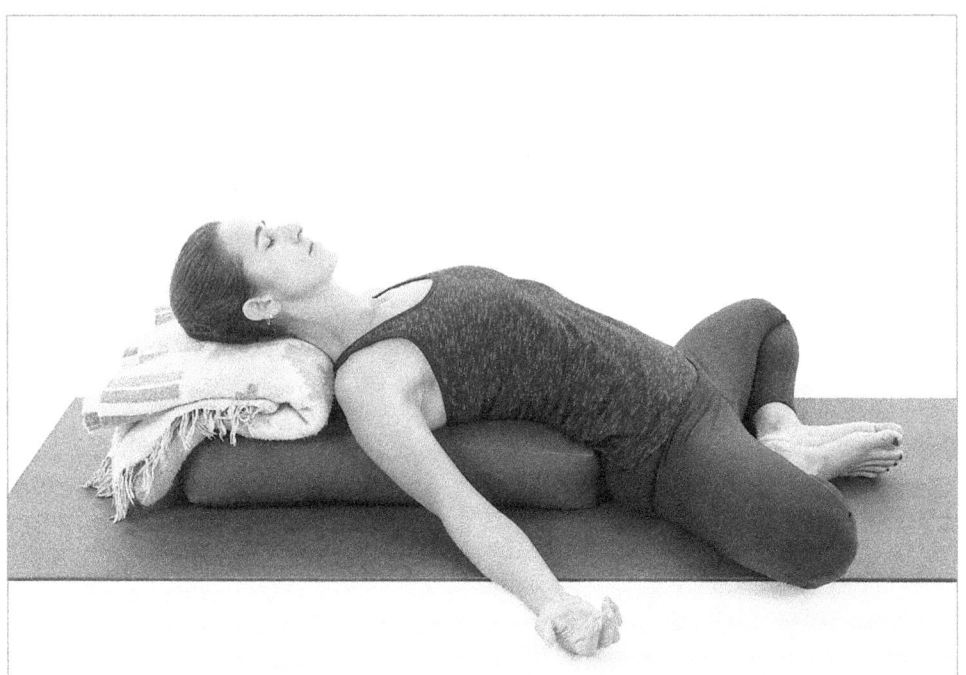

12.e Supta baddha konasana with props

but do not make it too tight; you will need a little leeway to lie back onto the bolster. When you lie back the belt will run across the top of your sacrum, around the outside of your hips, across your inner thighs, and around the outsides of your feet. Leave the end of the strap in an accessible position so you can tighten it after you recline (if necessary).

STEPS 3-5: On an inhale, lift your chest and extend your spine. Keep your front body lifted as you exhale and lower onto the bolster. Use your hands to support your descent but do not twist; go straight back onto the bolster. If you don't feel supported, come up and add more props. There shouldn't be any space between you and the props beneath you. Once you are settled, place a blanket under your head to expand your occiput as you did in *supta virasana*. Soften everywhere and breathe.

STEP 6: When you are ready to come out, straighten your legs and stay for one to two minutes before rolling to one side. If you are short on time, use your hands to support the outside of your thighs and bring your knees together. Place your feet on the mat and rest your knees together for a few moments before rolling to one side. If you used a belt, reach down and release the belt before coming out.

THE BOX

The box does not have a Sanskrit name because it's not a traditional pose. It was introduced to yoga by Dona Holleman, a senior Iyengar practitioner. It is also called "double pigeon".

The box opens your hips by eternally rotating both femurs (thigh bones) in their hip sockets. It is a much stronger external rotation than *baddha konasana*, and the stretch is centered more in your buttocks/outer hip than your groin. The top leg usually gets the stronger stretch but the bottom leg is still extremely important.

The primary contraindication is pain in your knees. If your knees are lifted, please use bolsters or folded blankets to support them. They should not be floating in space. If you feel pain in your knees or at the top of your shin bones when you exit the pose, your knees need more support. You can decrease the size of your props as your hips open, but please do not open your hips at the expense of your knees. It's not worth it.

Seated Hip Openers

1. Sit on the floor with your legs in front of you.

2. Bend your left knee and put your outer left calf on the mat in front of you with your left shin bone parallel to the front of the mat.

3. Use blankets or bolsters to fill any space between your left knee and the floor.

4. Bend your right knee and place your right outer heel onto your left inner knee. Make your right shin parallel to the front of your mat and bring your right knee directly above your left heel.

5. Use blankets or bolsters to fill any space between your right knee and your left heel.

6. Walk your hands behind your hips. Inhale and lift your chest.

7. Exhale and come forward over your legs. Rest your head in your hands and breathe. Stay three to five minutes *(12.f)*.

Seated Hip Openers

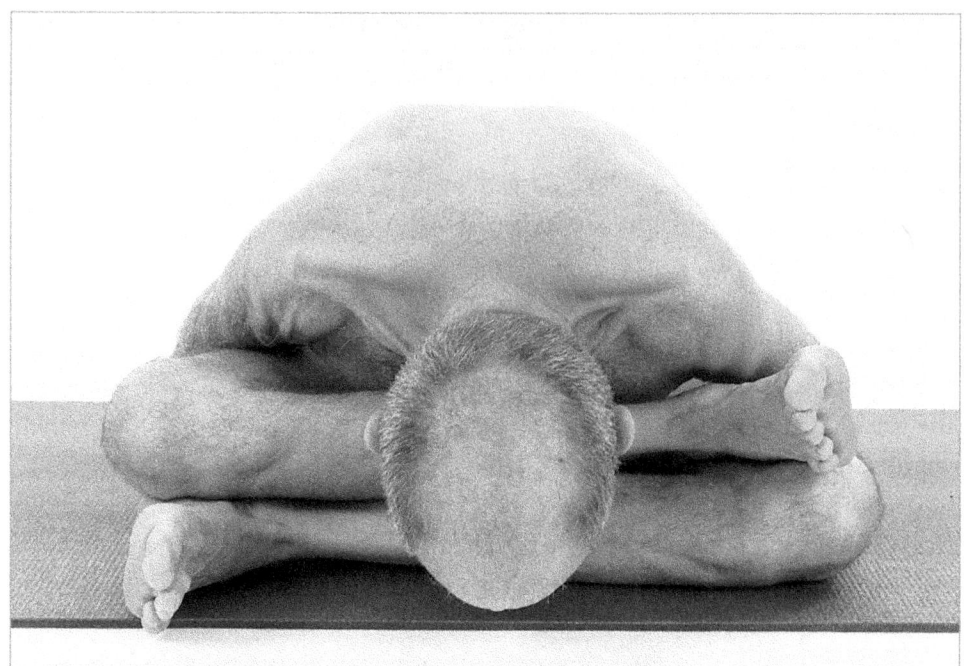

12.f The box with forward bend

8. Inhale to press up and exhale to straighten your legs before you switch sides.

STEPS 1–5: The setup is extremely important. The alignment is heel to knee and knee to heel. The toes are forward of the legs. When you look down to the space between your legs, there should be an even triangle with your pubic bone in the middle.

Use your hand to check that your right heel is completely supported: the flat part of your palm should be able to touch the pad of your right heel and the top of your left knee at the same time. This will put your right knee directly above your left inner heel. If there is space between them, or between your left knee and the mat, fill it with something soft and stable. There should be no strain or downward pressure on either knee. Flex your feet to protect your knees and extend your heels in opposite directions. Keep your inner heel skin taut as you move forward into the pose. If there is a lot of pressure on the outside of your left foot place a blanket underneath it for padding.

STEPS 6–7: If you can get your elbows to the floor, bend your arms and rest your forehead in your palms. If not, use props to find a way to be comfortable. Soften your jaw and release the tension in your hips. If there is any pain in your knees, give them more support. Do not tolerate pain in your knees!

If bending forward pulls on your lower back, rewind the pose. Stay upright or use a high prop to support your torso (e.g. the seat of a chair or a series of bolsters). Do not jeopardize your lumbar discs to open your hips.

STEP 8: Use your hands to gently press upright. Straighten your legs. Take a few moments to check in with your knees before you switch sides. If there is any discomfort in your knees or at the tops of your shins, you need to give them more support. Use a timer to ensure you spend the same amount of time on each side.

LITTLE HIP OPENER

This is not a traditional Sanskrit pose. It draws on the same anatomical actions as the box and *parsvakonasana*: externally rotating the femur to open your hips. We often include the little hip opener as a cool-down pose after a backbending sequence, as it helps decompress the lower back and reintegrate the pelvis.

1. Lie on your back and with your knees bent and your heels flat on the floor.

2. Place the outside of your right heel on top of your left knee. The bottom of your right heel should be in line with the outside of your left knee, identical to the position of the top leg in the box pose.

3. Flex your right foot and lift your left knee toward your chest.

4. Reach your right arm through the space between your legs and reach your left arm outside of your left leg. Clasp your hands together behind your left thigh or on the front of your left shin.

5. Hug your left knee toward your chest and encourage your right knee away from your right shoulder. Stay here two to three minutes *(12.g)*.

6. Release the clasp on your left leg and switch sides.

Seated Hip Openers

Seated Hip Openers

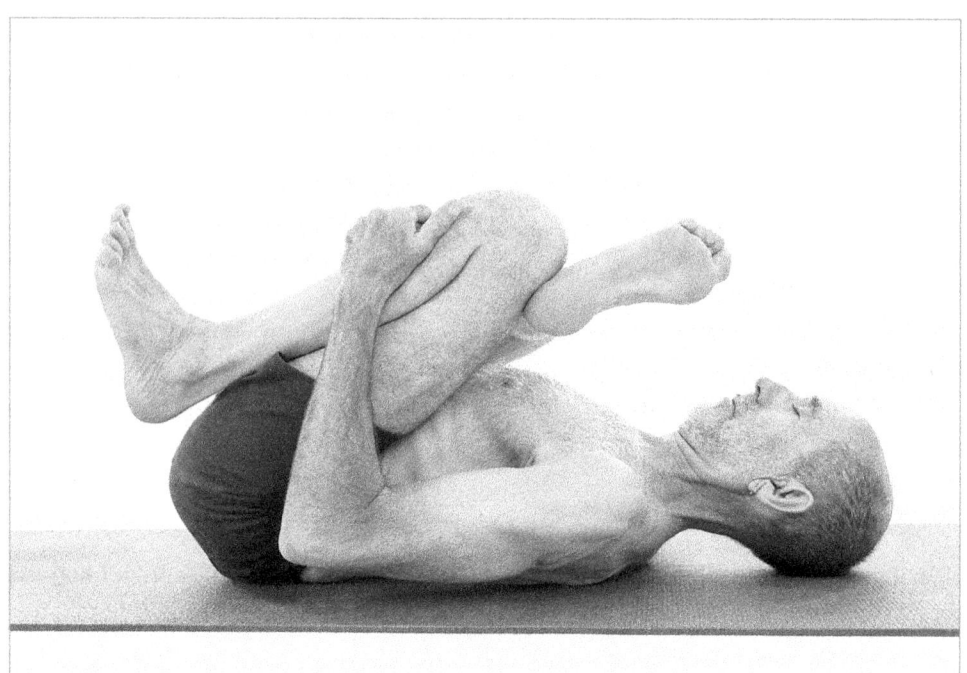

12.g Little hip opener

STEPS 1–3: Keep the right foot completely supported, just as you did in the box; do not allow your right foot to dangle off of your left knee. Flex your foot to protect the ligaments of your knee and ankle.

STEP 4: Begin by interlacing your fingers behind your left thigh, over your hamstrings. If that feels readily available, clasp your hands around the front of your left shin. Keep the back of your neck long and your throat relaxed. If you need to lift your chin to clasp your shin, put your hands back on your hamstrings.

STEP 5: Hug your left knee toward your chest and encourage your right knee away from your right shoulder. Resist the urge to push on your right knee; it's your hips that need to open, not your knee. Use *mula bandha* to keep your right sit bone tracking toward your left sit bone. Watch for any tension in your throat and jaw. If your chin begins to lift, loosen your arms and allow your left knee to move away from your chest until you can relax your throat. Find a place within the stretch that is both soft and effective, and stay there until your hips invite you to go further.

GOMUKHASANA

go·moo·kahs·ahn·nuh | *cow-face pose*

The pose commonly taught as *gomukhasana* is described in the Hatha Yoga Pradipika as *sankatasana*. Traditional *gomukhasana* is stronger than *sankatasana*; it sets the feet together underneath the hips to create a deep hip opener combined with a balancing pose. *Sankatasana* sets the feet outside of the hips, but for the sake of clarity, we often teach this variation as *gomukhasana* in our general classes. The "cow face" referenced by the Sanskrit name is formed by adding the arm clasp, but for restorative classes, we omit the hand clasp in order to focus on the primary anatomical intention: opening your hips.

Seated Hip Openers

Gomukhasana is felt strongly in the outer hip. It targets the piriformis muscle that stretches underneath the glutes (buttocks) between the sacrum and the head of the femur (thigh bone). The sciatic nerve typically runs underneath the piriformis, and a tightening in the muscle can exert a painful pressure on the nerve called sciatica. In some cases the sciatic nerve may run between two of the piriformis' three heads, giving the muscle even more leverage to squeeze the nerve. *Gomukhasana* and *supta gomukhasana* lengthen the piriformis by rotating the head of the femur in relation to the sacrum, thus relieving the pressure.

The primary contraindication is pain in your knees or ankles, and you have two options to relieve it: place a prop under your sit bones or place a prop under your knees. Some individuals find relief (and a deeper stretch) by elevating the hips, others respond better to elevating the knees. Experiment and see which arrangement best protects your anatomy while bringing you closer to the pose.

1. Sit on the floor with your legs in front of you.

2. Bend your left knee under your right knee. Set the outside of your left leg on the mat with your knee pointed forward and bring your left heel to your outer right hip.

3. Cross your right knee over your left and bring your right heel to your outer left hip so your right knee is on top of your left knee.

4. Place your right hand on the outside of your right knee and your left hand on the outside of your left knee. Gently push your knees in opposite directions to stack them on top of each other, directly in front of your belly button.

Seated Hip Openers

5. Place your hands on the soles of your feet. Inhale and lift your chest *(12.h)*.

6. Exhale and lean forward to bring your belly in contact with your thighs, and then lower your chest and head. Rest your chin over your knees or place a bolster in front of you to rest your head. If your hips begin to get light, walk your hands forward and use them to push back onto your sit bones. Stay here three to five minutes.

7. Inhale and press into your hands to sit upright. Let your head come up last. Uncross your knees and straighten your legs before switching sides.

STEPS 1–3: Keep your sit bones firmly on the ground for the duration of the pose; otherwise the pressure intended for your hips may migrate to your knees. If you find that crossing your knees pulls your hips off the ground, even slightly, put a blanket under your hips for support. If it is difficult to bring one or both of your heels to your outer hips, try Eddie's adjustment: get as far into the pose as

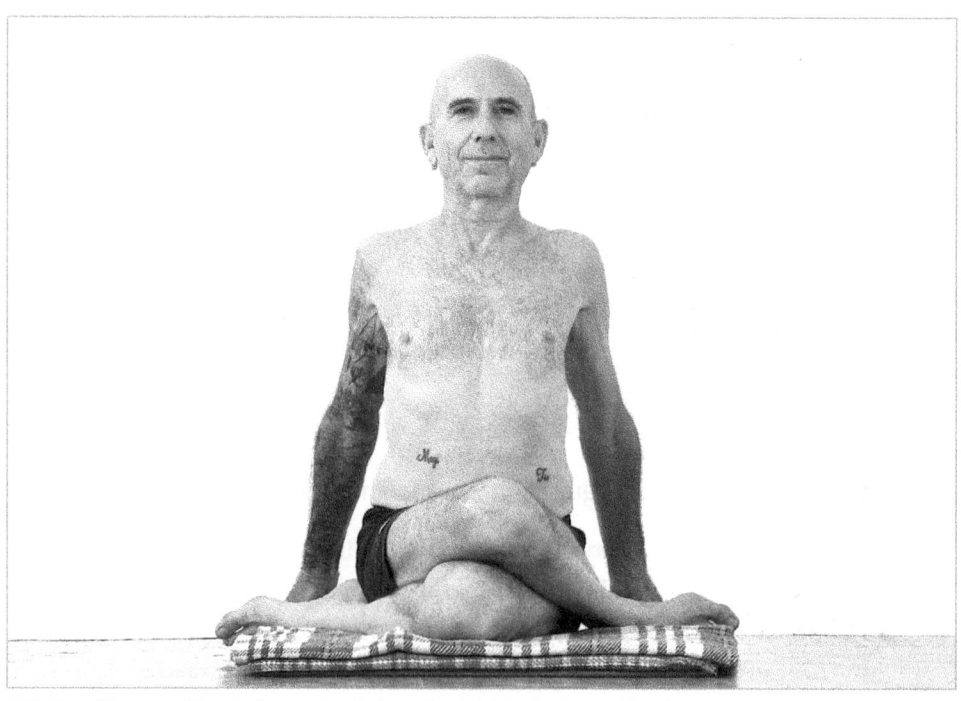

12.h Gomukhasana with spinal extension, before releasing into the forward bend.

you can and then lean to the right to bring your right heel to your outer left hip. Leaning rolls your pelvis in the direction of the external rotation and makes it easier to get your heel where you want it. Start with whichever leg is on top, as it's usually more problematic. Once the top leg is in position set your hips firmly on the mat and lean to the left to bring your left (bottom) heel to your outer right hip. If this adjustment helps keep your feet in place but makes your sit bones light, put a blanket under your hips for support. Be sensitive to any discomfort in your knees.

Seated Hip Openers

The mat should help keep your feet close to your outer hips, but if they begin to slide, use a belt around both ankles to keep them close. The belt is a strong but effective tool and Eddie used it for many years to heal his sciatica. Make the belt into a loop and place it around your right ankle (or whichever leg is on top), and then pull the loop around your back and wrap it around your left ankle. Set your knees on top of each other, and then tighten the belt to keep your ankles close to your hips. Be very sensitive to any discomfort in your knees.

STEP 4: This pose pulls strongly on the top leg, and if your piriformis is tight, it may be difficult to align your knees on the first try. Use your hands to stack your knees on top of each other, directly in front of your belly button. You can also pull your knees instead of pushing them; either one will work.

STEPS 5 & 6: The strong external rotation in your legs will begin to spin the soles of your feet toward the ceiling. Place your hands onto the soles of your feet and lift your chest, and then walk your hands forward to lower your belly onto your thighs. Lower your belly first, followed by your chest and head. Wrap your chin over your knees to rest your head, or bring your hands forward and rest your head in your palms. Stay here and breathe.

STEP 7: Inhale and come up to uncross your legs. Straighten your legs between sides and be sensitive to any discomfort in your knees and ankles.

SUPTA GOMUKHASANA
soup·tah go·moo·kahs·ahn·nuh | *reclined cow-face pose*

This variation of *gomukhasana* is done on your back. If your hips are very stiff, you may find it to be more accessible than seated *gomukhasana*. Individuals suffering from severe sciatica may prefer to start with *supta gomukhasana* to approach the piriformis from a less acute angle. The primary contraindication is pain in your knees. If there is pain in your knees loosen your arms to reduce the pull on your ankles.

Seated Hip Openers

1. Lie on your back and bend your knees into your chest.
2. Cross your right thigh over your left and separate your feet.
3. Hold your right ankle (or shin) with your left hand and hold your left ankle with your right hand.
4. Drop your heels toward your outer hips.
5. Soften your shoulders and be sensitive to any discomfort in your knees. Stay three to five minutes *(12.i)*.
6. To come out, release your ankles and switch sides.

Use your hands to hold your ankles or shins; holding your feet can strain the ligaments in your ankles. Resist the urge to yank on your ankles to get your heels down, and watch for tension in your neck and chest. If your upper body begins

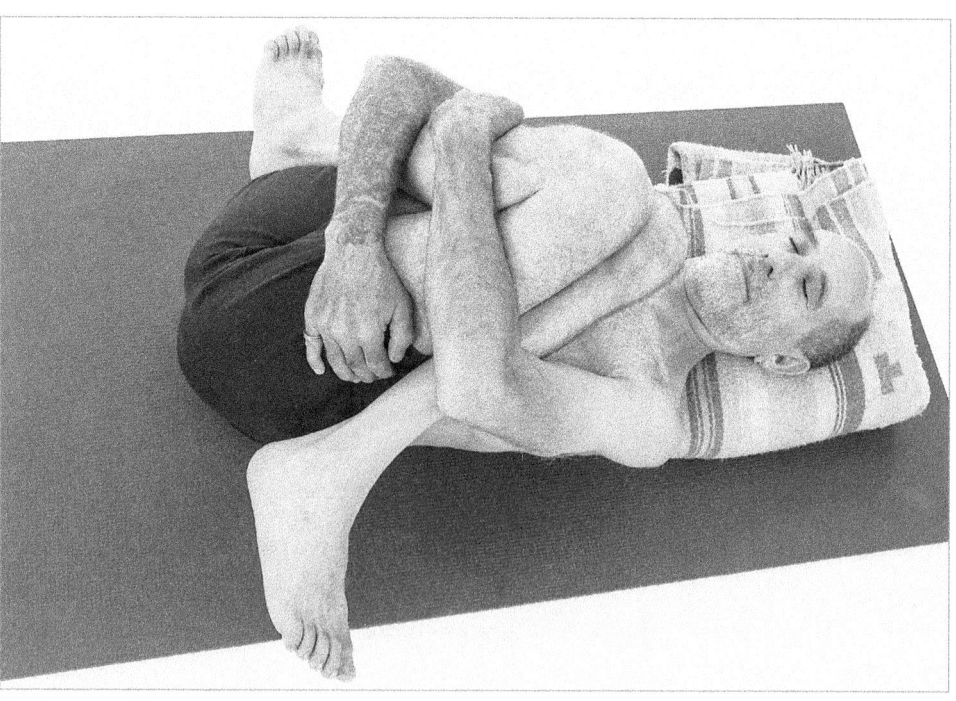

12.i Supta gomukhasana with props

to feel tense, you may be pulling too hard. Move slowly and remain sensitive to any discomfort in your knees.

THE BEACH POSE

We call this the beach pose because it starts by lying on your outer hip, like you're relaxing on a towel by the beach. We developed it in response to the way *eka pada rajakapotasana* (one-legged king pigeon pose) is being taught in America. *Eka pada rajakapotasana* is a magnificent backbend, but for some mystifying reason, many Americans prefer to teach it as a forward bend. We're okay with that as long as it is practiced with proper alignment, but without proper alignment it can be a very dangerous pose. If your hips are stiff, like most of the western world, the pressure and rotation intended for your hips will fall into the front knee, and as you should be well aware by now, knees are not supposed to twist. The beach pose is our answer to that problem.

Seated Hip Openers

1. Sit on the floor with your legs in front of you.

2. Bend your right knee and put your outer right calf on the mat in front of you with your shin bone parallel to the front of the mat.

3. Lean to your right side. Bring your elbow to the floor outside of your right thigh and rest your head in your right hand.

4. Use your left leg to put your right outer hip on the mat. There are two ways to get there:

    A. Bring your left foot to the floor outside of your hips. Press into your left leg to roll onto your outer right hip.

    B. Bring your left foot to the floor outside of your hips. Press into your left leg and lift your right hip off the mat. Grab the skin of your outer right thigh and pull it under, and then place your right outer hip down on the mat.

   Both actions externally rotate your right thigh and place your right leg at a 90° angle.

5. Keep your right leg perfectly still as you slowly walk your left leg toward the back of the mat and bring your torso over your front leg. Watch the skin of your right inner knee, and if it begins to roll

inward, press back onto the right outer hip to protect your knee.

6. Internally rotate your left leg and reach it toward the back of the mat.

7. Rest your head in your hands and breathe. Soften into your right hip. Stay three to five minutes *(12.j.1 and 12.j.2)*.

Seated Hip Openers

8. To come out, roll onto your outer right hip and then switch sides.

STEPS 1 & 2: The setup is similar to the box pose: bring the outside of your right leg into contact with the mat to create an external rotation, and flex your right foot to help maintain that alignment. In the box pose there may be space between your right knee and the floor, but in the beach pose, leaning to the side should eliminate any space under your knee.

STEPS 3 & 4: Lean to your right side and put your left foot on the mat, to the left of your left hip. Push into your left leg and use the sticky mat to roll the skin of your right hip under and down. If that doesn't work, press into your left leg and lift your right hip off the mat. Use your left hand to reach under your right hip and pull your right outer thigh down, and then place your right outer hip on the mat. Both actions will bring your right greater trochanter—the bony knob on the outside of your right femur bone—in contact with the mat. They will also roll the skin of your right inner thigh toward the top of your thigh, and you want to keep it there for the duration of the pose. If you see that skin beginning to roll inward, you've lost the external rotation and your knee is at risk.

STEP 5: Keep your right leg externally rotated as you move your torso forward and reach your left leg back. Move very slowly, and watch the skin of your right inner knee as you go. If the skin begins to roll inward, rewind the pose and reestablish the external rotation of your right thigh—you want to keep the rotation in your hips, not in your knee. Use your hands if necessary. If the skin above your knee moves in a different direction than the skin below your knee, your knee is twisting.

This is a slow, incremental process. You may not get your torso over your front leg on the first try, and you may not get your left leg all the way back either. Stay at the point where you can maintain the external rotation of the front leg, even if it means you are still leaning on your right elbow and your left leg is more to the side than back. Look carefully, move slowly, and stay connected to the

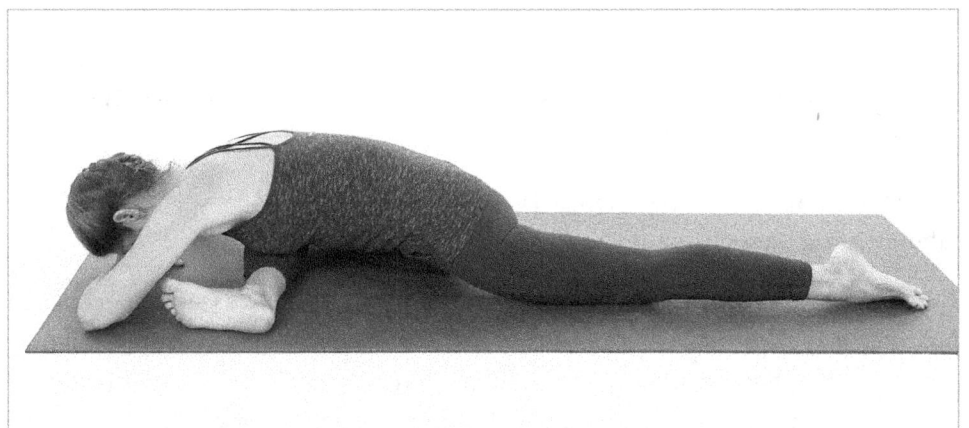

12.j.1 The beach pose

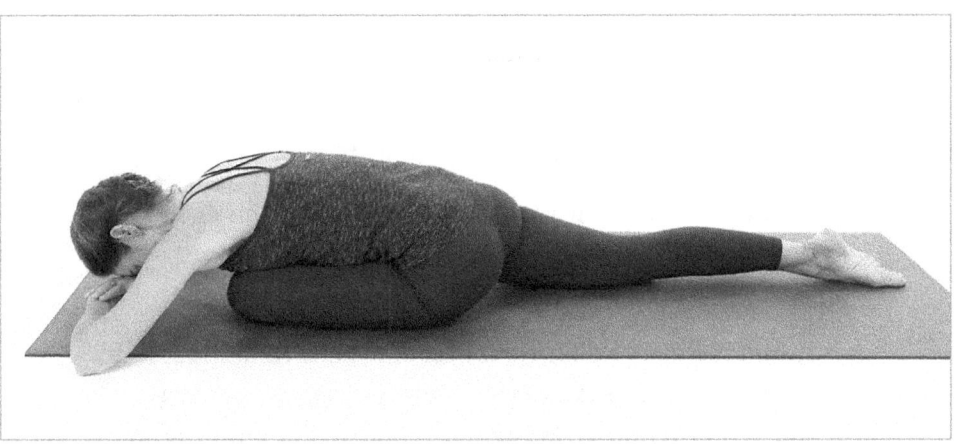

12.j.2 The beach pose

Seated Hip Openers

anatomical action of the pose, not to the image of the "full" pose. And if you can't move at all without internally rotating your right leg, or if your right hip lifts off the mat, you need to spend more time in the lunges. This pose might look easy, but seated forward bends can be more injurious to a stiff body than lunges and standing poses.

STEP 6: If you can get your left leg behind you give it a strong internal rotation. Curl your left toes under and lift your left knee off the mat. Internally rotate your entire leg and put it back down so your left outer knee rests on the mat. Roll the pinkie toe side of your left foot toward the mat. Do not allow the movement of your left leg to affect the alignment in your right leg.

STEPS 7 & 8: Wherever you are, find a way to rest your head and soften the tension in your right hip. After a few minutes, you may be able to move further into the pose without affecting your front leg. When you're ready to come out, press to the right and roll out of the pose. Switch sides.

JANU SIRSASANA (VARIATION)
jah·new sheer·saas·ahn·nuh | *head to knee pose*

Seated Hip Openers

Eddie prefers to teach this modification in most of his classes, especially in restorative applications where students spend several minutes in the pose. It protects the lower back by bending in the direction of the pelvis and uses bolsters to support the torso, thus removing any strain on the lumbar spine.

1. Sit on the floor with your legs in front of you.
2. Shift to the left side of your mat so your left leg is parallel to the long end of the mat.
3. There are two positions for the right foot:
   A. Modified: Place your right heel onto your left inner thigh, as close to your pelvis as possible. Point your right toes toward your left inner knee.
   B. Traditional: Place your right heel onto your right inner thigh, as close to your pelvis as possbile. Put your right toes onto your left inner thigh. Move your right knee behind you so the angle between your legs is wider than 90°.
4. Point your left toes straight up and bring your left inner knee to the mat.
5. Pull a bolster into your groin and place it in line with your torso (not your left leg).
6. Inhale and lift your spine. Exhale and come forward onto the bolster. Do not twist. If you need more height, get another bolster or blanket(s) to support your head. Stay three to five minutes *(12.k)*.
7. Inhale and use your hands to press up to seated. Move the bolster and release your right leg. Switch sides.

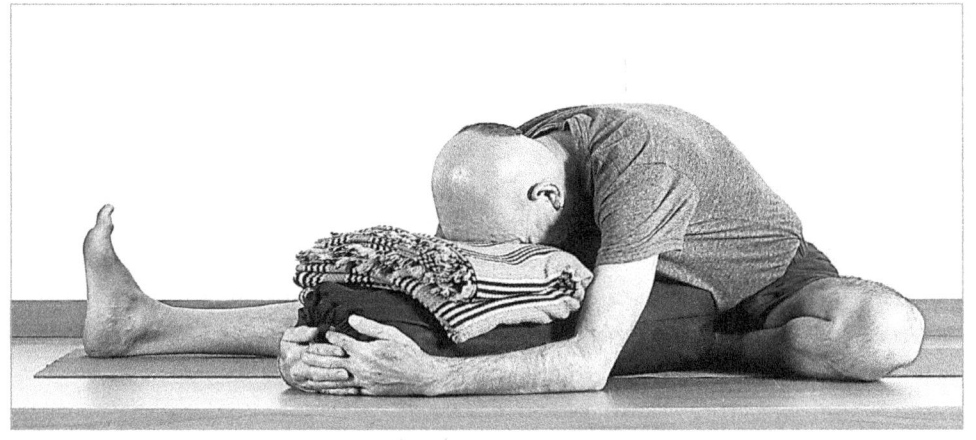

12.k Janu sirsasana

Seated Hip Openers

We teach two foot variations in *janu sirsasana*. They are both valid and valuable. You may find one serves you more than the other, but remember that your dark, difficult areas are just as important as the bright ones.

STEP 3A: Place the right heel onto the left inner groin, with the right toes pointed toward the left inner knee. If there is any pain in your right knee, put something under it.

STEP 3B: Placing the right heel on the right inner thigh broadens the pelvis and moves the right knee back. This will push the stretch more toward the left inner thigh than the right outer hip. It is generally more available when your hips are open. If there is any pain in your right knee, put something under it.

STEPS 4 & 5: In traditional *janu sirsasana*, the pelvis points one way, the spine goes another way, and the lower back can get caught in the middle. In this modification of *janu sirsasana*, the pelvis and the spine point in the same direction. The lower back is completely safe and the stretch stays in the hips and legs. The bolster should not be touching your left leg because your left leg is not pointed in the same direction as your pelvis.

STEP 6: Lie your torso straight down onto the bolster. If the bolster is not tall enough to support your chest and head, get another one. Get whatever it takes to be comfortable—even if it's the seat of a chair. Soften into the bolsters and breathe. Keep your left leg straight and press your left inner knee into the mat. If there is any pain in your right knee, put something under it.

STEP 7: On an inhale, press up to seated. Let your head come up last. Release your right leg and switch sides.

SUPTA PADANGUSTHASANA A
soup·tah pha·dan·goost·thas·ahn·nuh | *reclined big toe posture*

Seated Hip Openers

Supta means reclined, *padas* are your feet and *angustas* are your big toes, so *supta padangusthasana* means reclined big toe pose. It sounds simple enough, but grabbing your big toe without distorting your hips can be a pretty gargantuan task—even for flexible people. For that reason, we prefer to teach the pose against a wall with a belt to reinforce the principles of alignment. When done properly, this pose is one of the most effective ways to address an SI joint imbalance.

1. Lie on your back with your feet against the wall, toes pointed up and heels against the floor.

2. Scoot toward the wall so both knees are slightly bent. Lift your right leg and put the belt around your right foot, either at the arch or the big toe bone. Hold the belt with both hands.

3. Simultaneously straighten both legs. Keep your back in contact with the mat to keep your right hip in line with your left as you straighten.

4. Position your right heel directly over your right sit bone, or as close to it as possible. Straighten your leg, lift your inner ankle bone and extend your big toe bone. Press your foot upward as though it were pressing into the ceiling.

5. Shift your left heel slightly to the left and press your inner left knee to the floor.

6. Shift your outer right hip toward your inner left thigh to reinforce the action of *mula bandha*; move your sit bones toward each other to align your pelvis.

7. Press into both feet and straighten both legs. Lift your kneecaps, engage *mula bandha*, and soften your shoulders. Stay here five minutes or more *(12.1)*.

Seated Hip Openers

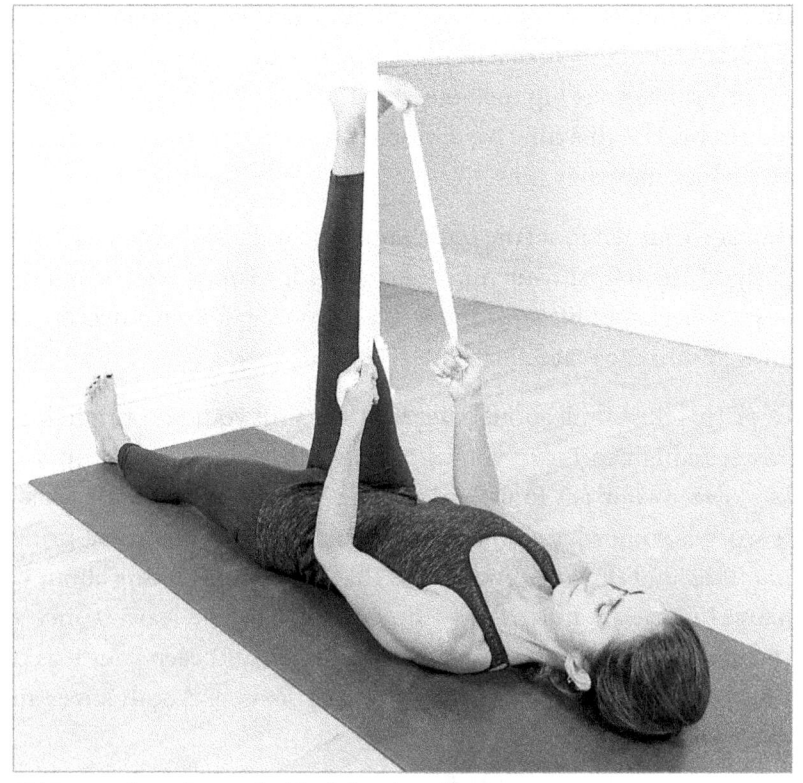

12.1 Supta padangusthasana A with a belt at the wall

8. Exhale and bend your right knee. Release the belt and scoot back toward the wall to switch sides.

Step 3 uses the sticky mat to help hold your hips in place as you straighten both legs. Without the sticky mat (and often even with the mat) your hips may shift in the direction of the right leg, similar to the way they shift toward the front knee in lunges: they are too stiff to let your leg extend freely so they recruit flexibility from your lower back to do the pose. Hold the belt with both hands in whatever way is comfortable—some prefer straight arms and others bend their elbows—and try not to clench your hands.

STEP 4: The most common mistake is bringing the right foot too far forward (being further back is okay, just keep your leg completely straight and work on those hamstrings). Bringing your foot toward your face usually comes at the expense of your pelvis: your right sit bone moves away from your left and *mula bandha* goes out the window. We're interested in pelvic integrity so please keep your right heel directly over your right sit bone and engage *mula bandha*. Look at your right foot and organize it as though you're doing a standing pose: spread your toes, press into your big toe bone and the center of your heel, and lift your inner ankle bone. Use this time to reinforce the architecture of your foot so it can carry you further into your hips.

Seated Hip Openers

STEP 5: Engage your left foot (the one against the wall) and organize it: shift your heel slightly to the left, spread your toes, press into your big toe bone and the center of your heel, and lift your inner ankle bone. Lift your kneecap and press your left thigh into the mat to straighten your leg.

STEPS 6 & 7: This pose is all about *mula bandha*. Shift your outer right hip toward your inner left thigh to move your sit bones closer together. Drop your right hip crease toward your left foot to lengthen the right side of your waist. Hopefully this work is somewhat familiar; it's the exact same alignment principles as *parsvottanasana* and the first few lunges. That's the coolest thing about yoga: the poses change but the alignment stays the same, so you can learn it once and take it with you. Soften your shoulders, engage your feet, and keep your legs perfectly straight. Stay here for three to five minutes, and then bend both knees and scoot toward the wall to switch sides.

SUPTA PADANGUSTHASANA B
soup·tah pha·dan·goost·thas·ahn·nuh | *reclined big toe posture*

This variation changes the orientation of your foot to address your groin and inner hamstring muscles. The *A* variation is similar to *parsvottanasana* and the *B* variation is similar to *trikonasana*.

1. Lie on your back with your feet against the wall, toes pointed up and heels against the floor.

2. Scoot toward the wall so both knees are slightly bent. Lift your right leg and put the belt around your right heel. Hold the belt with your right hand and put your left hand on your left thigh.

3. Simultaneously straighten both legs.

4. Position your right heel directly over your right sit bone, or as close to it as possible.

5. Shift your left heel slightly to the left and press your left thigh to the floor.

6. Shift your outer right hip toward your inner left thigh to reinforce the action of *mula bandha*.

7. Externally rotate your right leg so your toes point over your right shoulder. If this is very strong, stay here and continue to work your legs, feet, and *mula bandha*.

Seated Hip Openers

8. If you want to go further, begin to lower your right leg in the direction of your right toes. Keep the action of *mula bandha* in your pelvis and spin your thigh to the right to externally rotate your leg. If your leg is able to reach all the way down, your toes should touch the floor outside of your right shoulder.

9. Press into both feet and straighten both legs. Lift your kneecaps, engage *mula bandha*, and soften your shoulders. Stay three to five minutes *(12.m)*.

10. To come out, bring your right foot back over your hip and turn your toes to center. Exhale and bend your right knee. Release the belt and scoot back toward the wall to switch sides.

The setup is exactly the same as A, except for the belt: create a loop that goes around the outside of your ankle and comes down across your inner arch to secure your heel, and then hold it with your right hand only. Keep your left hand on your left thigh to encourage it toward the floor.

Externally rotating your right leg makes this a more difficult pose than A, in the same way *trikonasana* is more difficult than *parsvottanasana*. Please move slowly, and don't sacrifice your pelvis to get closer to the floor. The best things in life take time. The most common mistake is dropping the right leg in the direction of the right heel, which brings your foot outside of your right hip. That pushes the bony knob of your greater trochanter against the rim of your hip socket, and we don't want that. Dropping your leg in the direction of your right toes will spin your greater trochanter away from your acetabulum.

Continue to work your feet and legs. Reinforce the action of *mula bandha* to develop integrity in your pelvis. When you're ready to come out, bring your right foot back over your right hip and turn it to center before bending both knees and switching sides.

Seated Hip Openers

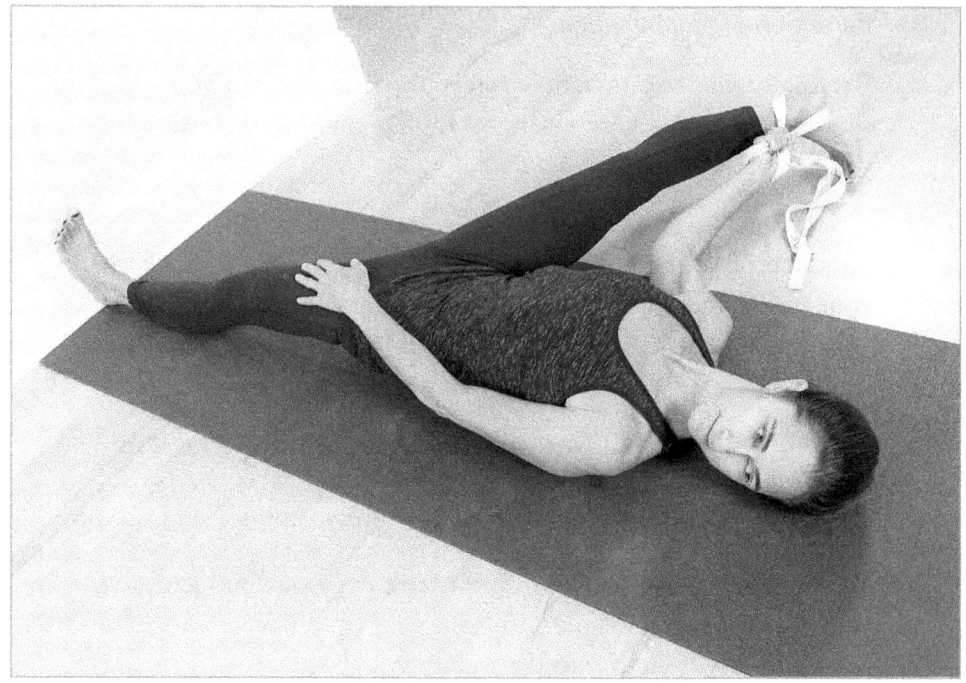

12.m Supta padangusthasana B with a belt at the wall

PRANAYAMA

Pranayama is the fourth limb of Ashtanga yoga's eight-limbed path. It is the study of breath and the effects of breath on the psyche, but in yoga, "breath" encompasses more than just respiration. *Prana* is the universal life force and *ayama* means to extend or lengthen so *pranayama* is truly an extension of your life force. It increases the *prana* being assimilated between your sinuses and your pituitary gland and thus has a profound effect on the hormones moving through your body. It is the first of yoga's internal limbs; a stepping stone on the long journey that starts with connecting your mind to your muscles and ends with connecting your mind to itself, or to the God within.

Pranayama provides a window into your psyche. It invites you to observe how controlling your breath can affect your thoughts and emotions and to use that knowledge to improve your life. It requires that you be comfortable, quiet, and still, which is one of the reasons *pranayama* comes after *asana*. *Asana* removes your physical congestion to achieve unrestricted spinal extension. It allows you to sit comfortably upright for long enough to explore introductory *pranayama* such as *surya bhedana*.

Asana strengthens your neurological passageways in preparation for *pranayama*. Standing poses are the real litmus test; if you are shaking in a one-minute *trikonasana* you are not ready for *pranayama*. Shaking in the limbs (also called *angamedjayatva*) indicates weakness in the nervous system. *Pranayama* increases the energy moving through the nervous system, and if your nerves are weak, it's like plugging a 120 volt lamp into a 220 volt system: pop, fizzle, lights out. That may sound like an empty threat—I mean really, how much damage can you do by breathing?—but we've seen serious injuries arise from pursuing *pranayama* too quickly. Wait until you can hold the standing poses for two minutes without shaking, and then start with simple practices like *surya* and *chandra bhedana*. There are no shortcuts in *pranayama*; start from where you are and be kind to yourself along the way.

Pranayama is best done in the morning before *asana*. If you prefer to do a restful *pranayama* after *asana*, such as *viloma*, be sure to take a long *savasana* between the two practices.

EDDIE:
When I was introduced to yoga, I felt like I had finally met the thing that would alleviate the pain in my life. I ran in the direction of that pain relief. I used to really do my practice, very deliberately, and I was very capable of doing it. But about 20 years into it, I realized yoga was really un-doing me. It was taking me apart so I could start to look at my true components and use *asana* to polish the lens of my being. It's like polishing a stone. When you start, you need really rough tools to chip away the impurities. As you progress, the tools become finer and finer. The physical postures are the sledgehammers, chisels, and sandpaper. *Pranayama* is the polishing cloth.

CONTRAINDICATIONS

You should never sweat above your neck in *pranayama*. Sweating on your brow, upper lip, temples, etc. indicates you are beyond your threshold; perhaps you are being too aggressive in your approach or the length and/or retention of your breath has moved beyond your capacity. Do not take these warnings lightly. We have seen people suffer for years after moving beyond their threshold in *pranayama*. Please stay in touch with your internal dialogue. If you feel trapped, anxious, or clammy, take a break. *Pranayama* should always be soft, cool, and relaxed because you're working with your nervous system.

PREPARATORY ASANA

These three poses use blankets and bolsters to cultivate a relaxed state while simultaneously opening your ribcage for *pranayama*. The blankets should be large and thick and the bolsters should be round; rectangular bolsters do not accommodate backbends in the same way. The goal is to cultivate an effortless state in your body and mind so be meticulous. Take the time to make yourself comfortable. Discomfort breeds distraction and distraction is, quite literally, a loss of connection and a waste of time.

Relaxation in *pranayama* works from the outside in, just as it does in *asana*. It starts with your skin, muscles, and bones and eventually moves inside to affect your subtle body and internal organs. It's easier to relax your face than your kidneys, so start with your face. Learning to relax tangible tissues in *pranayama* will refine your nervous system to help incorporate deeper, less accessible elements of your being, allowing you to release chronic tension in these deep tissues.

Double Bolster

Place two bolsters at the top end of your mat, about six inches apart, perpendicular to the mat and parallel to each other. The top bolster will be under your head and the bottom bolster will be under your sternum.

1. Rest your upper back (the area directly behind your sternum) on the bottom bolster. Place the back of your head on the top bolster. Your butt should be firm on the mat; if it is light, the bottom bolster is too far down your back.

EDDIE:
These poses point you toward your subtle body so you can learn to let it calm down. Stress is insidious in our world. We have trained ourselves to live with it. We accommodate it in all the layers of our being and have become desensitized to its crippling effect on our lives. Many of us can barely determine whether we are in a state of stress because stress has become a constant state. These poses open the door to your subtle body and allow you to work with the layers of stress that have enveloped your life. They will help you develop a subtle body relationship that is supportive, loving, and highly effective at releasing the toxic side effects of modern society. It sounds profound but it is really quite simple: find the position and be still. Look inside and soften. The stillness addresses agitation in your neurological body and the softness addresses agitation in your emotional body. This practice will ease you down to a simple, subtle, sensitive baseline of your being so you can detect and address stress when it enters your life.

2. Bend your knees and place your feet flat on the floor. Push into your legs and roll your shoulders over the bottom bolster in the direction of the floor. Keep the skin of your upper back in contact with the bolster so that the rolling action pulls your shoulder blades toward your lower back. The tops of your shoulders should be off the bolster, hanging in the space between the two bolsters.

3. Use your hands to bring the top bolster (the one under your head) as close to your shoulders as possible without supporting them. Raise your forehead slightly higher than your chin and then rest your head on the bolster.

4. Bend your elbows and release your arms out to the side, palms up.

5. Soften your body into the bolsters and relax completely. Stay in the pose for five to ten minutes *(13.a.1)*.

Pranayama

EDDIE:
Use your mind to scan your body for tension. It might be in your lips, your cheeks, your forehead, or your tongue; find it and soften it away from your being. As you learn to let go, the line between the bolster and your back will begin to dissipate. Give in to the prop. Let it mold your being into the shape of yoga.

Double bolster rolls your sternum and upper chest into a backbend supported by the round shape of the bolster. The tops of your shoulders are off the bolster, allowing gravity to bring them closer to the floor in order to open the topmost portion of your armpit chest. Placing your forehead slightly higher than your chin creates a gentle downward angle in your face and expands the occiput at the base of your skull. These two actions stimulate the parasympathetic nervous system, your internal catalyst of rest, relaxation, and nourishment.

If this pose hurts your lower back, bend your knees and place your feet on the floor. Bring your feet wider than your hips and let your knees fall together

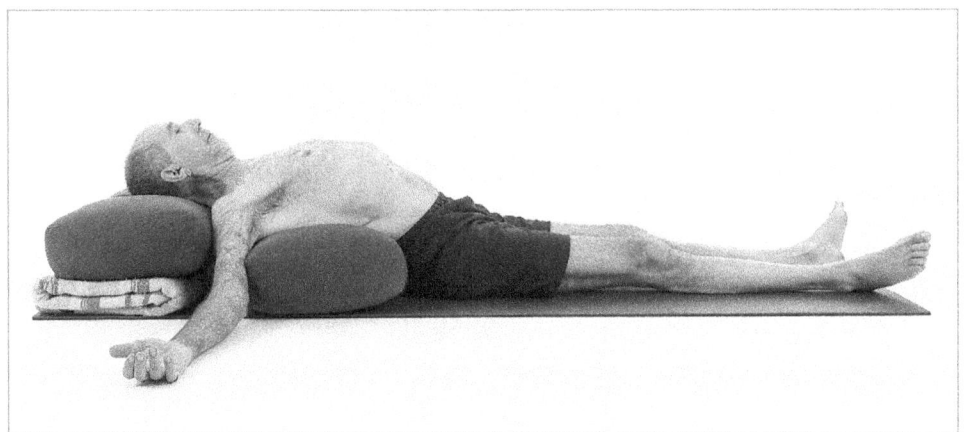

13.a.1 Double bolster

to release your lower back. Straightening your legs provides more leverage into your spine, but if you are in pain you cannot relax, and if you cannot relax the opening will not come.

To come out of the pose, bend your knees and put your feet on the floor. Roll to one side and push the lower bolster out from under you, leaving you on your side with your head on the top bolster. Stay on your side for a few moments and then use your top arm to press up to a seated position. Let your head come up last. Try to maintain softness and relaxation as you transition out of the pose.

Pranayama

Setu Bandha Sarvangasana with Two Bolsters

This supported variation of *setu bandha sarvangasana* requires two bolsters and a belt. The bolsters support your legs, pelvis and spine as your shoulders and sternum move toward the floor. It is similar to the action of double bolster: the skin of your upper back gets pulled down and your shoulders roll back to open your upper chest. This pose targets one of the most inflexible parts of the body: the upper ribcage and the upper lobes of your lungs that sit beneath them. Your topmost ribs are difficult to open because they sit underneath your clavicles; this pose uses the round end of the bolster to propel you toward this illusive anatomical treasure.

1. Place the bolsters end to end to form a single line. Sit on the bottom end of the topmost bolster with your feet on either side, facing the bottom bolster.

2. Fasten the belt into a loose loop and slide it over your legs. Separate your feet and turn them slightly pigeon-toed to internally rotate your thighs. Tighten the belt to maintain the internal rotation of your legs.

3. Lay back onto the top bolster. Push into your feet and slide your body up the bolster until the very top of your shoulders are resting on the mat, as in *setu bandha sarvangasana*. As you slide, maintain contact with the bolster to pull your shoulder blades down your back and open your upper ribcage. Stop when your head and the top of your shoulders are off the bolster. The bottom tip of your shoulder blades should remain in contact with it.

4. Straighten your legs onto the bolster. Bend your elbows and release your arms to the side, palms up. Stay for five to ten minutes *(13.a.2)*.

If there is pain in your lower back, use more belts to keep a strong internal rotation in your thighs. Place the second belt just past your mid-thigh so it is closer to your pelvis than your knees. Alternate the belts so they tighten in opposite directions; if you tightened the first belt from the left, tighten the second belt from the right. You can also place an additional belt around your big toes to keep them pressed together.

To come out of the pose, bend your knees toward your chest and loosen the belt. Be aware of the space between you and the floor as you roll off the bolsters and onto one side. Stay on your side for a few moments, and then use your top arm to press up to a seated position. Let your head come up last.

Cross Bolsters

Cross bolsters is done with two bolsters and a belt. The top bolster facilitates an opening similar to *setu bandha* with two bolsters—your shoulders wrap around the end of the bolster to open your upper ribcage—but in cross bolster, the lower bolster goes under you to create a backbend through the length of your body. It provides more leverage into your spine than the previous two poses, and if your lower back is sensitive, you may need to take additional steps to navigate that discomfort.

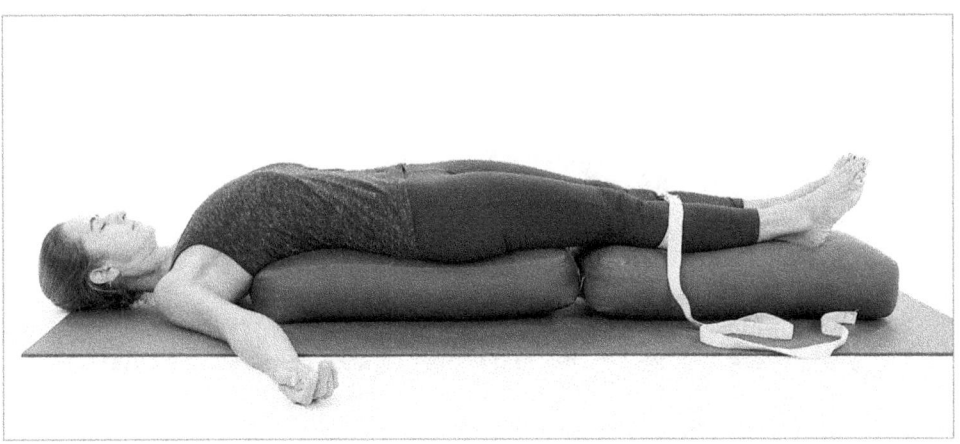

13.a.2 Setu bandha sarvangasana with two bolsters

Pranayama

1. Place one bolster in the center of your mat, parallel with the short end of your mat. Place the second bolster on top of the first one, parallel to the long edge of the mat. They should create a cross in the middle of your mat, hence the name cross bolsters.

2. Sit onto the cross formed by the bolsters, facing the lower end of the top bolster. Use the belt to internally rotate your legs as you did in *setu bandha* with two bolsters.

   A. If you have a very long torso, you may need to sit just below the cross.

3. Keep your feet on the floor and lower your torso along the top bolster.

4. Push into your legs to slide toward the top end of the bolster When your head and shoulders reach the floor, straighten your legs onto the bolster. Your torso, pelvis, and upper thighs should be supported but your head, shoulders, and heels will be on the mat. The top edge of the bolster should be at the bottom of your shoulder blades.

5. Bend your elbows and relax your arms out to the side or over your head. Breathe into the sides of your ribcage. Stay for five to ten minutes *(13.a.3)*.

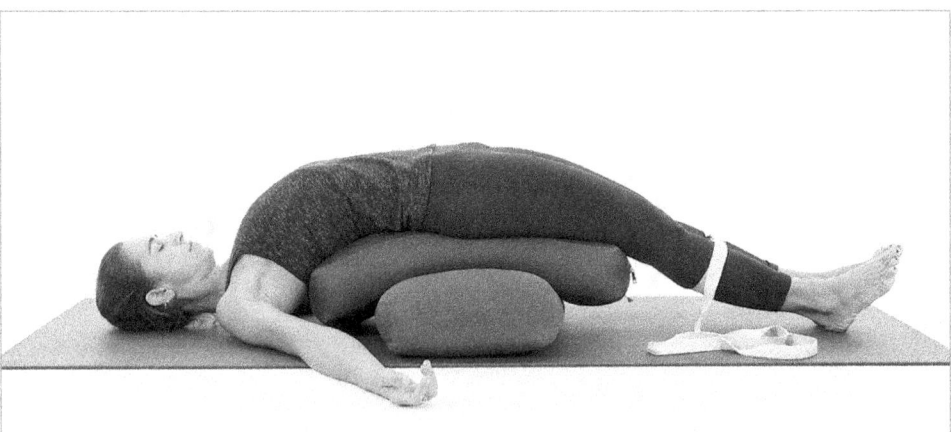

13.a.3 Cross bolsters

If you feel pressure in your lower back, lift your sternum in the direction of your chin to move the backbend up your spine. Bending your knees may also help remove pressure, but it makes the pose less effective. If you cannot get the pressure out of your lower back by internally rotating your legs and lifting your sternum, stay with *setu bandha sarvangasana* with two bolsters. Use your *asana* practice to continue developing flexibility in your pelvis and return to cross bolsters when it becomes more available.

To come out of the pose, bend your knees toward your chest and release the belt. Roll to one side and shift off of both bolsters. Stay on your side for a few moments, and then use your top arm to press up to a seated position. Bring your head up last and maintain your softness and relaxation as you transition out of the pose.

SURYA BHEDHANA AND CHANDRA BHEDANA
sir·ya bheyd·nah | *piercing the sun* · chawn·dra bheyd·nah | *piercing the moon*

Surya and *chandra* are Sanskrit for the sun and moon, and *bhedana* means to pierce through. *Surya bhedana* is piercing the sun and *chandra bhedana* is piercing the moon. The sun is represented in the right nostril, also called *pingala nadi*, so *surya bhedana* is inhaling through the right nostril and exhaling through the left nostril. The moon is symbolized in the left nostril, also called *ida nadi,* so *chandra bhedana* is inhaling through the left nostril and exhaling through the right nostril. These two complementary *pranayama* practices are used to cleanse the nervous system.

Surya bhedana is associated with solar energy: hot, active, and masculine. *Chandra bhedana* cultivates the moon energy: cool, restful, and feminine. They are often done on alternating days because they cultivate very different forms of bodily energy. If surya and *chandra bhedana* are an alternative daily practice, begin with *surya bhedana* on Sunday and *chandra bhedana* on Monday. Saturday is your day off.

We teach *surya* and *chandra bhedana* with *ujayii pranayama* because the sound of *ujayii* helps cultivate balance in your breath. Other traditions teach it with normal breathing. Regardless of what you practice, the breath of *surya* and *chandra bhedana* should be soft. Cultivate a slow, smooth acceleration on the inhale and a slow, smooth deceleration on the exhale, so that you arrive at the bridge between them in a soft way. There is no retention or holding of the breath. Nothing in *pranayama* should be forced or abrupt because you are trying to

Pranayama

EDDIE:
It is said that cleansing the nervous system requires a daily *pranayama* practice for at least two years. That is a huge commitment, so start small. Try to make it a sustainable practice because refining your nervous system will carry you gracefully through all the stages of your life.

facilitate mental, physical, and vibrational relaxation. Breaking your relaxation will agitate your physical tissues and take you further away from your subtle body.

Murghi Mudra

mur·ghee moo·drah | *gesture of the deer*

Pranayama

A *mudra* is a gesture or hand position that has symbolic meaning. *Murghi mudra* means gesture of the deer. It creates two points that are used to control the passage of air through your nostrils in *surya* and *chandra bhedana*. *Murghi mudra* is traditionally done with your right hand, though you may initially need to use your left hand to fold your right hand into position.

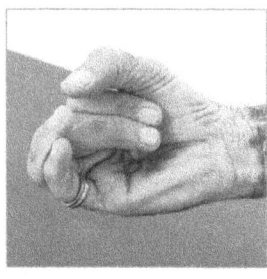

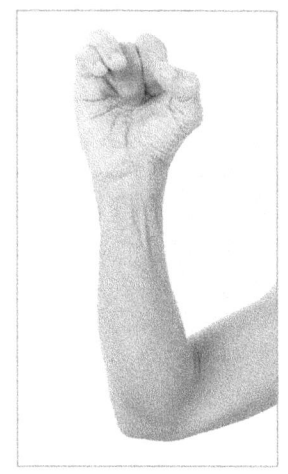

1. Fold your middle and index finger toward your wrist.

2. Bring your pinkie, ring finger, and thumb toward each other.

3. Touch the top pads of those three fingers together. The point of contact is right at the top of the fingertip, not on the side or front pads of the finger. Place your thumb in the middle of the other two fingertips so it maintains equal contact with both.

The *mudra* may be difficult to hold at first, but as with all things in yoga, exact placement is very important. Energy comes out of your fingertips and travels in the direction the finger points. When the top pads of these three fingers are truly aligned, the fingers themselves reflect that line and the energy it carries.

Surya Bhedana

Surya bhedana is inhaling through the right nostril and exhaling through the left nostril. The two points of *murghi mudra* are used to control these actions in a very specific way: they are placed just above the flare of your nostril, with the pinkie and ring finger on the left and the thumb on the right. The ring finger and thumb touch the skin immediately above the flare and the pinkie rests on the flare itself. Once you are in this position, shift your forearm to the left to close your right nasal passageway, and shift it to the right to close the left. Do not pinch or squeeze your nose; keep *murghi mudra* perfectly still as you shift your forearm side to side *(13.b.1)*. It is a very subtle movement with a tiny amount of pressure—just enough to close the passageway, not enough to leave a mark on your nose. It may be difficult to keep all this in your head at first, but with practice you'll become familiar enough to maintain all this detail within the overall subtlety of your *pranayama* practice.

Surya bhedana is always done in an upright seated positon. Gather whatever props you need to sit comfortably and settle in.

1. Find your seat and establish *ujayii pranayama*.

2. Set *jiva bandha* in your mouth and *jalandara bandha* between your chest and chin. If *jalandara bandha* is uncomfortable, simply bow your head and soften your throat.

3. Lift your right hand and create the shape of *murghi mudra*. Place *murghi mudra* accurately on your nose and close your eyes. Relax your left hand on your left thigh and soften both shoulders.

4. Exhale completely, and when you are empty, shift *murghi mudra* to the right to close your left nostril.

5. Inhale through your right nostril. At the top of your inhale, shift *murghi mudra* to the left to close your right nostril.

6. Exhale through your left nostril. At the base of your exhale, shift *murghi mudra* to the right to close your left nostril.

7. Inhale through the right and continue the cycle; breathe in through the right and breathe out through the left.

Continue *surya bhedana* for three to five minutes. There is no retention between inhale and exhale, just a slight natural pause that facilitates shifting *murghi mudra*. Do not force your breath or extend it beyond your capacity; allow the length of your breath to honor your natural respiratory cycle. If you begin to feel tension or anxiety creep into your breath, return to normal breathing and relax.

Chandra Bhedana

Chandra bhedana is inhaling through the left nostril and exhaling through the right nostril. All the other instructions are the same; simply reverse the direction of *murghi mudra* to change the flow.

Nadi Shodna

nah·dee showd·nah | *alternate nostril breathing*

Nadi shodna combines *surya* and *chandra bhedana* to balance the two hemispheres of your brain. *Surya bhedana, chandra bhedana,* and *nadi shodna* are the safest forms of *pranayama* because there is no retention.

Pranayama

1. Find your seat and establish *ujayii pranayama*.

2. Set *jiva bandha* in your mouth and *jalandara bandha* between your chest and chin. If *jalandara bandha* is uncomfortable, simply bow your head and keep your throat soft.

3. Lift your right hand and create the shape of *murghi mudra*. Place *murghi mudra* accurately on your nose and close your eyes. Relax your left hand on your left thigh and soften both shoulders.

4. Exhale completely, and when you are empty, shift *murghi mudra* to the right to close your left nostril.

5. Inhale through your right nostril. At the top of your inhale, shift *murghi mudra* to the left to close your right nostril.

6. Exhale through your left nostril.

7. Inhale through your left nostril, and at the top of your inhale, shift *murghi mudra* to the right to close your left nostril.

8. Exhale through your right nostril.

9. Repeat steps 5-8 and continue the cycle for three to five minutes. End by exhaling on the right side *(13.b.2)*.

VILOMA
vill·oh·mah | *against the hair*

Viloma means against the hair. It is the most physically accessible form of *pranayama* because it's done on your back over a folded blanket; you don't need to have open hips or even be able to sit upright. The blanket is layered over itself in an accordion-like fold to create a long, skinny ridge that is wide on the bottom and narrow on top, like an elongated pyramid (more Mesoamerican than Egyptian). Your spine is supported by the ridge of the pyramid and your ribs cascade down the sides to create lateral expansion in your lungs.

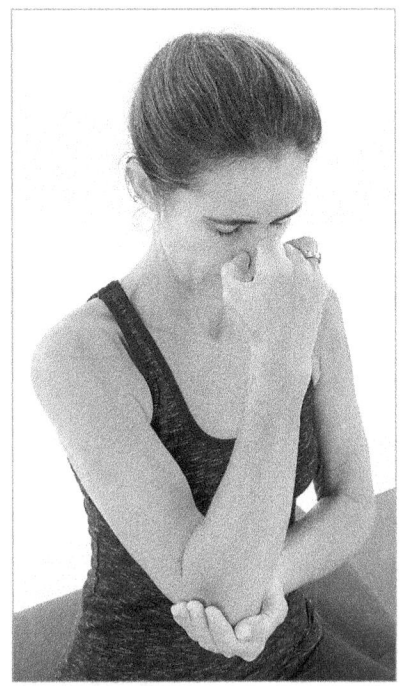
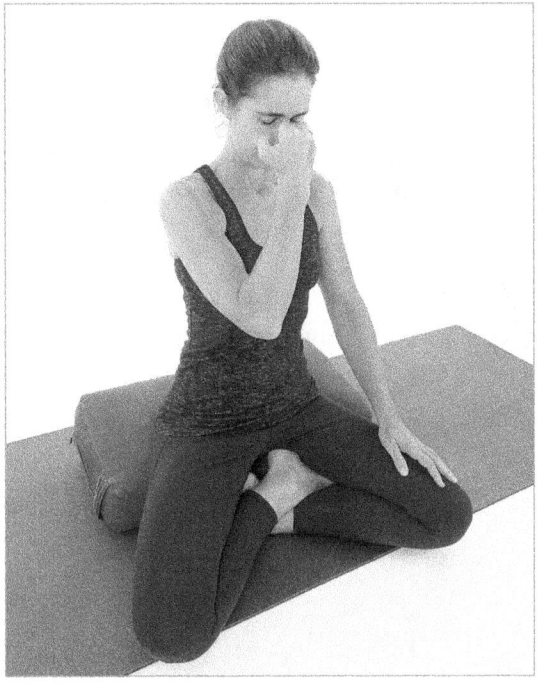

Pranayama

13.b.1 *Shifting murhi mudra*   13.b.2 *Nadi shodna*

Viloma divides the torso into three sections. The goal is to utilize the full pranic vessel from bottom to top. The bottom segment is from the pubic bone/pelvic floor to the navel, the middle is from the navel to the heart, and the top is from the heart to the clavicles. *Puraka* is Sanskrit for inhale and *rechaka* means exhale. *Viloma* usually starts with *puraka*: segmented inhales and uninterrupted exhales. Your breath pours into your torso like water into a cup, filling from the bottom up. The second part is *rechaka*: uninterrupted inhales and segmented exhales. Again, breath is expelled from your torso as from a cup: from the top to the bottom.

The retention between each segment is called *kumbaka* and it is considered the most important part of the practice. In fact, *pranayama* is often described as the study of the space between the breath. Begin with short, two-second *kumbaka*/pauses between each section and work up to five to six seconds. If you begin to feel anxious, trapped or uncomfortable at any point, simply return to normal breathing and resume the practice when you're calm. Remember: you're working with your nervous system. It's essential you remain calm, soft, and steady.

Begin with *puraka*:

Pranayama

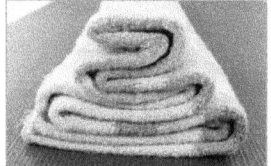

1. Open the blanket into a large rectangle. Lay an 8"-10" section of the wide end of the rectangle on the floor to create a base, and then fold a slightly smaller layer (7"-9") on top of that, in an accordion-like fold. Continue folding slightly smaller layers to create a long pyramid with a narrow (1"-2") ridge on top.

2. Sit on the floor at the bottom of the blanket and lie back, so the narrow ridge supports the length of your spine. Reach up and fold the top of the blanket over itself to support your head. Your forehead should be higher than your chin. Release your arms out to the side, palms up *(13.c.1)*.

3. Close your eyes and establish *ujayii pranayama*. Take several long, deep *ujayii* breaths with slight retentions (*kumbaka*) between the inhale and exhale.

4. Exhale all your air and pause when you are empty. Engage *mula bandha*.

5. Inhale from your pubic bone to your navel and pause (*kumbaka*).

6. Inhale from your navel to your heart and pause.

7. Inhale from your heart to your clavicle and pause. Hold your breath and scan your body to release any tension.

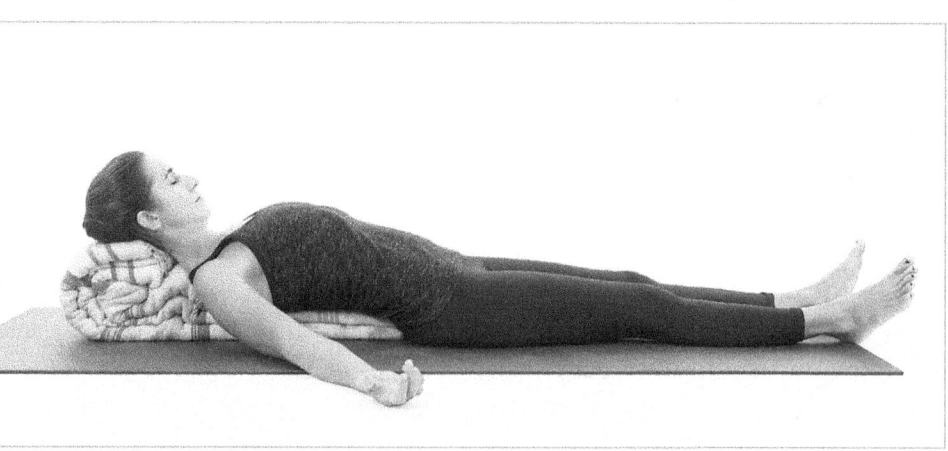

13.c.1 Viloma

8. Exhale in a smooth, uninterrupted breath, and pause at the bottom. Engage *mula bandha*.

9. Repeat steps 5-8 for three to five minutes.

Puraka is about fullness of breath. It brings you to the threshold of your pranic vessel and invites you to explore that fullness and, most importantly, to see how fullness affects your body and mind. Use the *kumbaka* between every section to observe your physical tissue and your mental fluctuations. Try to dissolve both tension and anxiety around the fullness of your breath. If you begin to feel anxious, or as though you are choking, return to normal breathing and resume the practice when you're sufficiently calm.

Rechaka begins from step 3 of *puraka*. If you are combining them into a single practice, take a full minute of regular *ujayii* breathing between each one.

4. Inhale completely and pause at the top.

5. Exhale from your clavicles to your heart and pause. Keep your chest lifted.

6. Exhale from your heart to your navel and pause.

7. Exhale from your navel to your pubic bone and pause. Stay empty and soften everywhere.

8. Inhale in a smooth, uninterrupted breath, and pause at the top.

9. Repeat for three to five minutes.

Rechaka is about emptiness but "empty" can be hard to find; it might feel like you've exhaled completely but there's often a little bit more to go. Use the final exhale, and the *kumbaka* that follows, to find complete emptiness and explore its effect on your body and mind. Most of us have a slightly different reaction to each practice; some find *puraka* to be easy and others are more comfortable with *rechaka*. Explore each one separately until you are comfortable practicing for three to five minutes, and then they can be combined into full *viloma pranayama*.

Begin at step 3 of *puraka*:

Pranayama

4. Exhale all your air and pause when you are empty. Engage *mula bandha*.

5. Inhale from your pubic bone to your navel and pause.

6. Inhale from your navel to your heart and pause.

7. Inhale from your heart to your clavicle and pause. Hold your breath and scan your body to release any tension.

8. Exhale from your clavicle to your heart and pause.

9. Exhale from your heart to your navel and pause.

10. Exhale from your navel to your pubic bone and pause. Stay empty and soften everywhere.

11. Repeat steps 4-10 for two to three minutes.

Return to normal breathing. Soften everywhere and observe the fluctuations of your body and mind. When you are ready to transition, bend your knees and separate your feet to rest your knees against one another. Put one hand on your heart and one hand on your belly, and let your breath breathe you. Be witness to your experience. Stay there for a moment and then roll to one side, off the blanket, and rest for a few more moments. Use your top arm to push up to a seated position, and let your head come up last.

8 LIMBS OF ASHTANGA YOGA

The Yoga Sutras of Patanjali describe yoga as a tree with eight limbs: *Yama, Niyama, Asana, Pranayama, Pratyahara, Dharana, Dhyana,* and *Samadhi*. The ultimate goal of yoga practice is *Samadhi*, a complete equanimity of being. The journey to *Samadhi* is long but well-traveled, and every part of the path is paved with practice.

YAMA AND NIYAMA

Yama and *Niyama* are rules of social conduct, similar to a yogic moral code. There are five *Yama*s and five *Niyama*s. In general, the *Yama*s apply to broad social conduct while *Niyama*s are more personal observances. Yogis are supposed to master the *Yama*s and *Niyama*s before practicing *Asana*, but if that were truly the case,there would be a lot less people doing yoga. Pattabhi Jois always said *Asana* and *Pranayama* should be the first two limbs because they cultivate the mental and emotional prerequisites of the *Yama*s and *Niyama*s.

Yama

The first *Yama* is *Ahimsa*. *Ahimsa* means nonviolence: *A* is a negating prefix and *himsa* means violence. Nonviolence is a fundamental social value of almost every world culture. Most of us learn to abide it as young children. As we mature, the concept of non-violence expands (hopefully) to include cultivating compassion toward all creatures, being watchful of your thoughts and gentle in your actions, and being non-judgmental toward others. The concept of *Ahimsa* takes these qualities a step further by turning them inward: *Ahimsa* encourages you to refrain from physical, mental, and emotional violence toward your Self, not just the outside world.

Most of us are harder on ourselves than anyone else. We beat ourselves up on a regular basis, whether through the direct ignorance of physical pain or the more indirect imposition of guilt, judgment, and self-defeating tendencies. Some of us choose to ignore physical discomfort until it becomes life-threatening; others choose to pursue toxic relationships and destructive patterns. Many of us do both. These negative emotions are hardwired into our daily lives and societal values, and that self-inflicted violence can seep into your yoga practice.

8 Limbs of Ashtanga Yoga

Ahimsa encourages you to uproot these destructive tendencies by becoming mindful of how you practice yoga. Do you force yourself into poses or push "through" pain in order to do a set sequence? Do you critique every personal anatomical restriction you find? These habits may seem innocuous but they encourage violence toward your Self and can turn this profoundly integrating practice into another opportunity for self-flagellation. Remember: what you do on the mat is what you do in your daily life. If you beat yourself up on the mat, you'll beat yourself up in life. If you can learn to love yourself on the mat, you can learn to love yourself in life. Cultivating *Ahimsa* is the first step.

Ahimsa can also be interpreted to include vegetarianism, but we don't think you have to be a vegetarian to start practicing yoga. There are no prerequisites to practicing yoga. Krishnamacharya (the father of modern yoga) said to eat the food that makes you happy and BKS Iyengar said you don't even have to quit smoking cigarettes to practice yoga. All you have to do is start the practice, and if the practice is effective all your unnecessary habits will fall away. In other words, an effective practice will create positive change in your life. If you are doing the poses and nothing is changing, you may want to reevaluate your practice.

The second *Yama* is *Satya*. *Sat* means true and *ya* is an emphatic suffix, like the word "yeah!" *Satya* is truth, emphatically stated. Living in truth means keeping yourself and your actions grounded in reality. Embracing reality requires honesty, integrity, and personal responsibility, and like *Ahimsa*, *Satya* encourages you to turn these values inward. Be honest with yourself and the people around you, especially when the truth is difficult. Resist the urge to hide behind defensive personality traits and useless mental distractions. Be yourself at all times and permeate your life with integrity and authenticity. It sounds like a simple task but it requires a huge amount of personal responsibility. It is easier to point a finger than look in the mirror but the mirror holds *Satya*; it holds the truth that lives behind your words, thoughts, and actions.

The third *Yama* is *Asteya*, which means non-stealing: *A* is a negating prefix and *steya* is stealing or coveting. *Asteya* refers to the physical act of taking items that don't belong to you, which is obviously wrong, but it also operates on a deeper psychological level. *Asteya* encourages you to avoid the sense of entitlement that convinces you it's okay to steal in the first place. Practicing *Asteya* is about being content with what you have. It implies a sense of grace; not pining for things beyond your control and learning to let go of physical, mental, and emotional baggage—grudges, guilt, and the piles of commercial, material clutter that saturate our modern life.

Asteya also urges us to give credit where credit is due and only take ownership of praise and acclaim you have truly earned. It encourages you to acknowledge the things in your life that came from other people, whether they are tangible or intangible, and to be grateful for them. Acknowledging your teachers is a way of respecting your lineage and honoring the fact that we are all connected on the path toward enlightenment. After all, gratitude is one of the most powerful forces on the planet. Simple acts of daily gratitude help connect the tiny thread of your being to the vast web of human consciousness. They give you a place in the cosmos.

The fourth *Yama* is *Brahmacharya*. *Brahmacharya* is usually associated with abstinence or celibacy but "abstinence" fails to capture its broader application to modern life. *Brahma* comes from Brahma, the creative deity of Hindu mythology. Brahma is the catalyst of action and creation; he represents the dynamic energy that makes us "do" everything. *Charya* means to walk or conduct, and it denotes spiritual teachers who walk the land spreading their wisdom. The *ya* is an emphatic suffix, as in *Satya*. In that sense, *Brahmacharya* means walking with Brahma; it is the practice of walking with, channeling, and containing the creative energy inside of you. It entails moderation in all your human appetites. It's about avoiding overindulgence and cultivating a sense of temperance in your life.

The fifth *Yama* is *Aparigraha*. *A* is a negating prefix, *par* means to fill, and *graha* is your dwelling; *Aparigraha* means non-hoarding. It warns against our human tendency to accumulate things we don't actually need, and it refers to both physical and mental hoarding. We can become attached to physical things like fancy clothes but we can also become attached to unnecessary thoughts and relationships. Practicing *Aparigraha* encourages you to avoid these possessive tendencies and to release your life from the shackles of mental and emotional clutter. It also urges you to become generous in your actions and in your spirit, thus turning your inert clutter into a positive force for others.

Niyama

The first *Niyama* is *Saucha*. *Saucha* refers to purity of body and mind, with a strong emphasis on personal hygiene. It's important to clean your body on a regular basis and it's especially important to be clean for your yoga practice. Doing

8 Limbs of Ashtanga Yoga

yoga is like going to a sacred temple; you shouldn't go to the temple dirty and you shouldn't leave it in disarray. But "clean" doesn't require a lengthy, indulgent shower or piles of expensive cosmetics. *Saucha* is more about being thorough than being elaborate. It refers to daily cleansing rituals that require little more than a bit of water, some soap, and a toothbrush (bonus points for a tongue scraper).

Saucha also implores you to eat clean food, wear clean clothes, and keep your mat clean. Yoga is a detoxifying practice. The things that are being detoxed may end up lying in a puddle underneath you, so please clean them up. Don't leave them there until tomorrow and don't impose them on the people around you. It's a matter of personal responsibility; you are responsible for **all** of you.

The second *Niyama* is *Santosha*. *Santosha* is "the ability to cultivate joy independent of external sources," otherwise known as contentment or equanimity. In short, you are responsible for your own happiness. You cannot expect others to make you happy, and in truth, expectations are the root of all suffering. If you follow the thread of any discontent back to its source, you will probably find an expectation. It could be a simple, subconscious expectation but it's there nonetheless, and when that expectation is not met we dissolve into frustration, anger, and disappointment. It can be as simple as the weather; a rainy day only becomes a disappointment if you expected sunshine. You planted the seed of your discontent and set yourself up for unhappiness, but if you remove that expectation you can better appreciate the rain. *Santosha* encourages you to approach life with this sense of unconditional joy; to be open to infinite possibilities and content with whatever life brings you.

The third *Niyama* is *Tapas*. *Tap* means to burn, and *Tapas* refers to personal practices that burn away the impurities of your being. It is the heat and intensity of yoga's transformative process, the fire that transforms dull to bright. The traditional interpretation includes daily austerities such as fasting and rigorous *asana* practice. These illuminating practices reach deep inside of you to pull out the *halahala*, which is the poison of our conditioned existence, all the toxic crap we ingest on a daily basis (physically and mentally). Harnessing the transformative fire of *Tapas* will burn through the *halahala* to release *amrita*, the nectar of the gods that lives within you. Failing to ignite your *Tapas* will cause you to cycle through the karmic wheel like a gerbil in a cage, restricted by your heavy *halahala* and unable to recognize your true Self.

The fourth *Niyama* is *Svadhyaya*. *Sva* refers to the Self and *dhya* is meditation or study. *Svadhyaya* is the emphatic, focused, relentless study of the Self. Traditional interpretations include chanting and the study of ancient scriptures, but meditation on the Self is paramount. Everything you need to know is already inside of you, you have just forgotten it. Yoga is the process of remembering those deep spiritual truths. It requires that you embark on a process of rigorous self-exploration, leaving no mental, emotional, or physical stone unturned. Observe your thoughts, habits, beliefs, and actions. Be willing to question the things you hold dear. But always temper *Svadhyaya* with *Ahimsa*, or nonviolence; in the process of self-discovery, be gentle with your Self and compassionate toward the truths you find within.

8 Limbs of Ashtanga Yoga

The fifth *Niyama* is *Ishvara Pranidhana*. *Ishvara* is a fulfiller of wishes (God) and *Pranidhana* means to bring forth. *Ishvara Pranidhana* means to constantly live with the awareness of the divine. It entails a complete surrender to the divine being within you, and it is our ultimate saving grace. You can always just give it up to God, regardless of your physical, mental, or emotional circumstance. God will always accept your love.

Ishvara Pranidhana is considered the final step of Bhakti yoga, the yoga of love and devotion. For many people, Bhakti is the easiest yogic path. You don't have to be brilliant or physically advanced to follow the path of Bhakti yoga; you just have to be willing to surrender to God. It is the sentiment encapsulated in the Beatles' "Let It Be" and the Christian concept of faith: let go of your need for reason and find peace in the divine. Most Westerners find this concept of surrender more difficult than the tangible physicality of *asana* (despite widespread love for the Beatles), but over time, even Westerners may become comfortable with the heart-opening practice of *Ishvara Pranidhana*.

The *Yamas* and *Niyamas* may seem lofty and abstract so it's helpful to see them as guidelines instead of absolutes. We've been doing this practice for over 30 years and we're definitely not perfect. We're human, and accepting our imperfections without judgement is the root of personal evolution.

ASANA & PRANAYAMA

The third limb of Ashtanga Yoga is *Asana*. *As* is "the place where you choose to reside," so *Asana* refers to the placement (postures) of your body and mind. *Asana* also commonly translates to "seat" because the seat is the posture of meditation, but *Asana* encompasses any yogic posture of the body and mind. All of the poses we present in this book are *Asanas* and the specific posture of your mind while practicing these poses is also an *Asana*.

The fourth limb is *Pranayama*. *Prana* is your life force and *ayama* means to lengthen or extend. *Pranayama* is the practice of extending your life force through the study of breath and subtle energy control. Yogis believe every life is measured by a set number of breaths, and each individual breath can be lengthened to extend your cumulative life force. "Extension" refers to the length of your breath and to your level of awareness within each breath. In other words, becoming fully present in each and every breath will literally lengthen your life. The more conscious you are of your breath, the more life you will have to live.

PRATYAHARA

Pattabhi Jois said the first four limbs of Ashtanga Yoga are external limbs and the last four are internal limbs. Everything in yoga follows this path: it moves from the outside in, from the periphery to the core.

The fifth limb of Ashtanga Yoga is *Pratyahara*. *Pratyahara* is the drawing inward of your senses. Your eyes, ears, nose, and skin receive constant vibrations from the world around you, even when your mind is trying to focus on something else. This incoming sensory stimulation causes an involuntary mental reaction that can distract you from the task at hand, and that mental distraction often causes a physical reaction. It happens in almost every yoga class: when someone walks in late, everyone looks toward the door—even though that newcomer has absolutely nothing to do with you or your practice. The sound and vibration of the newcomer grabbed your attention before you could even think about it because your senses are not yet disciplined in the art of *Pratyahara*.

Pratyahara is often described as a "withdrawal" of the senses, but "withdrawal" implies a complete absence, as though your senses had a simple on/off switch. *Pratyahara* is more about cultivating a sense of mastery over your senses, not simply turning them off. Withdrawing your senses might mean you ignore the urge to look up when someone enters the yoga room, but *Pratyahara* means you don't notice when someone walks into the yoga room. Every aspect of your being is focused on your practice. It's not a matter of simply ignoring the impulse, it's a complete mastery of the senses that create the impulse in the first place. All of those sense organs are still functioning—and with practice they will begin to function at a much higher level—but they're simply channeled inward instead of outward. They're fine-tuning your powers of self-observation, allowing you to feel, see, and hear what's inside of you instead of what is around you. This act of turning toward the Self is the preparatory stage for meditation.

DHARANA, DHYANA & SAMADHI

The three final limbs of Ashtanga yoga involve meditation. The end goal is *Samadhi*, or pure enlightenment, and *Dharana* and *Dhyana* are stepping stones along that path.

The sixth limb of Ashtanga yoga is *Dharana*. *Dharana* is extreme concentration on a single thing. It is the "training wheels" stage of meditation. It requires that you can sit comfortably (thanks to *Asana*), breathe consciously (*Pranayama*), and contain your senses (*Pratyahara*). But once you are quiet, seated, and ready to meditate, your mind suddenly becomes the loudest thing in the room. It is inundated with thoughts and images, and often overcome with an anxious need to escape the act of meditation by moving, fidgeting, or otherwise distracting yourself from the monumental task at hand. *Dharana* acknowledges this anxiety and provides an important tool to address it: an object on which to focus your meditation. The object can be something tangible, such as a *mala* (prayer beads), or audible, such as your breath or a *mantra* (the repetition of a *mantra* is called *japa*). These objects provide a constant, repetitive reminder to stay focused in the face of your mind's internal distractions.

8 Limbs of Ashtanga Yoga

The practice of *Dharana* also involves the concept of *ekagraha*. *Eka* means one and *graha* means pointed; *ekagraha* is the single-pointed focus of your mind. *Dharana* is the ability to maintain that single-pointed focus with all of your being. It teaches you to concentrate on the single object of your meditation as though it were the only thing in the entire universe. This laser-sharp focus is the stepping stone to *Dhyana*, which is broadly interpreted as "meditation."

Dhyana is a more advanced stage of meditation than *Dharana*. *Dharana* focuses all your awareness on a single object but you are still an individuated being that is 1) aware of your meditation and 2) separate from the object of your meditation. *Dhyana* takes you a step further by dissolving the act of meditation; it distills your awareness down to the Self (your consciousness) and the singular object of your meditation. At this stage, the object of your meditation has evolved past the introductory objects used in *Dharana* (prayer beads or *japa*) to focus on God—God meaning the divine power or whatever name is personally significant to you. *Dhyana* removes everything between you and God, including

8 Limbs of Ashtanga Yoga

your individuated ability to meditate on God. The entire universe is simply you and God, flowing toward each other in an unbroken current.

The final limb of Ashtanga Yoga is *Samadhi*. *Sam* means even and *adhi* means to adhere or stick together. *Samadhi* is enlightenment or super consciousness. It is the final stage of meditation. It removes the separation between you and God, thereby dissolving the individuated ego and merging the Self with the divine. *Samadhi* is stepping into the awareness that God is inside of you and inside of all things. Everything is connected. There are no true barriers among us, only the false barriers maintained by our individuated consciousness.

Many of us get glimpses of *Samadhi* in our practice; a feeling of unrestricted connectivity to the world around you, as though the walls of your consciousness have dissolved to reveal an infinite and intrinsically accessible universe. These glimpses are just tiny sips of *amrita*, but they provide enough nourishment to keep us steady on the path toward internal and external peace.

THE YOGA SUTRAS OF PATANJALI

From the Outside In

Krishnamacharya praised *asana* for providing health and guidance but he cautioned that the poses can also lead us astray. "Mastering" the physical poses can inflate your ego instead of transcending it, leading you to associate spiritual evolution with physical fitness. There can certainly be a correlation between the two but being able to put your foot behind your head doesn't mean you're an evolved person. There's more to it than that. After all, your body is transient. Your physical capability can and will disappear so you must remain humble. Don't use yoga to worship at the altar of your immaculate physique; use it to explore your Self. The poses are designed to penetrate your consciousness, and if they're not getting past your physical tissues you are not doing yoga, you're just participating in a circus act.

The Yoga Sutras are the bridge between yoga's external instructions and internal philosophy. They are the roadmap that illustrates the path to *Samadhi* and provides tools to navigate the challenges you will inevitably encounter. The Sutras also carry the lineage of yoga across the millennia by linking the teaching to the teacher and the teacher to the student. It is a circle that leads us back to our shared human consciousness. This is often the piece that alienates people because it is interpreted as the "religion" of yoga, but we do not think the Sutras are religious. Yoga is a life support system and the Sutras are simply its underlying philosophy; they can be understood and ingested regardless of your religious beliefs.

HISTORY

The exact age of the Yoga Sutras is not known. Some say they were written 1,500 years ago, some say 5,000, and others believe they are much older than that. The most interesting thing about them is not their exact age, it's how incredibly relevant they still are today. They are written proof that the human psyche has not changed very much in the last couple centuries, perhaps a millennia. We are still generally insecure and prone to selfish, ego-centric behavior, and we need constant spiritual guidance to avoid total self-destruction. That may seem depressing but it's also extremely comforting to know you're not alone. The

NICKI:
Guruji said yoga is an internal process; everything else is just a circus act.

The Yoga Sutras of Patanjali

path of spiritual evolution is not walked by isolated individuals, it is shared by centuries of dedicated practitioners who came before you and millions of practitioners currently on their way. It is also reassuring to know we all face the same internal struggle, regardless of our tribe. The Yoga Sutras are proof that all who walk this path have shared its challenges, and every one of them has left their footsteps to guide you.

The Sutras are simple aphorisms, but to a beginning practitioner they may seem to be written in code. They are purposely aloof because they were considered sacred language; their inherent power needed to be protected from all but true practitioners. If you pick up the book and read through them without an *asana* practice, they'll remain flat, lifeless words on paper. In fact, I (Nicki) spent years falling asleep to different translations—they were endlessly boring. But it wasn't the book or the translation, it was me. I wasn't ready yet. But after a few years of practicing yoga, everything fell into place. *Asana* gave me the code to unlock the meaning hiding in those simple words.

There has been a lot of literature in the past few years aimed at discrediting yoga's roots by attacking the validity of the Sutras and their disciples. It's disheartening, but ultimately it's completely irrelevant. We don't need a book or a date to validate yoga. The validity of this practice is written in our bodies and minds and in those of our students. Don't worry too much about how old the Sutras are or where they came from. Let this practice be felt and understood in your Self, and you will understand its true worth on the path of human evolution.

FORMAT

The word Sutra implies transcendental information: *su* means "to link" and *tra* means "in order to transcend." Pattabhi Jois described the Sutras as *shastras*, meaning both "sacred phrase" and "weapon." The *shastras* are words that have the power to cut through illusion and delusion.

The Sutras are short aphorisms—small words with huge meaning—which makes them easy to memorize and repeat. They were designed to be passed from teacher to student through *kirtan* chanting (call and response). Chanting the Sutras forms a *mantra*; *manas* is your mind and *tra* is to transcend so a *mantra* is that which helps you transcend your mind. Call and response chanting (*kirtan*) is also a form of *pranayama*, where an entire Sutra is chanted over the course of a smooth, complete exhale.

There are 196 individual Sutras divided into four books called *Padas*. *Pada* means feet. Only three of the 196 Sutras directly relate to *asana*. The remaining 193 Sutras are about what's going on in your head, the place where most of our suffering occurs.

The first book is called *Samadhi Pada*. The root word is *Samadhi*; the elusive 8th limb of Ashtanga yoga. *Samadhi Pada* explains why you should do yoga. It defines yoga and describes the lofty ideals and beneficial qualities that can be achieved through its practice, but it doesn't really tell you how to get there. The second book, *Sadhana Pada*, is about the practice of yoga. Sadhana actually means "practice." It explains how to move from a state of constant distraction to one of pure concentration and explains the obstacles you may encounter along the way. It has the most relevant, practical information for introductory students and also contains the only three Sutras that directly relate to *asana*.

The Yoga Sutras of Patanjali

The third book is called *Vibhuti Pada*. Vibhuti means "transcending and negating Earth-based consciousness." It describes the supernatural powers (*siddis*) that can be gained through the practice of yoga, such as reading minds and stopping your heartbeat. *Vibhuti Pada* suggests continual refinement of your consciousness will allow you to tap into these powers, but it also warns they can become a dangerous distraction. A blind pursuit of these powers puts your ego above your true Self; in other words, power corrupts. Krishnamacharya also cautioned that most practitioners are unlikely to access the *siddis* in a single lifetime so we're better off focusing on the simple, tangible benefits of refining our consciousness. Regardless of how you feel about supernatural powers, *Vibhuti Pada* can serve as a reminder to look beyond your limited physicality and find the greatness that resides within.

The fourth and final book is called *Kevalya Pada*. *Kevalya* means "isolated and absolutely pure," and it is reserved for the most advanced practitioners. It describes a stage of consciousness where the mind serves the master (Self) instead of the other way around. It is complete mastery of your mind, where consciousness rests on itself. For most of us—myself included—it's a long way away. Thankfully, it's the process that matters.

SANSKRIT

The written form of Sanskrit is called *devanagri*, or the language of the angels (*Devas*). The individual letters are called *maitrika*, which means little mother. Those words combine to a simple but wonderful meaning: Sanskrit is an angelic language transmitted by the mothers of the world. Sanskrit is considered to be the most perfect, precise grammatical language in existence. All attempts to record Sanskrit words in English are a gross transliteration so the exact spelling is somewhat irrelevant. None of them are really right or wrong. The Sanskrit spelling in this book simply represents the transliterations that make sense to us.

Sanskrit is a language of internal response, one that is both vibratory and implosive. English, in contrast, is very explosive; the sounds originate in the front of your mouth and act like little projectiles, shot straight from your mind to its target. If the target doesn't understand the sound often gets louder. Sanskrit, in contrast, is internal. The sounds originate deep in your throat and are broadcast in every direction like wavelets from a drop of water. They ripple through you and around you, and the vibrations they create affect you more than the people around you. Speaking Sanskrit is like gently drumming a gong into a powerful spiritual crescendo.

Chanting Sanskrit has been described as profound internal medicine. It is said to bestow *deva dristhi*, or the angelic gaze. We usually begin all *kirtan* (call and response) by chanting *aum* three times to create vibrational space for the Sutras. The full name of *aum* is *aum pranava*; *pra* means to draw forth and *nah* is the eternal cosmic vibration. *Aum* is believed to be the first sound uttered in the universe; it represents the birthing of our cosmic existence.

PATANJALI

Patanjali was a Sanskrit grammarian, an Ayurvedic physician and a Yogi. He is credited with creating the first substantial books on each of these subjects and the yoga Sutras are his book of yoga psychology. All of his works indicate he is not the source of the knowledge contained within; he is simply tasked with its transmission. There is a wealth of fascinating research surrounding Patanjali as a historical figure but we prefer to honor the image of Patanjali as it was presented to us: with a strong dose of cultural relativism and a touch of the mystical unknown.

The Story of Patanjali

Hindu tradition has many rich and varied stories regarding Patanjali. This is our personal favorite, partially because it's the first we learned and partially because it mirrors the mythology of many world religions. Yoga is about dissolving the

The Yoga Sutras of Patanjali

NICKI:
I once had a fellow teacher tell me my Sanskrit pronunciations were weird. It bugged me so I asked Guruji if they were right or wrong. He laughed. He told me all Westerners pronounced Sanskrit incorrectly; we were simply not born with the right mouths to properly make those sounds. But he was very happy we were trying. He said as long as we are sincere and speak the words with love in our hearts, the Sanskrit is correct. His words are a reminder to avoid our human inclination to be overly critical of ourselves and others. The simple act of opening your mouth to speak these words is a huge step in the right direction.

barriers we erect within ourselves and between our earthly communities, and every little bit helps.

The three main gods of Hindu mythology are Brahma, Vishnu, and Shiva. Brahma is the creator, Vishnu is the sustainer and Shiva is the destroyer. Together they maintain the balance of the universe: birth, life, and death. Shiva is known as the Maha Yogi, or "great" yogi. He spends most of his time in deep meditation at the top of Mt. Kailash and becomes quite angry when disturbed. He is called upon to rectify mankind's most dire situations, but for everyday drama, Vishnu (the sustainer) does most of the work. Vishnu is often shown reclining on a couch made of his serpent avatar, Adishesha. Together they float through the ocean of milk, a vast, murky sea that symbolizes our consciousness. Patanjali is an avatar of Vishnu and this is his story.

The Yoga Sutras of Patanjali

The story of Patanjali begins at a time when the world had slipped out of balance. The gods had become quite lazy; Hindu gods often mirror our own self-indulgent human behavior and their godliness is revealed when they manage to address it with profound spiritual wisdom. But without the gods' spiritual guidance, the world had fallen into chaos. Both civilization and language were in decline. Mankind went to Brahma for help, who in turn took them to Vishnu.

Vishnu looked down from his heavenly realm and immediately realized something needed to be done. He closed his eyes with the intention of meditating on the issue, but he quickly fell asleep. As he slept, his body grew heavier and heavier. Adishesha struggled under the weight until he could no longer carry him. The serpent finally shook himself to wake the sleeping god, and Vishnu explained that he had experienced the most amazing vision. He had seen Shiva dancing *tandvah*, a sacred dance that symbolizes the karmic destruction of evil. *Tandvah* was too sacred to be seen, even by Vishnu, so Adishesha was immediately excited. He wanted to see it for himself. Vishnu replied that Adishesha would be called upon to serve in some way, and in return for his service, he would be shown the sacred *deva dristhi*, or angelic visions or gaze.

Vishnu went to Shiva, who was meditating at the top of Mt. Kailash. Shiva was angry at being disturbed but quickly realized Earth was in serious trouble. He decided it was time to deliver *devanagri* to mankind, and he put Vishnu in charge of that important task. *Devanagri* means language of the angels; it is the written form of Sanskrit.

Vishnu went back to Adishesha and tasked him with this important transmission. Together they looked toward Earth for a worthy individual to provide

264

The Yoga Sutras of Patanjali

Adishesha with a human form, and they immediately saw Gonika. Gonika was a humble, devout woman who desperately wanted a son. Every day she went to the river to ask the gods for their blessing and knelt near the water with her hands in *anjali mudra*. One day while Gonika prayed, Adishesha hopped off the heavenly plane and landed in the space between her clasped palms. Gonika opened her hands and watched the tiny serpent turn into a man, who was named Patanjali. Patanjali means "one who falls into open or folded hands." Patanjali explained he was an avatar of Vishnu and Gonika was to be his mother. Gonika was overjoyed. She took him back to the village to be raised with her Brahmin family.

Patanjali began to spread the sacred teachings of *Devanagri* (Sanskrit), Ayurveda, and Yoga. Students from all over the world flocked to him for wisdom. As his popularity grew he asked his disciples to erect a screen in front of him so he could teach with anonymity. He taught larger and larger audiences from behind the screen and, though his students couldn't see him, all remained enthralled. All of his students received exactly what they sought, despite the fact that everyone came with different levels of understanding and experience.

One day a student decided to peek behind the screen. What he saw blew his mind: Patanjali was no longer fully human. He had taken his divine serpent form, but instead of a single head he had a thousand heads of white light hovering above his thickly coiled body. Each head was transmitting a steady stream of light to an individual student in the room, providing that individual student with exactly what they needed to recognize the divinity within.

Patanjali's thousand heads of shining light symbolize yoga's deeply individual nature. You might be doing the same pose as the other 50 people in the room, but you're definitely not having the same experience as those other 50 people because you're you. You are completely unique. You're learning exactly what you need to be learning right now and it's completely different from the person next to you. Yoga doesn't always give you what you want, but if you stay open to the process it will always give you what you need. And if the individual process is effective all of us will arrive at exactly the same place: complete freedom of body, mind, and spirit.

NICKI'S 10 FOUNDATIONAL SUTRAS

There are many fantastic books that describe the Yoga Sutras in detail so we'll limit this discussion to the 10 Sutras we find to be the most personally significant. The first five are from the first book (*Samadhi Pada*) and six through ten are pulled from various sections of the second book (*Sadhana Pada*).

1.1 Atha Yoga Nushasanam

> ATHA: Here; now; in this exact moment; the moment all other moments have brought us to
>
> YOGA: Union; to yoke; being from the root; to bring together the seemingly polar opposites of our being
>
> ANU: The smallest incremental measurement; the tiniest grain, thread or essence of your being
>
> SHASANAM: (from shastra) the sacred teachings; the weapon to pierce our consciousness

The Yoga Sutras of Patanjali

Here, now, in this exact moment of which all other moments are comprised, we choose to follow, along with the thread of our being, the teachings of yoga.

Less poetic interpretations will simply say, "Now begins yoga," but Sanskrit can be so much more interesting. Every moment of your life has led you to this point: the point where you decide to follow the sacred path of yoga. Following yoga truly amounts to following your Self because yoga is already inside of you; it is stamped onto the smallest grain of your being. But following yoga is a choice, and many others will choose instead to toil in the darkness. The word "*atha*" also implies you are about to undertake some serious work that should not be underestimated.

1.2 Yogah Chitta Vritti Nirodhah

> YOGAS: Union; to yoke; holding the reigns; joining together
>
> CHITTA: Your individuated consciousness; everything you have ever seen, done, or thought; the compilation of impressions and experiences that make you who you are (*chit* means to collect)
>
> VRITTI: The fluctuations and agitations of the mind
>
> NIRODHAHA: A positive state of mind; quiet, calm lucidity; the state that exists after the agitations and fluctuations subside

Yoga is the intentional quieting and calming of all the self-limiting, self-judging, self-defeating tendencies of our individuated consciousness (mind).

This Sutra is often referred to as the beginning and the end; all 196 Sutras begin here and return to this point.

The Yoga Sutras of Patanjali

CHITTA. *Chitta* is your individuated consciousness. It is a collection of your past experiences and your impression of those experiences, and it makes you completely unique. There are four aspects of *chitta*/consciousness: *manas*, *ahamkhar*, *buddhi* and *chitta*.

The first aspect of *chitta* is *manas*. *Man* is your mind (it literally means "to think") and *as* means to breathe so *manas* is your thinking apparatus. *Manas* is your mind as a sense organ; the part of your consciousness that is alive. It has five "input" organs called the *jnanendriyas* that gather sensory information and five "output" organs called *karmendriyas* that create action. The *jnanendriyas* are the eyes, ears, nose, mouth, and skin/touch; the *karmendriyas* are the hands, feet, mouth, sexual organs, and anus. Together, the five *jnanendriyas* and five *karmendriyas* form the ten doors of your consciousness. These two sides of *manas* (sense and action) govern most of your physical, tangible interaction with the world around you. Observing these ten doors can shed light on how your Self—the essence that resides inside the *manas*—interacts with, responds to, and is affected by the world around you.

The second form of *chitta* is the *ahamkhar*. The *ahamkhar* is your ego; *aha* means "I am" and *khar* means "to do." *Ahamkhar* is the part of your consciousness that sees you as separate from the world around you. It usually manifests around age two, with the adamant assertion of "me" and "I." This individuation is an important part of human development. It's not inherently evil; in fact, the ego's desire for attention and accomplishment often provides the driving force behind action. It's the reason we do many of the things we need to do. But the ego's primary objective is self-preservation, and it can easily dominate other forms of consciousness. It refuses to be subjugated, is prone to judgment, and is almost never satiated. In that light, the *ahamkhar* is a manifestation of the veil that separates you from your divinity. It represents the person you think you are, not who you really are.

The third form of *chitta* is the *buddhi* mind. It is derived from the word *budh* or Buddha, which means to be awake, to know, and to understand. *Buddhi* is the part of your mind that gravitates toward morality and spiritual truth, otherwise known as your conscience. It is often described as the "over mind" because it can see beyond selfish human needs, i.e. beyond the *ahamkhar*/ego. The practice of yoga is intended to awaken and bring forth the *buddhi* mind from behind the cloud of your *ahamkhar*. Once awakened, the *buddhi* mind will guide your thoughts and actions in the direction of spiritual wisdom instead of personal gain.

The fourth form of *chitta* is called *chitta*, and it refers to the subconscious mind. *Chitta* is like a massive secret storage facility holding all the layers of your being. It contains your life's deepest imprints; the thoughts, emotions, and memories that condition your daily existence but are not involved in your daily thought process. It represents everything that gets swept under the rug in your daily march toward stability and productivity.

The *chitta* is the part of your mind most hidden from you but it affects all other aspects of your mind: it informs the actions and motivations of the *ahamkhar*; causes strong bias in the *jnanendriya*s (senses); and restricts expression in the *karmendriya*s (action). Only the *buddhi* mind is not subject to *chitta*'s strong lens, but it lives behind *chitta*'s deceptive coloring until it is liberated through the practice of yoga. Yoga is a process of digging through the *chitta*'s closely-guarded contents to uncover the roots of your personality and thus bring forth the *buddhi* mind from behind the *chitta*'s strong biases.

The four forms of *chitta*/consciousness exist simultaneously at all times. The dominance between them varies from person to person; some of us are more morally inclined and others are more ego-driven. The practice of yoga can shift this dominance over the course of a person's lifetime. The goal is to have your *manas* influenced by the *buddhi* mind instead of the *ahamkhar* and the *chitta*. Operating from the *buddhi* mind allows your decisions to be influenced by a strong moral conscience with the knowledge that your individual actions are part of a larger spiritual construct. Until that happens, your *manas* will be influenced by the stored patterns and habits of the *chitta*, combined with the selfish needs of the *ahamkhar*. In other words, your life choices will be based on the fear and pain of your past experiences, combined with an egotistical need for self-preservation.

VRITTIS. *Vrit* means to whirl, revolve, and spin wildly out of control. The *vrittis* are our knee-jerk reactions, our senseless impulses, and our tendency to lash out when we feel threatened or hurt. They're the inflammatory words and actions

The Yoga Sutras of Patanjali

The Yoga Sutras of Patanjali

we later regret. These quick, senseless outbursts are part of our everyday human experience but they rarely have a positive connotation. In fact, they almost always bring us pain.

Yoga seeks to curb the *vritti*s by improving our patience, compassion, and powers of self-observation. We learn these principles in *asana*; the poses provide a framework to see and unravel our physical restrictions. They teach us to pay close attention to detail, and with enough practice, we can turn this attention inward to unravel the mental and emotional restrictions that create our *vritti*s. So when we're telling you to lift your kneecap in *trikonasana*, we're actually teaching you how to better observe and communicate with your Self. The goal is to become conscious enough to catch your *vritti*s before they manifest into words or actions. Eventually, you may even be able to catch the thoughts that create the *vritti*s, and then the behavioral patterns that create the thoughts, and on and on until you have erased that deep-seated insecurity from your being.

Curbing your *vritti*s doesn't mean your life will become free of conflict or that you should stop standing up for yourself when you're attacked. Life is not always fair or compassionate, and conflicts need to be addressed. Managing your *vritti*s simply means you take the time to examine your thoughts and emotions—including your role in their creation (remember those expectations!)—and present them in a non-threatening, non-defensive way. It's another aspect of personal responsibility; you cannot constructively address a conflict unless you fully understand the way(s) you have contributed to it. This is extremely important in your most personal relationships: your partner(s), children, and close friends. It is the underlying sentiment behind Pattabhi Jois' adage that "the highest form of yoga is being in a relationship and having children." These relationships are closer to you than anything else and observing them offers the most direct path to personal evolution.

Quick disclaimer: doing yoga will not magically make you a better partner or parent. You are still human, and your behavioral patterns are hard-wired by a lifetime of past experiences. We have been doing yoga for decades and we still slip into *vritti*s; we say things to each other, and to our children, that we immediately regret. But yoga has taught us to better see the truth of our actions, instead of our perception of our actions, and empowered us to take personal responsibility for that truth. It has taught us to acknowledge our transgressions, to make amends quickly and unconditionally, and—most importantly—to forgive ourselves and the people around us. And the best thing about yoga is it doesn't start with the lofty goal of observing your thoughts and *vritti*s, it starts with the extremely tangible goal of observing your body in *asana*. Training your mind to develop a relationship with your kneecap cultivates the same powers of self-observation that allow you to understand your role in your own suffering and in that of the people you love.

NIRODHAHA. *Ni* is a negating prefix and rodha is derived from Rudra, the Hindu God of Storms. Rudra is the embodiment of our tempestuous nature. His wild hair and fierce disposition illustrate the state of our mind when it is governed by the agitating force of the *vritti*s. They whip through your mind like a storm over the ocean, making it choppy, rough, forceful, and destructive. The practice of yoga calms the storm to create a state of *nirodhaha*; it removes the ripples from your mind so your consciousness is clear, calm, and smooth.

1.3 Tada Drasthu Svarupe Avasthanam

> **TADA:** Here it is; there; then
>
> **DRASHDAHU:** From *drish*, which means "to see"; the witness; they who see from within
>
> **SVARUPE:** *Sva* is the Self and *rupe* is a form or manifestation; the true manifestation of our Self
>
> **AUVASTANAM:** *Auva* is coming down; *sta* is to stand firmly; *nam* is to love, revere and respect; being firmly established; to dwell or reside; to radiate (also the root of the word "avatar")

It is only once we are living yoga as it is defined that we can recognize and reside in our true self; that of God (the see-er).

The previous Sutra describes the practice of yoga (in a nutshell) and this Sutra explains what happens if we're able to achieve that practice. When we begin to live our yoga as described—i.e. remove the *vritti*s to reveal a state of *nirodhaha*—we will be able to recognize our true Self; the fact that God, the see-er of all things, lives within us. But this process is up to you. No one can show you the true divinity within, you must discover it through your own practice.

1.4 Vritti Sarupyam Itaratra

VRITTI: The fluctuations and agitations of the mind; our patterns and behavior

SARUPYAM: To put together with; to be attached to the form

ITARATRA: of the night; refers to the subconscious; not being able to see ourselves

The Yoga Sutras of Patanjali

When we are not in that state of yoga, our tendency is to not only identify with the vrittis but to project them.

NICKI: I used to blame my parents for a lot of my behavior. Once I had kids, I saw them demonstrating that same negative, defensive behavior I attributed to my parents. It forced me to realize all my undesired behavior actually belongs to me, not my parents, and if I don't deal with those *vritti*s now I'll project them onto the most important people in my life. In short, we have to take personal responsibility for our words, actions, and emotions to break the patterns that cause us pain.

This Sutra warns us what will happen if we don't have the tools to achieve the practice of yoga: we will be governed by our *vritti*s. We'll identify with their negative, disruptive energy and carry it through our daily lives. Worse yet, we will often project those *vritti*s onto everyone and everything around us.

Projecting negativity is the complete opposite of taking personal responsibility. It is endemic in our Western world. We project our insecurities, pain, and anger onto everyone around us because we're unwilling (or unable) to look at those emotions and deal with them ourselves. It's increasingly common to blame someone else for everything we see, think, feel, and experience, and it's not just the bad days or catastrophic events. *Vritti*s can wrap themselves around your entire personality. They can become embedded in your life.

One example of toxic projections that hits particularly close to home is when students say a particular teacher "hurt them" in yoga and blame the teacher for their injury. We're sympathetic, but unless that teacher was physically pushing you toward the injury, they didn't actually hurt you. You hurt yourself. You pushed past your early indications of pain, which only you can feel, and continued to follow general instructions despite your personal needs. You also chose to study with that particular teacher and attend that particular class. It's easy to see yourself as a victim, but in truth, you are responsible for your pain. If you do not recognize the subconscious decisions that put you there you'll probably continue to get hurt.

Just to be clear, managing your *vritti*s isn't about beating yourself up for things you cannot control. Taking personal responsibility doesn't mean you're inherently evil or always at fault. You shouldn't seek to internalize pain you did not create or to let the guise of "personal responsibility" shield you from sorrow and grief. Sometimes you truly have no control over your circumstance, and the emotional processes that arise from trauma are completely natural and valid. But it's important to recognize that there doesn't have to be any blame to create resolution. Guilt and shame are *vritti*s too. They're stagnant, corrosive emotions.

Managing your *vritti*s is more about analyzing the destructive mental gymnastics we put ourselves through and breaking the thought patterns that govern our lives. It's about beginning to unravel our own story by finding the truth beneath our thoughts and actions and moving forward with patience, intelligence, and compassionate self-observation.

The Yoga Sutras of Patanjali

1.5 Vrittayah Panchatayyah Klista Aklistah

VRITTAYAH: The *vritti*s

PANCHATAYYAH: *Pancha* means 5; fivefold

KLISTA: Painful

AKLISTAH: Seemingly non-painful

There are five painful vritti*s and five seemingly non-painful* vritti*s.*

This Sutra divides the *vritti*s into two categories: five that do not seem painful but can create unintentional suffering and five that are definitely painful. The next Sutra (1.6) goes on to describe the five seemingly non-painful *vritti*s, which are correct knowledge, delusion, imagination, sleep, and memory. The five painful Sutras are described in detail in the second book (*Sadhana Pada*) as the *klesha*s, which are ignorance, egotism, attachment, aversion, and fear of death. The painful ramifications of the last five *vritti*s are pretty obvious but the five non-painful ones leave much more room for interpretation.

The first one, correct knowledge, encourages us to retain our capacity for critical thinking. We need to acknowledge that all knowledge can be biased. The things we "know" to be true are the result of a specific circumstance and social construct. The walls in which that knowledge was built may prohibit you from understanding truths that arise from a different social construct, so it's important to look behind the curtain. Leave room in your mind to ingest the fact that "correct" knowledge may be completely wrong. Holding stubbornly to false "correct" knowledge will almost certainly bring you pain.

Imagination is another tricky one to decipher. What could possibly be wrong with daydreaming? There's nothing inherently wrong with it, but if left unchecked, it creates a corrosive mental escape from the present. You are living in this moment, right now, whether you like it or not. If your imagination is always spiriting you away from the here and now, you're less likely to acknowledge and address the challenges of your present circumstance. In that sense, imagination facilitates an aversion from pain; it's a kind of mental antalgia. And as we learned in *asana*, avoiding pain in the present creates more pain in the future. To look at it in a more uplifting light, the happiness you pursue in your imagination will never manifest if you don't stay present to create it.

Delusion, sleep, and memory are a little more straightforward. Delusion is an extension of knowledge and imagination: clinging to "correct" knowledge and imagination can create a state of delusion. Living in delusion may not seem painful until the walls of that suspended reality come crashing down around you. The painful side of sleep is also pretty easy to understand: rest is good, but too much sleep results in lethargy and sloth. The painful side of memory comes from our imperfect human thinking apparatus; your mind has a powerful ability to distort the facts of the past. Your brain is not a computer (thank goodness), and failing to recognize the fallible nature of your mental filing system will almost always bring you pain.

These five seemingly non-painful *vritti*s remind us that even seemingly innocuous things can lead us astray, which underlines the importance of the next foundational Sutra (which is actually in the next book, *Sadhana Pada*).

2.10 Te Pratiprasava Heyah Suksmah

> TE: These
>
> PRATIPRASAVA: The involution; *prat* is in opposition to; *prasava* is to draw forth
>
> HEYA: to abandon; to abstain; to desert
>
> SUKSHMAH: subtle; minute; delicate; sweet

When the obstacles do not appear to be present, don't think for a minute that they are truly absent. Go inside and be vigilant; pay attention to the details and remember what you already know.

This is one of our all-time favorite Sutras. The moment you think you "know it all" is the most dangerous moment of all. That false assertion contains the seed of true ignorance. If you don't uproot that seed immediately, the toxic fruit can take you all the way back to the most crude, basic state of human nature; a state of ignorance, egotism, and false superiority. These moments of false understanding require the utmost vigilance. We must develop the patience to look closely at ourselves, inside and out, to find the truth of our situation. You cannot know unless you truly see; you cannot act unless you truly know; and you cannot change unless you truly act. You must look closely at yourself to unravel the patterns that create your circumstance.

This Sutra is directly related to *asana*. If you've taken a class with us, you've probably heard it. We even have it on our T-shirts. We use it to remind our students to actually look at themselves to see, in a very physical sense: is your leg truly straight? Are your quadriceps truly engaged? You have to check, check, and check again. You won't really know what your body is doing unless you take the time to look at it. Functioning on assumptions is ineffective and dangerous. This constant vigilance might seem tedious but it's really a fantastic opportunity to spend some quality time with you. Look at yourself, see what's there, and then learn to love it—all of it.

The Yoga Sutras of Patanjali

NICKI:
Humans have the unfortunate habit of believing what we think, whether or not it's true.

2.16 Heyam Duhkham Anagatam

HEYAM: To be avoided; abandoned

DUKHA: Suffering; literally a "bad axle hole" that prohibits a wheel from turning

ANAGATAM: Not yet come; the future

The practice of yoga gives us the tools to alleviate and avoid our future suffering.

The literal interpretation of this Sutra paints a pretty fantastic picture; without yoga, you'll be like a wheel with a bad axle hole: unable to turn and thumping painfully along. That's obviously a bit extreme, but we are living proof that yoga can keep you moving gracefully into the future. The diseases of modern aging stem from congestion, stagnation, and overindulgence; we eat too much, stress too much, and don't move enough. Yoga addresses all of those issues in a fantastic way and in doing so will help alleviate your future suffering.

The Yoga Sutras of Patanjali

Practicing yoga will not allow us to avoid all of our suffering. The first noble truth, as taught by Buddha, is, "In life, there is suffering." It is an inevitable part of our human experience, but yoga provides tools to decrease the depth and duration of your present and future suffering. This applies to suffering in your physical form and your mental/spiritual/emotional form. *Asana* and *pranayama* banish stagnation, congestion, and pain from your body, and as BKS Iyengar said, pain in the body is disease that has not yet manifested. Yoga allows you to remove it from your body now, before it removes you from this earth. The refined mental state achieved in *asana* and *pranayama* teaches you to be fully conscious in every moment, and that evolved consciousness allows you to make decisions in the present that positively affect your future. It's compressed evolution.

2.46 Sthira Sukham Asanam

> **STHIRA:** Steadiness; strength; endurance; stability
>
> **SUKHAM:** Ease; sweetness; the root of the word "sugar"
>
> **ASANAM:** pose; posture of the body and mind

Asana is a state of effort without tension and a state of relaxation without being dull.

This is probably the most widely known Sutra in modern yoga. The eloquent interpretation above comes from TKV Desikachar, and we have always found it to be perfectly concise. The outer form of a yoga pose is just anatomical geometry; the true quality of *asana* is defined by the state of your body and mind. If you're in *trikonasana* but your kneecap is sluggish and your mind is wandering, you're not doing *asana*. The opposite is also true: if you're holding *trikonasana* while gasping for breath and clenching your jaw, you're not doing *asana*. *Asana* is achieved by striking a perfect balance between seemingly-opposite qualities: strength and softness; action and ease; steadiness and dynamism; sun and moon. These energies complement and complete each other. Cultivating one without the other will create an imbalance in your practice, and when a system is imbalanced, it will eventually collapse.

2.47 Prayatna Shaithilya Ananta Samapattibhyam

> **PRAYATNA:** To bring forth the sincere effort; *pra* is to bring forth and *yatna* is sincere, persevering energy; effort

The Yoga Sutras of Patanjali

SHAI: Finding stillness; derived from *shanti*, meaning "peace"

THILYA: To loosen or slacken

ANANTA: The serpentine/kundalini energy; the latent or potential energy that lies coiled at the base of your spine

SAMA: Even; equal

PATTHIBH: Assuming the original form; the completion; the conclusion

YAM: An emphatic affirmative suffix

Relax the intensity of your effort and meditate on the endless energy within because this process never ends.

This is another of our favorite yoga-class Sutras because it's so incredibly relevant. *Asana* challenges your physical body as a means to stir your psyche, and that churning often generates physical, mental, and emotional intensity. It's easy to get lost in that intensity; to grit your teeth, furrow your brow, and surrender your mind to a deafening roar of thoughts and emotions. That intensity may appear to be part of the process, but this Sutra reminds us that intensity is something we ascribe to the process. It is not a necessary ingredient. The clenched jaw and mind-numbing static will not bring you closer to the *asana* or to your Self. The quiet energy of spiritual growth lives deep underneath that surface noise, and it's this calm, sincere energy that will bring you forward on the long path to freedom. And if it wasn't this *asana* that provoked your intensity it would be something else: your job, your spouse, your children; the list is endless. If it wasn't this practice it would certainly be something else. Use this opportunity to harness the persevering current that lives beneath the intensity of your effort.

2.48 Tatah Dvandvah Anabhighatah

TATAH: Therefor; it follows

DVANDVAH: To divide

ANABHIGHATAH: The stopping or cessation of the disturbances

When we can relax the intensity of our effort, it is then that our mind is truly free of disturbances.

The Yoga Sutras of Patanjali

If we can achieve the directives of the two preceding Sutras (steadiness and ease; relax the intensity of your effort) the seemingly opposite duality of body and mind will finally merge into a single divine entity free of disturbances. BKS Iyengar called it, "perfection in action and freedom in consciousness."

This Sutra tells us it doesn't matter how we come to yoga—old, young, rich, poor, unhealthy, etc.—as long as we come with sincerity, this place is open for us. Yoga is available to all who have sincere effort, and for those individuals, it will make the impossible possible.

FUNCTIONAL ANATOMY

The anatomical concepts presented here are broad generalizations. The bones and tissues we describe may not perfectly reflect the shape of your body because you are completely unique. Our goal is to explain the anatomical foundations of posturally integrated movement, and we'll keep it as simple as possible. Anatomical concepts will not be explained in their entirety, they will be explained only as they relate to yoga.

This information is not intended to diagnose or cure a disease or injury. If you think you have a serious injury please consult a physician. Yoga may have fantastic tools to help address your injury but yoga cannot help unless you know what's going on in your anatomy. Western medicine has some of the best diagnostic tools on the planet, especially when it comes to bones and muscles. Get an X-ray or MRI to figure out what's going on in your body, and once you have an accurate diagnosis, consult an experienced yoga instructor to identify which of yoga's many tools are appropriate for your situation.

FORM VS. FUNCTION

The study of anatomy in yoga brings up a fundamental question: does form follow function or does function follow form? Was your anatomical shape created by your patterns, your life choices, and your physical and emotional behavior or have the circumstances of your life, your decisions, your behavior, and your emotions been dictated by your anatomical shape?

We believe form follows function. Making a conscious decision to use your body differently will absolutely change its shape. Eddie watched it happen in his spine. At 28 years old he had bone spurs and slipped discs. Now, at 66 years old, he has no bone spurs and no slipped discs. His discs look healthier at 66 than they did at 28. His spinal pathology was completely altered with absolutely no allopathic intervention, only the precise and deliberate practice of yoga.

BONES

Your skeleton is a compromise between movement and stability. Areas of your body that need to move, like your neck and shoulders, sacrifice stability in favor of movement. Areas that need to be stable, like your hips and ribs, sacrifice movement in favor of stability. It is an evolutionary blueprint that has served

Functional Anatomy

us well for thousands of years, and yoga supports its core anatomical principles through the use of integrated structural alignment.

Bones and the Piezoelectric Force

The piezoelectric force is an electrical current that accumulates solid material in response to pressure. In your bones, the "solid material" is calcium and the "pressure" is how you use your bones. Piezoelectricity moves through a bone in the direction of the force you put through it. Using a bone in the same way all the time (i.e. your movement patterns; the way you walk, stand, lean, etc.) solidifies the force line and causes calcium to accumulate in the direction of the force. When the force line is anatomically indicated the piezoelectric force strengthens the natural density of the bone. When the force line is not anatomically indicated the piezoelectric force can cause painful calcium deposits called bone spurs.

Bone spurs are a product of pressure, repetition, and time. They can develop on the bones of any joint that is pressurized in an anatomically incorrect direction. Bunions are a perfect example. The bones in the front of your foot are designed to press weight through your big toe bone, in the direction of your big toe. If your big toe is pushed toward your little toe (perhaps by a pair of beautiful stilettos), the force line goes out the side of your big toe bone instead. Piezoelectricity follows this line and lays down calcium on the outside of the bone, i.e. on the inside of your foot. This calcium builds up to create the bunion, bringing inflammation and extreme pain to the big toe bone of your foot.

Yoga will change the piezoelectric forces acting within your body. Arranging your skeleton in the direction of yoga changes the force lines running through your bones, which changes the direction of calcium buildup in your bones. It can halt the development of bone spurs and begin to assimilate displaced calcium back into your body. It is further proof that form follows function; the precise placement of your bones will absolutely change the shape of your body.

SPINAL ANATOMY

Your spine is composed of four integrated segments. It is important to understand how each of these four segments is designed to move and the indications and contraindications that apply to each.

Foundational Terms

Flexion is a forward bend and **extension** is a backbend.

The **articular face** of a bone is the exact place where one bone interacts with another bone. It's where your bones communicate their motion. The shape of the articular face determines the nature of the conversation, i.e. how each bone moves in relation to the other.

Functional Anatomy

Condyles and **processes** are knobs, bumps, or ridges that extend off the main body a bone. They are usually located on or near the articular face of a bone.

Vertebrae are the individual bones that make up your spine. "Vertebra" is a single bone and "vertebrae" is plural.

There are 24 vertebrae in the top three segments of your spine: the **cervical**, **thoracic**, and **lumbar**.

There are eight to nine fused vertebrae that form your **sacrum** (five to six vertebrae) and **coccyx** (three to four vertebrae).

The sacrum and coccyx are located underneath L5, the last lumbar vertebra. The sacrum is the back of your pelvis and the coccyx is your tailbone.

There are four natural curves in your spine. The **cervical spine** (neck) curves toward your front body, the **thoracic spine** curves toward your back body, the **lumbar spine** curves toward your front body, and the **sacrum** curves toward your back body. The forward (inward) curves are called lordosis and the backward (outward) curves are called kyphosis.

Vertebra

Vertebrae are the individual bones that make up your spine. Your 24 individual vertebrae are divided into three sections based on their shape, location, and function:

Functional Anatomy

Seven cervical vertebrae (C1 – C7) make up the cervical spine that forms your neck;

Twelve thoracic vertebrae (T1 – T12) make up the thoracic spine that forms your chest and ribcage;

Five lumbar vertebrae (L1 – L5) make up the lumbar spine that forms your lower back.

The sacrum and coccyx are located below your lumbar spine, underneath L5. The sacrum is a triangle-shaped bone that connects your spine to your pelvis. It simultaneously serves as the base of your spine and the back of your pelvic girdle. The coccyx is your tailbone. It sits below your sacrum and is pointed toward the base of your pelvis.

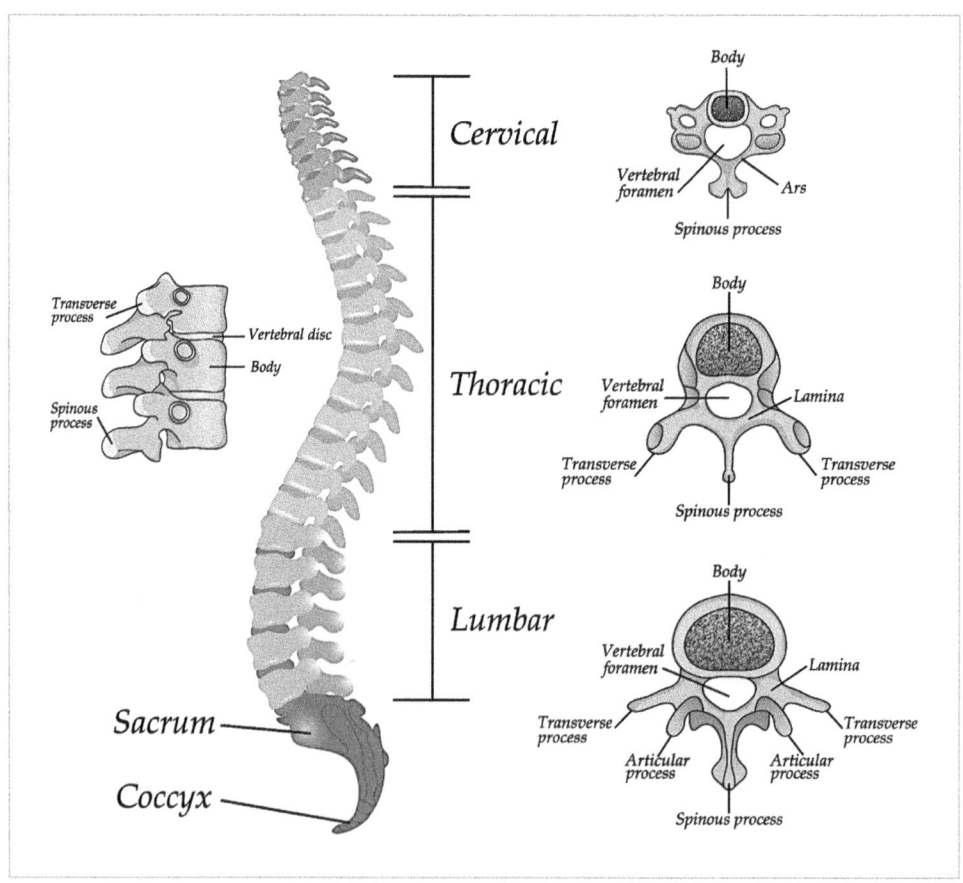

16.a Segments of the spine and sample vertebra from each section.

The top two vertebrae of the spine are called the Atlas and the Axis (C1 and C2). They are completely unique, and we'll discuss them in the cervical section. The remaining 22 vertebrae (C3 – L5) differ in their shape and function, but they have a few common structural components we'll describe below.

BODY. The body of each vertebra is a hard, flat disc, like a miniature hockey puck. It is situated on the inside of your spine with the front edge pointing toward your front body. The discs are small and relatively thin at the top of your spine and become thicker and broader as you go down; the body of a lumbar vertebra (in your lower back) is twice as large and thick as the body of a cervical vertebra (in your neck). Positioning the thickest vertebrae at the bottom of your spine provides stability and shock absorption near your hips and legs.

The cylindrical walls of a young vertebral body are straight up and down, and some may even bulge outward like a water balloon squished between two plates. They bulge because their bone tissue is full of fluid, and fluid is synonymous with youth. As you age, your bones dehydrate and begin to shrivel. The walls of the vertebrae become concave like an eroded sandstone cliff. The body responds to this erosion by putting down calcium at the edges of the vertebral body, along the top and bottom edges of the cliff. These calcium deposits can develop into sharp bone spurs at the edge of the vertebral body, at the exact point where the bone touches your intervertebral discs. A vertebral bone spur is like a large, jagged tooth that pushes into your sensitive discs and makes every movement extremely painful.

SPINOUS PROCESS. The spinous process is a bony protrusion that sits on back of each vertebra. It extends off the vertebra's round body like a dorsal fin and forms the bumpy ridge that makes your spine visible on your back. The shape of each vertebra's spinous process determines the amount of extension it can safely support; i.e. how much that vertebra can tilt in a backbend. Short, horizontal spinous processes allow for a lot of extension; long, vertical spinous processes are more restrictive. Together, the spinous processes create an overlapping locking system that keeps your spine from folding over backward. They prohibit you from doing a fully reversed forward bend, such as a backward *uttanasana*. But their varying shapes do allow for limited amounts of extension in each part of your spine, and together they facilitate healthy backbends like *urdhva dhanurasana*.

The shape and angle of the spinous processes change radically from one spinal segment to the next. The length and slope of each spinous process either

Functional Anatomy

facilitates or restricts extension for that vertebra and helps determine the anatomically indicated movement for that spinal segment. A long, steeply sloped spinous process rests on top of the spinous process of the vertebra below it, and this overlap restricts extension; the vertebra can only tilt a little bit before it locks into place against the spinous processes above and below it. But a short, moderately sloped spinous process will not overlap, and that vertebra can tilt much further; the next spinous process is further away so it can lift and lower without running into another bony locking mechanism.

VERTEBRAL FORAMEN. The vertebral foramen is a hole behind the round body of each vertebra. It sits toward the back of your spine, between the body of the vertebra and the spinous process (i.e. between the hockey puck and the dorsal fin). Your spinal cord threads through this hole, and that's one of the main reasons we care about safe spinal movement. Your spinal cord provides instructions to every part of your body. Vertebrae are like specialized armor for the cord and its intricate network of nerve roots and branches, and pushing vertebrae in the wrong direction can endanger this precious cargo.

TRANSVERSE PROCESSES. The transverse processes extend off the side of each vertebra like wings, with one on either side of the vertebral foramen. They are behind the body of the vertebra and roughly perpendicular to the spinous process (behind the hockey puck and on either side of the dorsal fin). They provide muscle attachments for the paraspinal muscles, a tight muscular network that crisscrosses your spine to create stability and movement. The transverse processes are like a set of handlebars that allow your paraspinal muscles to steer each vertebra and facilitate movement in your spine.

INTERVERTEBRAL FACET JOINTS. Each vertebra articulates (communicates) with the next vertebra in line at the intervertebral facet joints. The shape and position of the intervertebral facet joints determine the way each vertebra can move in relation to the next. They differ from the spinous processes because they can influence the flexion, extension, and twisting capacity of each vertebra and are thus the most important determinants of safe spinal movement.

The intervertebral facet joints are located on the articulating processes of each vertebra, which are little knobs that extend off the top and bottom. The articulating processes on the bottom of each vertebra reach down to touch the articulating processes on the top of the next vertebra, and the place where they overlap forms the intervertebral facet joints. There is a set of left and right articulating processes on the top and bottom of each vertebra, meaning there are four articulating processes (two top and two bottom) for each vertebra and two intervertebral facet joints between each set of vertebrae (left and right). To illustrate: the top left articulating process of one vertebra overlaps with the bottom left articulating process of the vertebra above it, and the place where they overlap is the left intervertebral facet joint for that set of vertebrae *(17.c.2)*.

Functional Anatomy

Intervertebral facet joints are usually located between the vertebral foramen (spinal column) and the spinous process, but their exact position changes for each segment of your spine. In the cervical spine (neck), they are located toward the front of the spine, close to the body of the vertebra. In the thoracic spine (ribcage) they are located on the sides of the vertebra, roughly between the body and the spinous process. In the lumbar spine (lower back) they are toward the back the vertebra, closer to the spinous process itself.

The shape of the intervertebral facet joints determines how each vertebra can move in relation to the next vertebra in line. They govern flexion, extension, and rotation and are thus more comprehensive than the spinous processes (which really only restrict extension). In general, the facet joints in the cervical spine (neck) facilitate the greatest range of motion, followed by the facet joints in the lumbar spine (lower back). The thoracic facet joints (ribcage) are tightly overlapped, providing the least range of motion from one vertebra to the next.

INTERVERTEBRAL DISCS. There are intervertebral discs between each set of vertebrae, beginning at the bottom of the Axis (C2). The discs are wedged between

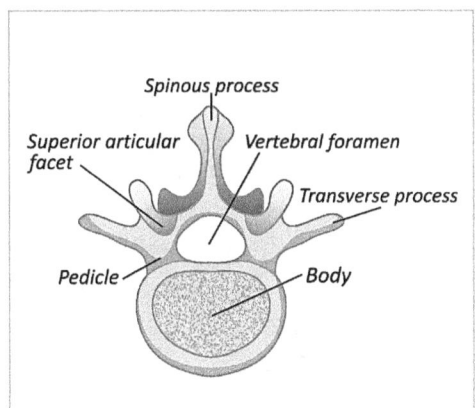 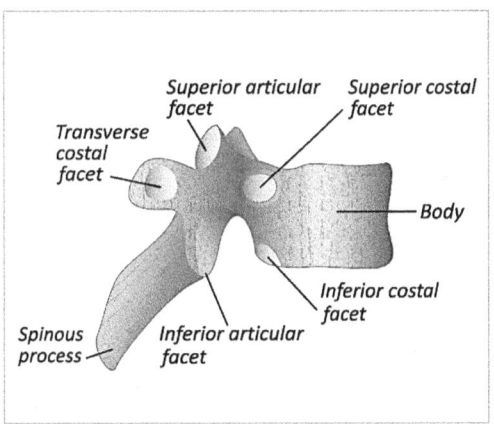

16.b Thoracic vertebra from the top (l) and side (r). Note the superior articular facet (l) and inferior articular facet (r). These two articulating processes connect to create a single intervertebral facet joint.

the body of each vertebra like a jelly donut between the hockey pucks. The size and shape of each disc match the size and shape of its surrounding vertebral bodies: the cervical discs in your neck are small and relatively thin, and the lumbar discs in your lower back are large and thick.

Functional Anatomy

Intervertebral discs are a type of white connective tissue. They have two major components: an outer membrane and an inner nucleus. The outer membrane is composed of strong circular ligaments wrapped in alternating layers to create a fibrous ring. This ring holds the shape of the disc together and helps limit its movement. The nucleus is inside of this ring and is filled with an elastic gel. The gel provides shock absorption between each vertebra, and cumulatively it prevents the jarring effects of locomotion from reaching your brain. The discs also function as ligaments between each vertebra as they allow for a small amount of movement while simultaneously holding them in place.

Intervertebral discs do not usually protrude beyond the cylindrical walls of the vertebrae that contain them. That said, most discs have a very slight natural bulge that reflects the spinal curvature of the surrounding vertebrae. The cervical spine curves toward the front body so cervical discs are slightly thicker at the front than the back. The thoracic spine curves toward the back body so thoracic discs are slightly thicker in the back than in the front. The most pronounced bulge is in the lumbar spine, which has the largest intervertebral discs and the strongest spinal curvature. The lumbar discs bulge toward the front of the vertebra more than any other type of disc and this natural bulge makes them more susceptible to injury.

Intervertebral discs are subject to a number of injuries. The most common are bruising/protrusions and herniation/slipped discs. Bruising happens when the disc receives uneven pressure, either from abrupt movement in the surrounding vertebrae or from a long-term muscular imbalance. Bruising can cause the disc to develop an unnatural bulge called a protrusion. It's like stepping on one side of an inflatable inner tube; the pressurized area gets squished and air is pushed to the opposite side. That bulging protrusion can put painful pressure on nerve roots that extend out from the spinal cord, and that pain can radiate out to the body part controlled by that nerve root. The fibrous outer membrane of the disc remains intact, but it will eventually weaken under the pressure of a sustained protrusion.

A herniation/slipped disc occurs when the fibrous outer membrane ruptures and the nucleus releases some of its inner gel-like fluid. The disc does not actu-

Segment	Cervical	Thoracic	Lumbar
Body Part	Neck	Chest & Ribs	Lower Back
Vertebra	7	12	5
Curve	Front Body	Back Body	Front Body
Flexion (forward bend)	Yes	Limited	Yes
Extension (back bend)	Yes	Limited	Yes
Twisting	Yes	Yes	Limited

Functional Anatomy

ally "slip" from its place between the vertebrae, but the loss of fluid causes a significant deflation inside the disc and a subsequent swelling outside the disc. That swelling can put pressure on your nerve roots, and the tear itself releases inflammatory chemicals that can cause severe pain even if the rupture does not directly affect your nerves. It is the most serious and painful type of disc injury.

Spinal Movement

Your vertebrae are designed to protect your spinal cord and intervertebral discs. It's important to know how they are supposed to move and, perhaps more importantly, how they are **not** supposed to move. The "safe" direction for each spinal segment is determined by the shape of its intervertebral facet joints and spinous processes. We will review each segment of the spine individually in the following section, but the general directions are outlined in the chart on the following page.

The table makes it seem pretty straightforward: your chest is stiff and your lower back is bendy. But yoga is all about balance. Your lumbar spine is naturally predisposed toward flexion and extension but that doesn't mean you should focus all your backbends in your lower back. In fact, the segments with the least bony restrictions are usually the most likely to get hurt.

Functional Anatomy

SAFE SPINAL MOVEMENT. Movement in the spine is a sum of all its parts; there is not a lot of movement in any single joint but cumulatively they achieve a fantastic range of motion.

Cumulative movement can be illustrated in the simple act of turning your head to the right. Visualize your head on a 360° circle, where looking straight forward is equivalent to 0° and looking over your right shoulder is 90°. Your top two vertebrae, the Atlas (C1) and Axis (C2), account for 50% of your head's total movement; they bring you to 45° without moving any other part of your body. The intervertebral facet joints between each additional vertebra add a little bit more rotation: the movement between C2 and C3 gets you from roughly 45° to 53°, and the movement between C3 and C4 brings you to 61°. This incremental rotation continues down the cervical spine, so that when you reach C7, you're at a full 90° turn. No individual vertebra could achieve that much movement on its own but together they allow you to look directly over your right shoulder.

Yoga seeks to spread each anatomical movement among as many vertebrae as possible. Sharing spinal movement harnesses the cumulative capacity of all your vertebrae and creates the most effective expression of each pose. Sharing spinal movement also creates the safest expression of each pose by allowing your intervertebral discs to evenly absorb the force and pressure of each action. Forcing movement into a smaller set of vertebrae has the opposite effect: if one segment of the spine is locked in place, the remaining segments have to work twice as hard to achieve the desired movement. This creates a "hinging" action between the individual vertebrae and forces the pressure of each movement into a smaller number of intervertebral discs.

Take the above example, where the vertebrae of the cervical spine work together to look over your right shoulder. If the middle vertebrae of your cervical spine are stiff the remaining vertebrae will have to pick up the slack. Pressure always looks for the weakest link, and in this case, the "weakest" link is the most flexible vertebrae: the Atlas and the Axis. These two vertebrae have the least bony restrictions against movement. To accomplish the task of looking over your right shoulder, they will begin to move far beyond their normal range of motion. It's the same kind of recruiting we mentioned earlier in the book: your body recruits flexibility from C1 and C2 to compensate for stiffness in the rest of your neck. These two bones may absorb an additional 15° or 20° of rotation that was supposed to come from the vertebrae below them, and in the long run, this recruiting can damage the structural integrity of C1 and C2.

SEGMENTS OF THE SPINE

Cervical Spine

There are seven vertebrae in the cervical spine. They are the smallest vertebrae but they have a huge responsibility: they connect your skull to your spine and provide your head with a fantastic range of motion.

OCCIPUT, ATLAS AND AXIS. The base of your skull is called the occiput. At the bottom of the occiput, where your head connects to your spine, there are two narrow ridges called occipital condyles. These condyles run from front to back and are roughly parallel to each other. They nest into two corresponding grooves on top of the Atlas (C1), which is the topmost vertebra in your cervical spine. The occipital condyles and the corresponding grooves in the Atlas allow your skull to smoothly slide back and forth, like a wheel on a track. They facilitate flexion and extension, i.e. the movement of nodding your head to say, "Yes." The Atlas also has wide transverse processes to provide lateral (side to side) stability for the broad circumference of your skull. It operates just like the Atlas of Greek mythology: it carries the weight of the world on its broad shoulders.

The bottom of the Atlas has two condyles that nest into corresponding grooves on the Axis (C2). These condyles are organized in a ring to facilitate rotation, i.e. the movement of looking left and right and shaking your head to say, "No." The Axis also has a vertical peg that extends up through the open ring of the Atlas, called the dens, and it further enables the Atlas to swivel on top of the Axis.

The Atlas and the Axis have a very different shape than the rest of your vertebrae. Most vertebrae have a flat bony disc in the middle that forms the vertebral body, but the Atlas and Axis are hollow. Their vertebral bodies are more like a ring than a hockey puck, and the top of the spinal cord runs through this ring and into the base of your skull. In other words, the Atlas and the Axis have a large vertebral foramen that takes the place of their vertebral bodies.

To recap: the joint between the occipital condyles and the Atlas facilitates the "yes" movement of your head. The joint between the Atlas and the Axis facili-

Functional Anatomy

Functional Anatomy

tates the "no" movement of your head. The combined movement between these three structural components accounts for roughly 50% of your head's total range of motion. There are no intervertebral discs between the Atlas and the occipital condyles or between the Atlas and the Axis. Intervertebral discs begin in the space between the Axis and C3.

CERVICAL SPINE: C3 THROUGH C7. The shape of your cervical vertebrae (neck) facilitates more movement than any other part of your spine. The articular processes do not completely overlap on a vertical or horizontal plane so the intervertebral facet joints are broad and gently sloped. They don't have a strong locking mechanism on either side; they can twist, fold, and extend with very few bony restrictions. The spinous processes of the cervical vertebrae are equally accommodating; they point almost straight back, and each one has a small notch at the end that allows it to nest deeper into the next one *(17.d.1)*. The deeper the notch the more each spinous process can tilt up or down before it runs into the next spinous process and the higher you can look without moving the rest of your body.

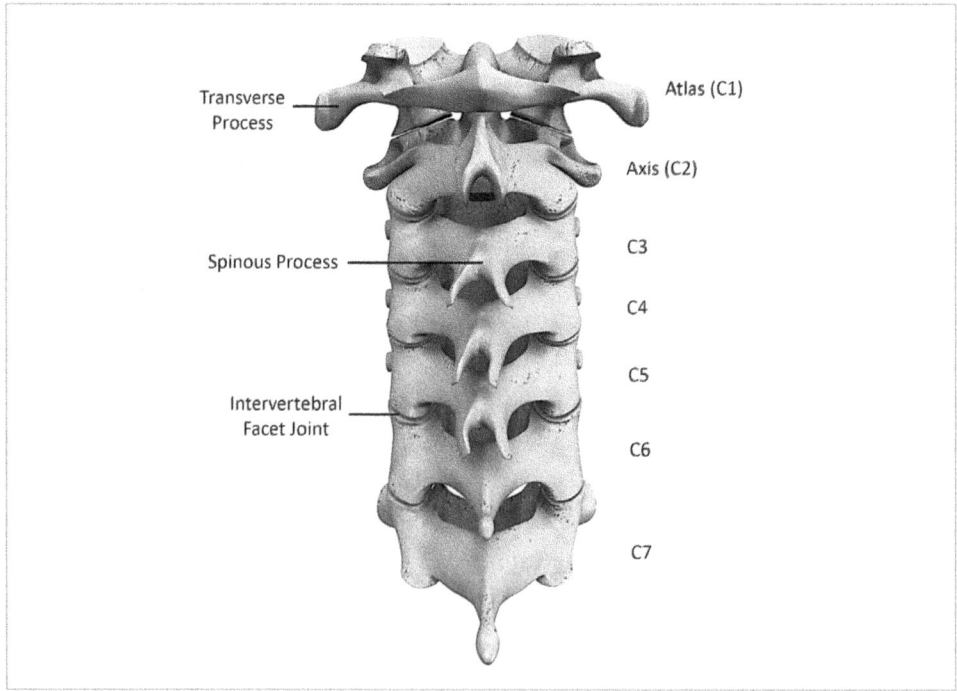

16.c Cervical spine, posterior view. Note the unique shape of the Atlas and Axis (top two vertebrae) and the deep notches in the spinous processes.

The spinous processes of the middle cervical vertebrae, C3 and C4, are the most steeply sloped of all the cervical vertebrae. They do the most to restrict extension (backbends) in the cervical spine; they are the lynchpin that keeps your neck from flipping backward when you look up. But they are also shorter than the other five cervical vertebrae, leaving those other vertebrae lots of room to tilt up and down. This extra space, combined with the unrestricted facet joints and the notches in the end of the spinous processes, allows your neck a truly amazing amount of extension.

The spinous process of the last cervical vertebra, C7, is almost horizontal. It points straight out behind you and often protrudes more than any other vertebra. It's the bone you can feel sticking out at the very base of your neck.

MOVEMENT IN THE CERVICAL SPINE. The cervical spine's fantastic range of motion dramatically improves your reaction time to the world around you. It allows you to quickly look over your shoulder and see what's sneaking up behind you. If you had to turn your whole body around to look behind you, you might not see that tiger until it's too late.

Unfortunately, the same structural freedom that makes your life easier also makes it easy to injure your neck. The relative ease of flexion and extension makes the cervical spine prone to hyperextension and hypermobility. The most structurally stable vertebrae are the middle ones, C3 – C5, so it's usually the vertebrae above and below them that become hypermobile. Hypermobility can put uneven pressure on your intervertebral discs, and over time, putting too much uneven pressure on a disc will weaken its outer membrane. Disc ruptures are most common in the discs between C5 and C7 and a rupture in this area affects the nerve roots leading to your arms and hands.

The Atlas and the Axis (C1 and C2) don't have an intervertebral disc between them (intervertebral discs start between the Axis and C3), but too much movement between them can weaken their ligaments and lead to subluxation. Subluxation is a slight dislocation that pushes the vertebra out of line in relation to its neighboring vertebrae. It can be extremely painful, and it can also have huge consequences for your nervous system.

If your cervical spine is capable of that much movement, should you avoid it completely? We certainly don't think so. As always, we think you should use yoga to cultivate balance. Use your practice to keep your entire neck supple and moving freely because stiffness in one vertebra may force other vertebrae to

Functional Anatomy

Functional Anatomy

become hypermobile. Stiffness also poses its own long-term threats: congestion, disintegration, and disease. But it is equally important to move your neck with intelligence. Moving quickly in a direction that is already stiff or painful can injure your discs and the nerves that surround them. Always move slowly and keep your throat soft to avoid bringing tension into your movement. When turning your head in a pose like *trikonasana*, keep your chin low to maintain lots of space at the back of your neck. Do not force movement or pressure toward the base of your skull, and never move in the direction of sharp, hot pain.

Thoracic Spine

There are twelve thoracic vertebrae. Each one is attached to a set of ribs to form your ribcage, the protective cage that houses your heart and lungs. The ribcage and thoracic spine work together to provide stability for these vital organs, and as such, they are not designed to accommodate very much movement.

THORACIC SPINE: T1–T11. The thoracic vertebrae have more bony restrictions than any other spinal vertebrae. The thoracic intervertebral facet joints operate on a vertical plane roughly parallel to the front of your body. They're like a pair of curved sliding glass doors: each one can turn left or right in relation to the next, allowing the vertebrae to twist quite well. But this vertical overlap strongly restricts flexion and extension. To illustrate: the bottom articulating process of T1 is directly behind the top articulating process of T2. When T1 tries to tilt up in a backbend it runs into the top of T2, and this bone-on-bone restriction stops the backbend from going further. Most of the thoracic joints can facilitate a tiny bit of extension via cumulative action but it's more restricted than any other part of your spine. It's like trying to open a sliding glass door by picking up the bottom of the door; you can probably get it to move a little bit but not enough to get through.

The spinous process of the first thoracic vertebra (T1) points straight back, similar to the last vertebra of the cervical spine (C7, the one that sticks out at the bottom of your neck). This angle allows for a brief continuation of the flexion and extension of the cervical spine, but the spinous processes of T2 - T4 begin to slope downward at a rapid rate. The spinous processes of the middle thoracic vertebrae (T5 - T8) are more steeply sloped than any other spinous processes, standing almost straight up and down. This strong overlap provides very little space for flexion or extension in the center of your upper back. That restriction

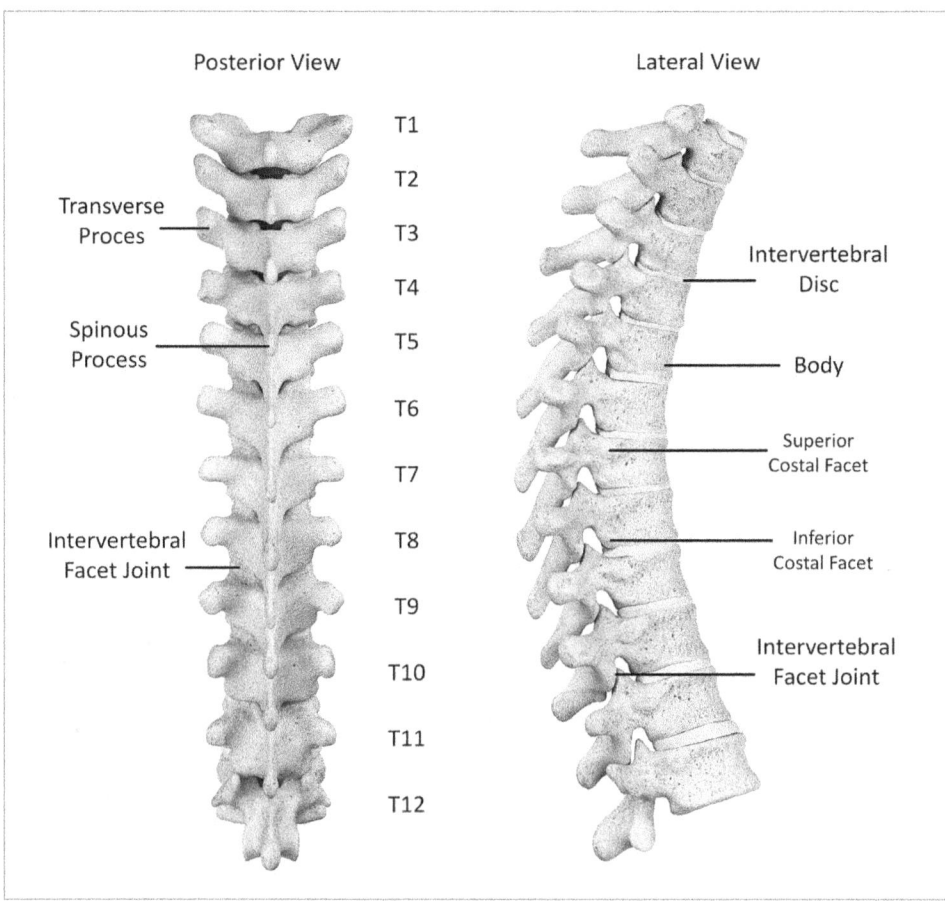

16.d Thoracic spine, posterior and lateral view. Intervertebral facet joints are posterior-facing and easiest to view in the lateral image. Costal facets provide attachments for rib bones.

is reinforced by your ribs, which are connected to the sternum (breastbone) in your front body. The sternum keeps the ribs in place and the spinous processes keep the vertebrae in place, so there's not very much movement on either side of the ribcage. It's a pretty solid piece of your anatomy.

The angle of the spinous processes eases slightly as you move from T8 to the top of T12, gradually allowing more flexion and extension between the vertebrae. The ribs connected to these bottom five vertebrae are called the "false ribs" because they are not directly connected to the sternum. The top three are only connected to the costal cartilage of the ribs above them and the bottom two sets are called the "floating" ribs. They are connected to their corresponding vertebrae (T11 and T12) but do not have any connection to the rest of the ribs. They

Functional Anatomy

can move further away from your ribcage than the other "true" ribs, and that freedom provides a little more flexion and extension than the preceding thoracic vertebrae.

THORACIC SPINE: T12. The last thoracic vertebra, T12, represents the most dramatic structural change in the length of your spine. The intervertebral facet joints at the top of T12 mirror the preceding thoracic vertebrae; they facilitate rotation and restrict extension. They can twist but they aren't very good at backbends. The intervertebral facet joints at the bottom of T12 are completely different. They have no bony restrictions against flexion or extension, but they restrict rotation. They can backbend like crazy but they aren't very good at twisting. It's as though the bone has split personalities: the top is thoracic and the bottom is lumbar. The top will twist but doesn't bend; the bottom will bend but doesn't twist.

This drastic shift makes T12 the most readily accessible "hinge" in your spine. In a backbend, the bottom half of the bone (lumbar) does most of the bending while the top (thoracic) stays straight. This "hinge" creates an acute angle instead of an even arc, and the backbend becomes compressed and angular instead of broad and rounded. The pressure of the backbend gets pushed into the disc between T12 and L1 instead being shared throughout the length of your spine.

In a twist, the top of the bone is free but the bottom is locked. The top (thoracic) can twist magnificently but the bottom (lumbar) cannot twist at all; the

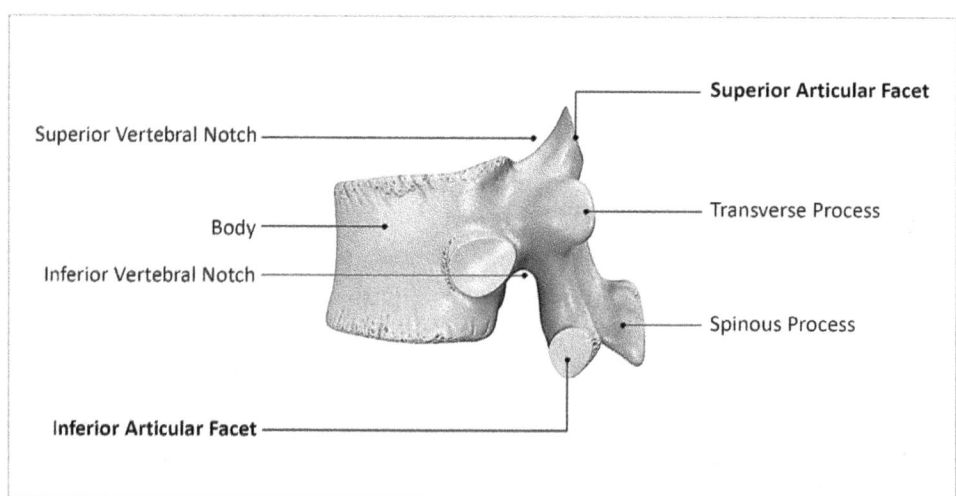

16.e Vertebra T12, lateral view. Note the superior articular facet faces straight back, consistent with the thoracic spine, but the inferior articular facet faces to the side, consistent with the lumbar spine.

shape of the five lumbar vertebrae strongly limits rotation. If the pelvis is also locked in place—i.e. students have been instructed to keep their hips or knees level—the pressure of the twist moves straight into the sacroiliac joint.

T12 is the most bi-polar bone in your body, and to further complicate things, there are ribs attached. They are the smallest ribs in your body but they are present nonetheless. The only saving grace of this anatomical blooper is that the floating ribs can help you identify hinging in T12. If there is a rapid, angular descent from the floating ribs to the pelvis in a backbend like *urdhva dhanurasana* (upward facing bow) you may be hinging in T12. The floating ribs can also come into play in *adho mukha svanasana* (downward facing dog). Instructing students to "contain" their lower floating ribs in downward dog keeps them from sagging into T12, and it also reinforces the natural curvature of the thoracic and lumbar spine.

RIBS & TRANSVERSE PROCESSES. The transverse processes (wings) of the thoracic spine are larger than the transverse processes of the cervical spine because they have a bigger job to do. Each thoracic transverse process has two additional facet joints that provide attachments for a rib bone. One joint is on the inside of the transverse process and faces the front body; the other is near the base of the transverse process and faces the side body. This set of joints accommodates two ribs for each vertebral bone: one on either side of the vertebral body. They support the head of the ribs from the front and the back, allowing for a lot of lateral movement (side to side) without the danger of dislocation. The front end of each "true" rib is also held in place by strong cartilage that connects to the sternum, which creates even more front-to-back stability in the ribcage.

MOVEMENT IN THE THORACIC SPINE. Thoracic facet joints are very well suited to rotation, i.e. twists. They cannot create as much rotation as the cervical spine but they are far more capable than the lumbar spine. Twists that originate in the thoracic spine and expand through the cervical spine are anatomically indicated. The ribcage is also well suited to lateral expansion (horizontal; out to the side), which happens when you breathe. You can increase this capacity through the practice of *pranayama*. The accordion-fold blanket used in *viloma* is particularly well suited to encouraging lateral expansion through the ribcage.

The thoracic spine has the strongest bony restrictions against extension, i.e. against backbends. The spinous processes and the intervertebral facet joints create bony restrictions that prohibit each vertebra from extending in relation to

Functional Anatomy

the next vertebra in line. Paradoxically, these bony restrictions make it the safest place to push your backbends. BKS Iyengar pushed backbends into the middle of the thoracic spine because it is the most difficult place to bend, and hence the safest place to bend. The spine is like specialized armor for your discs and spinal cord, and the thoracic vertebral armor is especially thick and effective. It's very difficult to bend them enough to endanger their precious cargo. The cervical spine and lumbar spine don't have the same bony restrictions and will easily bend more than they should.

Pushing backbends into the middle thoracic spine will also help prohibit you from hinging in T12. Hinging between T12 and L1 is responsible for a tremendous amount of injury in yoga, especially in flexible women. Learning to balance the bend on both sides of T12 will create a healthy, even, sustainable practice.

Lumbar Spine

The five vertebrae of the lumbar spine are the largest vertebral bones in your body. They also have the largest intervertebral discs and virtually no bony restrictions against flexion and extension. This combination makes the lumbar spine one of the most flexible places in your body but also one of the most vulnerable.

LUMBAR SPINE: L1 – L5. The intervertebral facet joints of the lumbar spine are perpendicular to your front body; a full 180° pivot from the thoracic facet joints above them. The articulating processes are stacked side-to-side instead of front-to-back, and this orientation allows them to flex and extend freely: the vertebrae can tilt forward and back without running into each other. But when they try to rotate, they hit a wall. The articulating processes on top of L2 sit directly outside the articulating processes on the bottom of L1, creating a barrier on either side. When L1 tries to turn, it immediately runs into the wall created by L2.

The spinous processes of the lumbar spine continue the easy flexion and extension established by the lumbar facet joints. They point straight back, and the relatively large amount of space between them allows the vertebrae to tilt pretty far back before they run into each other. That freedom translates into a radical backbending capacity in your lower back.

LUMBAR DISCS. Lumbar discs are the largest intervertebral discs in your spine. They are significantly thicker in the front than in the back because the strong curvature of the lumbar spine causes them to bulge toward your front body. The discs between L3 and the sacrum have the biggest bulge, and this natural bulge

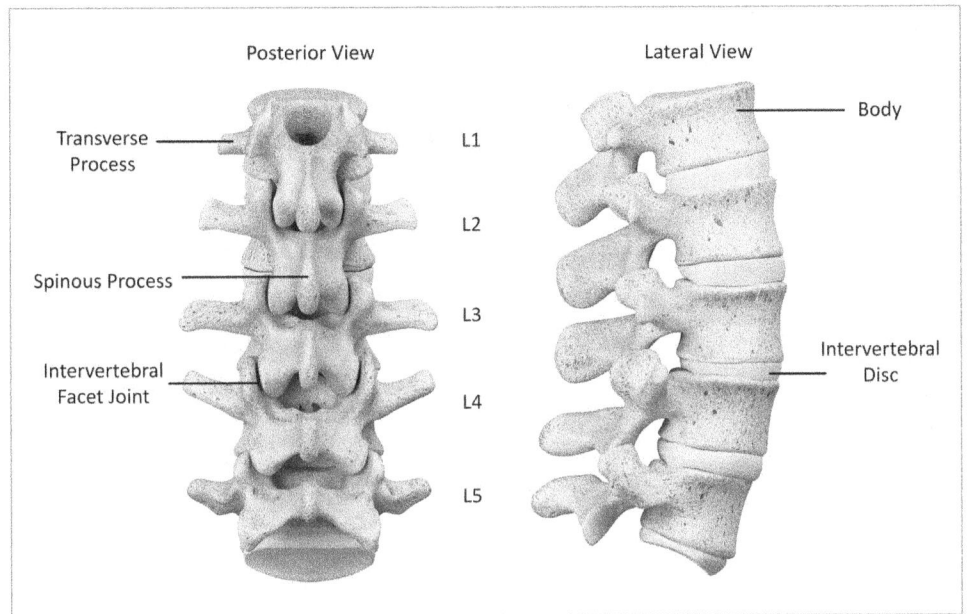

16.f Lumbar spine, posterior and lateral view. A typical lumbar curvature is more lordotic than the curve displayed in this image, with discs that are significantly thicker in front than in back.

Functional Anatomy

makes them more susceptible to injury than any other intervertebral discs. The primary culprit is a combination of flexion and rotation, i.e. twisting in a forward bend.

MOVEMENT IN THE LUMBAR SPINE. The lumbar spine is very, very capable of bending. The lack of bony restrictions allows each vertebra lots of space to extend. Some yoga practitioners may be getting close to a 90° angle from their lumbar spine alone, but your lumbar spine should not be doing all your bending. Pushing backbends into your lumbar spine can jeopardize the integrity of your lumbar discs, and more importantly, it will prohibit you from developing flexibility in the rest of your spine. Backbends are always safest when they are shared; when the force and direction of movement are spread among as many vertebrae as possible.

The lumbar spine is strongly restricted against rotation, but it can accommodate a minimal amount of rotation via cumulative action. Each vertebra can turn a tiny bit, and together the whole segment can turn ever so slightly to the right or left. The cumulative movement is aided by the extra lumbar facet joint on the bottom half of T12; there are only five lumbar vertebrae but there are six sets of

Functional Anatomy

lumbar facet joints. But even with that extra joint, lumbar rotation is much more restricted than thoracic rotation. The lumbar can only achieve a tiny fraction of the range that the thoracic can support, which makes the T12 transition especially problematic. The top of T12 will twist but the bottom will not, and nothing underneath it will twist either.

The most dangerous movement for your lumbar spine is a combination of flexion and rotation, i.e. twisting in a forward bend. Flexion moves the front of the vertebral bodies closer together and pushes the natural bulge at the front of the disc toward the back of the spine. Rotation then pushes it to the side, toward a section of the disc membrane that is significantly narrower than the frontal membrane; the strong lumbar curvature means the membrane is thicker and wider in the front than in the back. Over time, this repeated shift can weaken the disc membrane and cause a painful protrusion. It's like stepping on an inflated inner tube, except that the inner tube is already lopsided. Repeatedly pushing a bubble of compressed air into the narrowest section of the tube will eventually cause that section to lose its elasticity. With additional force and frequent repetition, the vertebral bodies can impose enough stress on the disc membrane to cause a painful protrusion or a complete rupture.

Unfortunately, many practitioners contract their abdomen in twists, which shortens the front body and pushes rotation toward the lower back. They are using strength to deepen the rotation instead of developing length in the spine. It's the dangerous infiltration of conventional exercise physiology; if we're not contracting, we're not working out. But bearing down in a twist is anatomically equal to the most dangerous action for your lower back: a combination of rotation (turning to the side), flexion (bending over), and weight bearing (lifting something heavy).

Bearing down in twists becomes especially problematic when the pelvis is locked. Contracting the front body pushes the twist toward the lumbar spine, but the lumbar vertebrae cannot twist. The twist cannot go up (because the spine is bearing down) so the next available structure is the sacrum. The sacrum is the base of your spine and one of three bones that form your pelvis. It is a large and relatively stable bone, but if the pelvis is locked and the spine is forced to twist, the sacrum can begin to shift. It's particularly dangerous when the femur bones are involved: i.e. when students are instructed to hold their knees level in a twist. Locking the thigh bones into the pelvis creates a pressurized torque against the twist, and the two opposing directions will inevitably come to a head at the sacrum. Shifting the sacrum sets off a problematic antalgic response we'll discuss in the next section.

The safest way to twist is to allow your pelvis to move in tandem with the limited rotation of your lumbar vertebrae. Allowing the pelvis to rotate spreads the twist along the length of your spine and leaves your SI joint happily balanced within the structure of your pelvis. It will harness the cumulative capacity of all your spinal vertebrae and keep your bones working together instead of against each other.

The Sacrum and Sacroiliac Joint

The last lumbar vertebra, L5, sits on top of the sacrum. The sacrum is a triangle-shaped bone comprised of four to six fused vertebrae. It forms the back wall of your pelvic girdle. There is an intervertebral disc between L5 and the sacrum but there are no discs within the sacrum itself. The sacrum curves toward your back body to balance the curve in your lumbar spine, and it ends at the coccyx (tailbone).

The sacrum is one of three bones that make up your pelvis. The other two are the left and right ilium, two very large crescent-shaped bones that form the majority of your pelvis. The sacrum and the ilia meet at the sacroiliac joint (SI joint). There is an SI joint on either side of your sacrum; the left SI joint is where it meets the left ilium and the right SI joint is where it meets the right ilium. The ilia arc forward from the SI joint to create the sides of your pelvic girdle, more commonly understood as your hips. They come together in the front at the pubic symphysis, which is your pubic bone. This "bone" is actually a joint held together by a strong, short ligament. The pubic symphysis combines with the two SI joints to allow a very limited amount of movement in the pubic girdle.

MOVEMENT IN THE SACRUM AND SACROILIAC JOINT. Your sacrum is the base of your spine. It's not supposed to move very much because movement can destabilize everything above it, i.e. the rest of your body. Shifting your sacrum is like twisting the bottom of a tightly coiled spring; the pressure doubles back on itself, and the spring (your spine) gets shorter, tighter, and less resilient. The sacrum does naturally move during childbirth but that movement is only supposed to happen when you're in labor. Many flexible women can unintentionally create a similar movement, and pushing further in that direction can cause serious injuries.

Functional Anatomy

The sacrum is more at risk than most people realize. The articular faces of the SI joints are too large and stable to dislocate, but with enough pressure (and repeated applications of pressure) the sacrum can shift within the structure of the pelvis. The pelvic bones are locked together so a shift in the sacrum causes the left and right ilium to shift as well. The ilia can shift forward and down or up and back to mirror the imbalance in the sacrum. For example, if the top of the sacrum tips forward and to the left, the left ilium will shift forward and down and the right ilium will move up and back. The left frontal hip bone will now be slightly lower than the right frontal hip bone. This shift can create a painful pinching in the sacroiliac joint, and it also sets the foundation for a corresponding spiral in the entire spine.

Destabilizing the sacrum sets off an alarm in your body. It immediately activates the neurosympathetic reflex, your body's most primal defense mechanism. This reflex bounces defensive messages between your muscles and your spinal cord, instructing everything near the sacrum to brace itself against further movement. The psoas and the quadreatus lumborum on the destabilized side become hypertonic to prohibit further movement, and these muscles pull on the lumbar vertebrae. That pull shortens one side of your lumbar spine and sends a ripple effect up your spine as the rest of your body seeks to balance itself in response to the muscular lockdown.

This subconscious anatomical balancing act is an antalgic reaction. Antalgia is your body's natural ability to compensate for pain through posture and motion. Your skeleton will change its shape and function to avoid pain and the imbalances that create it. Destabilizing your sacrum will cause the rest of your body to twist away from the imbalance, and this antalgic response can create a scoliotic spiral through the length of your spine.

Coccyx

The coccyx is your tailbone. It is comprised of three or four fused vertebrae and sits at the very bottom of the sacral curve. The end of your coccyx points toward the base of your pelvis, usually toward the pubic symphysis at the front of your body. It is a very small bone but it plays an important role as the skeletal and energetic base for the bowl of your pelvis.

MOVEMENT IN THE COCCYX. Your tailbone is like your sacrum: it's not supposed to move. It should always be pointed toward the base of your pelvis because it **is** the base of your pelvis. There is no yogic action that points your tailbone away from your pubic bone/pubis. Your tailbone moves toward your pubis in backbends, it moves toward your pubis in forward bends, and it moves toward your pubis in twists. You should never try to "lift" your tailbone. Attempting to lift your tailbone puts pressure on your SI joints and can force the top of your sacrum to dive toward your pubic symphysis. This movement is called "nutation" and it's only supposed to happen during childbirth.

PELVIC ANATOMY

The pelvis is formed by two large sets of fused bones. The left side of your pelvis is formed by the left ilium, ischium, and pubis, and the right side of your pelvis is formed by the right ilium, ischium, and pubis. These two sets combine with the sacrum to create a bowl-shaped cavity that contains your rectum and reproductive organs, commonly known as the pelvic girdle. The ilia (plural for ilium) are two large, crescent shaped bones that create the back and sides of your pelvis. The sacrum runs between the left and right ilium to create the "true" back of your pelvis, but it takes up less space on your back body than the left and right ilium. The crescent ridges of the ilia extend above the sacrum and reach out on either side of your spine to form the broadest part of your hips. They are most visible at the ASIS (Anterior Superior Iliac Spine), otherwise known as your frontal hip bones or those two bony knobs on the front of your hips. You may also be able to feel the rim of the iliac crest on your back and side body, in the space below your waist. The upper rim of the ilia represents the broadest part of your pelvis—the top opening of the pelvic bowl. The walls of the ilia angle inward from this top rim to create a narrower opening at the bottom of your pelvic girdle than at the top.

The pubis is the bony ridge that reaches forward from the ilium to create the front of your pelvis. It sits below and in front of the ilium and forms the front wall of the hip socket. The left and right pubis are joined at the pubic symphysis, which is a cartilaginous joint controlled by a thick ligament. The resulting structure is commonly referred to as your pubic bone, the angular bone that protrudes just above your genitals.

The ischium is at the bottom of the pelvic girdle and it creates the back and bottom walls of the hip socket. It connects the bottom of the ilium to the back side of the pubis, underneath and inside of the pubic bone. The most important element of the ischium is the ischial tuberosity, a circular loop of bone that extends down to create your sit bones (or sits/sitz bones). The front half of this bony loop is formed by the bottom of the pubis and the hole in the middle allows nerves and blood vessels to pass into and out of the pelvis.

Sits Bones / Ischial Tuberosity

The ischial tuberosities are called the "sit bones" because you sit on them. They are covered by your gluteal muscles (butt) when you stand upright, but when you sit down, the gluteus shifts backward and the ischial tuberosities come into contact with the chair. They also create a muscle attachment for your hamstrings, and this attachment is the primary lever for muscular interaction between your pelvis and the back of your legs. It allows you to stretch your hamstrings by rotating your pelvis—an action utilized in poses like *uttanasana* and downward dog—but it can also allow stiffness in your legs to affect the natural tilt of your pelvis.

Pain near the ischial tuberosities is often called "yoga butt." Yoga butt is a painful overstretching of the tendon that attaches your hamstrings to your sit bones, and it often comes from bending your knees in a static forward bend like *uttanasana*. *Uttanasana* stretches the hamstrings by rotating the pelvis around the thigh bones. If your hamstrings are too stiff to straighten your legs, it may seem appropriate to bend your knees. Unfortunately, bending your knees moves the action of the stretch higher up the back of your legs toward the sit bones. The stretch migrates from the broad center of your hamstrings to the narrow sheath of your tendon, forcing the tendon to stretch more than the muscle. The result is a nagging, persistent pain just under your sit bones.

Pelvic Tilt

Your pelvis has a natural tilt that stabilizes the base of your spine. The tilt varies slightly from person to person, but in general, a healthy natural tilt is slightly forward and down. This puts the pubic symphysis just below the bottom tip of the tailbone (or directly across from it, depending on the length of your tailbone), and positions the bulk of your torso over the broadest part of your pelvis. We generally refer to this slightly forward (anterior) tilt as a "neutral" pelvis, even though it is technically not neutral on a horizontal plane.

ANTERIOR & POSTERIOR TILT. An anterior tilt of the pelvis is a forward tilt that is more exaggerated than a "neutral" tilt. It is usually caused by stiffness in the

Functional Anatomy

quadriceps and/or psoas that pulls the front of the pelvis toward the front of the legs. It is the anatomical equivalent of sticking your butt out behind you, and it is also known as a hyperlordosis or swayback. This forward tilt places the pubic bone far below the tip of the tailbone, as though your pelvic bowl was pouring out in front of you. This tilt exacerbates the strong natural curvature of your lower back and can cause a painful hyperextension of the lumbar discs. It also depresses the front of your pubic bone and buries it deep into the stiffness of your inner groin.

A strong anterior pelvic tilt often causes a corresponding imbalance in the rest of the spine: the exaggerated curve in your lower back is mirrored by an exaggerated curve in your upper back. Your butt sticks out behind you, your abdomen and floating ribs extend forward, and your chest moves backward to keep your shoulders over your hips. These exaggerated curves decrease your overall spinal extension—i.e. make you shorter. They also concentrate your weight and shock absorption capacity into a smaller number of intervertebral discs.

A posterior tilt is when the pelvis tips backward. It is usually caused by extremely tight hamstrings. Tight hamstrings pull on the ischial tuberosities at the bottom of the pelvis and cause the entire pelvic girdle to tip backward. It is the anatomical equivalent of tucking your butt underneath your hips. This places the pubic bone above the tip of the tailbone, as though the pelvic bowl were pouring out behind you. It reverses the natural curve in your lower back and often causes a corresponding hunch in your upper back: your butt moves forward, your abdomen and floating ribs move backward, and your shoulders move forward to stay over your hips. The resulting curve in the upper body is also known as hyperkyphosis or hunchback.

Movement in the Pelvis

The pelvic girdle has three functional joints (aside from the hip socket): the left and right SI joints and the pubic symphysis. These three joints create a tightly pressurized bowl. If one part of the bowl moves, the other two have to move as well. The sacrum is the most likely to shift, and it forces the three fused bones on either side to pivot in the same direction (as mentioned in the previous section). All your external-body indicators become slightly off balance: one frontal hip bone is higher than the other; one sit bone is further forward than the other; and the pubic bone may point ever so slightly to the left or right. The respective

Functional Anatomy

angles of the hip sockets will change as well, which can affect the way each leg articulates with the pelvis.

If the SI joint is destabilized, for whatever reason, you may be able to use the pubic symphysis to help put it back into place. The pubic symphysis is the front gate of the pelvis. If the two back gates (SI joints) are stuck in place, you have to wiggle the front gate to get in. The best way to wiggle the front gate is with *baddha konasana* (bound angle pose). *Baddha konasana* places the soles of your feet together as you simultaneously 1) externally rotate your legs and 2) tip your pelvis forward (anterior rotation). This screws the heads of the femur into the hip sockets, and as they externally rotate, they pull the heads of the pubis away from each other. The energetic separation of the pubis encourages an opening in the pubic symphysis. The pubic symphysis will not actually separate because it's an incredibly strong ligament, but this action can create enough movement to release pressure in the joint. Releasing pressure in the pubic symphysis can relieve pressure in the SI joints, and relieving pressure in these joints will begin the long process of coaxing the bones of your pelvis back into alignment.

HIP ANATOMY

The hip joint is where your leg inserts into your pelvis. The joint is formed by the three fused bones of your pelvis (left and right, respectively), and the actual hip socket is called the acetabulum. The part of your leg that connects to your pelvis is the femur or thigh bone.

Femur and Acetabulum

Your femur is the biggest bone in your leg and the longest, strongest bone in your body—unless you're an orangutan. It's a long, narrow shaft with bony knobs at the top and bottom. The protrusion at the bottom forms the top of your knee and the protrusion at the top has two parts that help attach it to your pelvis. The largest of these is called the greater trochanter, and its bumpy surface provides muscle attachments for your pelvis and legs. It sits at the outermost point of your hip, near the top of your femur. There is also a small knob on the inside of the femur bone called the lesser trochanter, and it too plays an important role in the musculature of the pelvis.

Your femur inserts into your pelvis at the acetabulum, which is the circular depression that creates your hip socket. Acetabulum is Latin for "a small cup for serving vinegar" and it aptly describes the circular socket that "cups" itself around the round head of the femur. The narrow neck of the femur and the greater trochanter sit just outside of the hip socket, and in a normal posture the greater trochanters point straight out on either side of your hips.

Labrum

The head of the femur and the cup of the acetabulum are both rimmed with a thick layer of lubricating cartilage. The cartilage that surrounds the acetabulum is called the "acetabular labrum," or "labrum" for short. Labrum is Latin for "edge of a vessel" or "rim." This cartilage is designed to deepen the acetabulum and keep the head of the femur in place. It creates a seal for the hip joint and also maintains the protective fluid that keeps the joint working properly. It is directly involved in any movement that shifts your leg bone within your hip socket, which is pretty much every pose you will do in a yoga class.

The labrum is thinnest at the front of the hip socket and thus more susceptible to injury in the front than the back. The labrum is also only partially vascularized, meaning there is blood flow to only about one third of the entire structure. This lack of blood flow makes it partially "white" tissue, similar to a ligament, and particularly difficult to heal.

Your labrum can be at risk during twists, especially if the lever of the twist (the bent knee) is allowed to internally rotate. When you bend your knee (flexion) and move it toward the midline of your body, the neck of the femur grinds against the rim of the acetabulum. These two bones can pinch the labrum between them and create micro-tears that weaken the cartilage. Labrum injuries can also arise from an imbalance in the muscles that surround your pelvis, and more specifically, from a hypermobility in the hip joint itself. This is mainly a factor in lunges; without the stabilizing action of *mula bandha*, hypermobile individuals can sag into their frontal hip socket. If the extended hip socket is externally rotated, the head of the femur can pull the labrum away from the hip socket. These injuries are more common in women than in men, partially because of female pelvic anatomy and partially because women are more likely to be hypermobile.

Labrum injuries can be difficult to diagnose and treat, but they are rarely acute injuries; they don't come from doing any single pose just once. They come from repetitive wear and tear and from a conscious decision to ignore the early signs of injury. If you feel pain deep in the front of your groin when you are doing yoga, or after you finish your practice, please pay attention to that pain—just as

Functional Anatomy

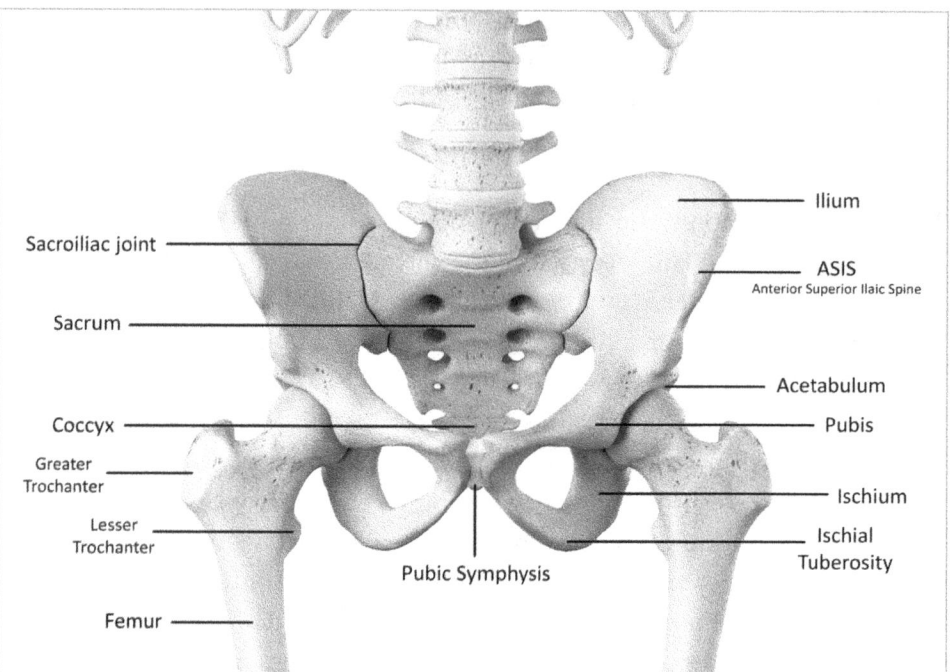

16.g Pelvic girdle and hip socket.

you should pay attention to pain in any of your joints. The stretch and "pain" of lunges and other hip openers should be in your muscles, not in your joints.

Movement in the Hip Socket

The thigh bone and hip socket form a ball-and-socket joint, which is the most stable kind of joint in your body. It can flex, extend, and rotate in several directions. The most basic actions are flexion and extension, i.e. lifting your leg in front of you and reaching it behind you. Many yogic actions also involve rotation of the ball within the socket to create internal or external rotation of your leg, and these actions usually have a much more specific anatomical goal.

EXTERNAL ROTATION OF THE FEMUR. Externally rotating your femur is an important part of most standing poses, for several reasons. First, externally rotating your femur protects the medial hamstring muscles of your inner knee. The tendons of the medial hamstrings wrap around the inside of your knee and attach to your tibia bone (lower leg). When you bend forward in a straight-leg standing pose like *parsvottanasana*, stiffness in your groin and hamstrings makes your leg internally rotate. Internal rotation brings the tendons of the medial hamstrings closer to the ground than the rest of your thigh. The tissue closest to the ground bears the strongest part of the stretch, but tendons are not supposed to stretch; muscles are supposed to stretch. Externally rotating your leg rolls the vulnerable tendons out of harm's way and points the center of your hamstrings straight down to bear the brunt of the stretch.

External rotation of the femur is also important in poses that use side-angle flexion—i.e. bending laterally at a sideways angle. Side-angle flexion occurs when the pelvis and the front leg are pointed in opposite directions, such as in *trikonasana* and *supta padangusthasana B*. These poses move the femur closer to the outside of the pelvis, and they can eventually bring the rim of the acetabulum into contact with the neck of the greater trochanter (that bony knob at the top of the femur, outside of the hip socket). Allowing the greater trochanter to push into the acetabulum wears down the cartilage of the joint and can eventually erode the bone of the hip socket itself. Externally rotating the femur rolls the greater trochanter away from the iliac crest, so the bony knob points behind you instead of out to the side. This prohibits the greater trochanter from grinding against the edge of the acetabulum, and in the long run that simple action may save you from a hip replacement.

INTERNAL ROTATION OF THE FEMUR. Internal rotation is primarily used to balance length in the inner and outer leg. It is important in poses that involve flexion with the legs together, such as *uttanasana* (standing forward bend) and *paschimottanasana* (seated forward bend). Most of us are shorter on the inside of our limbs than on the outside, and when we bend forward, our big toe bones get sucked back toward the congestion in our hips. Internal rotation counters that stiffness by lengthening the inseam of the leg and pushing the big toe bones forward. Internal rotation also encourages the legs to act as a single body, which is helpful in poses that require the legs to do a lot of lifting, such as inversions.

KNEE ANATOMY

Your knee sits at the intersection of your thigh bone and lower leg. Skeletally, it's where your femur bone meets your tibia and fibula. The knee is held together by ligaments and tendons, and the space between the bones is filled with a cartilaginous meniscus. The meniscus has a similar role to that of the intervertebral discs, but in contrast to the discs, it does not fill the entire space between the bones. It has two crescent-shaped bows that buffer the inside and outside of the knee (left to right), and the space between these two crescents is crisscrossed by ligaments.

There are four main ligaments in your knee. The two "collateral" ligaments (Medial Collateral Ligament or MCL and Lateral Collateral Ligament or LCL) run on the inside and outside of the knee (left side and right side) to provide protection against side-to-side movement. The two "cruciate" ligaments cross in the center of the knee to control the movement of your lower leg. The PCL (Posterior Cruciate Ligament) is primarily responsible for bending your lower leg (flexion) and the ACL (Anterior Cruciate Ligament) stops your lower leg from bending toward your quadriceps (hyperextension). The ACL is unique because it does not attach bone to bone; it attaches your thigh bone to the meniscus of your knee. It's one of the only places in the appendicular skeleton where a ligament attaches to soft tissue instead of bone, and it's probably the only piece of anatomy we find somewhat questionable. Everything else makes perfect sense but that connection is just a little bit wonky.

Functional Anatomy

You don't really need to know all these ligaments but you should definitely try to protect them. Never tolerate pain in your knees. Pain in your knees is a warning from the ligaments, meniscus, and tendons that hold it all together, and they're not known to cry wolf. When they speak up, you should always pay attention.

Movement in the Knee

Your knee is only designed to flex. It can bend and straighten but it is not designed to extend beyond straight. If the lower leg moves closer to the femur in a forward direction, i.e. the leg becomes bowed, the knee is hyperextended and its ligaments are at risk. Your knee is also not designed to twist. Always keep your knee pointed in the same direction as your toes. If it's pointed in a different direction, it's twisted.

The best way to protect your knee is to develop a relationship with your patella. The patella is your kneecap. It's a thick, circular-triangular bone that sits in front of your knee joint. The top of the patella is connected to the quadriceps and the bottom is connected to the front of the tibia. Engaging your quadriceps lifts the patella and slides it into the notch between the femur and the tibia, where it acts as a stabilizing peg between these two moving parts. It protects the structure of the knee by preventing the lower and upper leg from twisting against each other. Unfortunately, the patella is only effective when the leg is straight.

Knees can be at risk in the transition from flexion to extension, e.g. as you exit a bent knee standing pose. Bending your knee loosens its ligaments and can allow a slight twist to develop between your lower and upper leg. In most bent knee standing poses, such as *virabhadrasana B* (warrior 2), the toes and the lower leg are pointed forward in an external rotation. The femur also points forward as you enter the pose, but once the knee is bent and the ligaments relax, it can begin to internally rotate. Your knee may begin to track toward the midline of your body, moving tissue above the knee in a different direction than tissue below the knee. Straightening your leg in this position pushes these two opposing directions into the knee and puts excessive torque on its ligaments.

Your knee should always point in the same direction as your toes. It's extremely important to watch this alignment in bent knee poses, especially as you straighten your leg to exit the pose. In *virabhadrasana B*, that usually means moving your knee away from the midline of your body to keep it pointed over your toes. And if your knee cannot achieve the proper alignment of the pose, please adjust your foot to reflect the direction of your knee. Your knees are more important than "proper" alignment. Struggling to maintain proper alignment in the face of a strong restriction is more likely to hurt your knee than open your hips.

SHOULDER ANATOMY

Your shoulder girdle is like a set of football pads placed over the structure of your ribcage. The back of the pads is formed by the scapulae (shoulder blades), and the front and top of the pads are formed by the clavicle bones (collarbone). The shoulder joints sit just underneath the edge of the pads on either end.

Clavicle and Scapula

Clavicles are the horizontal bones that run along the top of your chest. There are two separate clavicle bones, one on either side of your chest, and they connect to the sternum in the center of your chest. The two bony knobs underneath the base of your throat are the heads of the left and right clavicle bones. The long, ridged bone underneath them is your sternum. The clavicles wrap over the top rib of your ribcage to create the top of your shoulder girdle, and then they reach toward your back body to connect with your shoulder blade. The clavicle and shoulder blade connect at the acromion, which it is a long, bony process that

Functional Anatomy

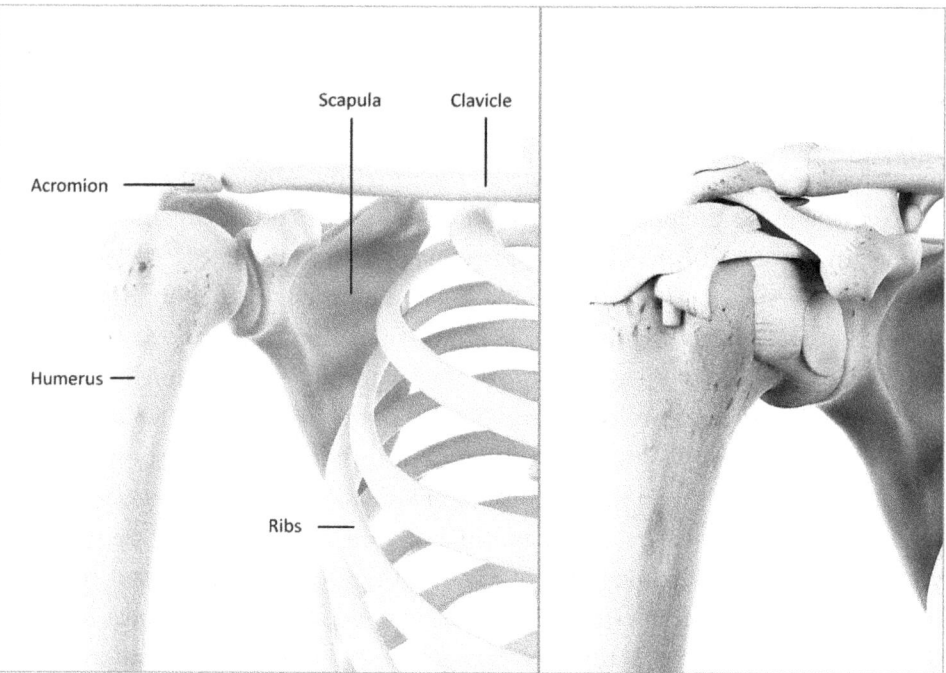

16.h Bones of the shoulder joint (left) and ligaments of the rotator cuff (right). Note that the origin and attachment of the shoulder's ligaments allow the joint to loosen with internal rotation and tighten with external rotation.

extends above the rest of the shoulder blade and hangs over the top of the shoulder joint.

The scapulae (shoulder blades) sit flush against your ribcage on your back body with one on either side of your thoracic spine. They are shaped like inverted elephant ears: the bottom tip of the ear points toward your hips and the thick bony part of the ear (where it connects to the elephant's head) sits at the top corner to form your shoulder joint. The broadest part of the ear fans out in the direction of your spine and is curved to reflect the curve of your ribs. The scapula is suspended behind the ribcage and shaped to accommodate it, but it does not have any bony connection to the ribcage or the thoracic spine. This freedom allows your shoulder blade to pivot laterally and to slide up and down to support movement in your shoulder joint.

Shoulder Joint

Your shoulder is a ball and socket joint that connects the head of your humerus (upper arm bone) to the topmost corner of your scapula. The socket is called the glenoid fossa, but it's more of a crescent-shaped depression than a true cup. The round head of the humerus rests against this depression like a golf ball on a tee, which is far less stable than a "true" ball and socket joint like your hip joint. The face of the glenoid fossa has a rim of cartilage (labrum) that strengthens its feeble grip on the humerus, similar to the way the acetabular labrum deepens the hip socket. There are also two bony processes at the top of the scapula that hang over the shoulder joint to stabilize it from above, but there are no bones underneath it. This poor articulation makes your shoulder joint the most mobile joint in your body and renders it susceptible to dislocation in a downward direction.

Movement in the Shoulder Joint

Stability in your shoulder joint comes from a network of strong connective tissues. The primary stabilizers are the joint capsule and the rotator cuff. The joint capsule encircles the entire shoulder joint from the top edge of the scapula to the neck of the humerus. It is a loose connective sheath that acts as a "passive restraint," allowing the bones to move apart in small increments while prohibiting them from moving too far apart. The main ligaments of the shoulder joint operate within this joint capsule. Most originate at the top or front of the joint and insert low on the head of the humerus, which gives them a slight downward spiral. Internally rotating the humerus moves the two ends of the ligament closer together and makes them loose. External rotation does the exact opposite; it moves the two ends further apart and tightens the ligaments, which tightens the joint capsule.

There are four muscles that form the rotator cuff and they work together to lift your arm. All four originate on the scapula and insert into the head of the humerus to create a direct relationship between your arms and your shoulder blades. They are inseparable. You have to lift your shoulder blades to fully extend your arms. They are anatomically required to lift in the direction of your head in a pose like downward dog. You cannot fully extend your arms while depressing your shoulder blades, and attempting to do so forces the muscles of your rotator cuff to work against one other. It is anatomically contraindicated.

Your shoulder is most at risk during internal rotation and extension. Internal rotation loosens the joint capsule and makes it easier for the humerus to separate from the scapula. External rotation tightens the joint capsule and screws the humerus tighter into the scapula.

CONNECTIVE TISSUE

Connective tissue holds your body together. Every part of your anatomy is wrapped in its protective sheath: all of your joints, muscles, bones, ligaments, and nerves. It's like a giant sheet of saran wrap that envelopes every part of your being. Your other bodily tissues connect specific things: ligaments connect bones to bones, tendons connect bones to muscles, and fascia connects muscles to muscles. Connective tissue is less specific. It touches everything and allows every part of your body to be connected in some way.

Your connective tissue is the most fluid at birth. As you age, it is subject to the same congestion and dehydration that affects all of your tissues. Dehydration makes your tissue shrink, tighten, and become more brittle. It squeezes the fluid out of your organs and bones and makes you drier, shrunken, and more congested. Doing yoga will help reverse this dehydration by stretching, expanding, and lubricating your connective tissue. It will help keep you fluid, and fluid is youth.

Connective tissue is strongly affected by heat. Developing internal heat makes it open and malleable. You can generate internal heat by doing poses in a dynamic way, such as in surya namaskar A.

Ligaments

Ligaments are the connective tissues that hold your joints together. They're composed of tightly attenuated collagen fibers, and people with lots of collagen fiber tend to have stronger ligaments. People with less collagen fiber have more vulnerable ligaments, and they may be prone to hyperextension, a permanent stretching of the ligaments that define a given joint. Ligaments are called "white" tissue because there is no blood flowing through them. Blood is your body's primary repairman for damaged tissues. If there's no blood flow to a particular body part, that part is very difficult to repair.

Ligaments provide structure and direction in all the places where bone meets bone, from your tiny intervertebral facet joints to your massive hip joint. Their natural length determines the normal range of motion for each joint. If the bones of a joint are pushed beyond their natural range of motion, the ligaments will be forced to stretch. Ligaments cannot bounce back like muscles. Once they extend beyond their natural range of motion, that new hyperextended position becomes the new range of motion for that joint. Hyperextension can create per-

Functional Anatomy

manent instability in a joint, and with enough time and pressure the joint may extend to a point that causes serious damage to the bones and connective tissues holding it together.

Hyperextension can be difficult to manage. Most people who are prone to hyperextension don't feel pain until the joint has pushed far beyond its normal range of motion, and at that point, it may be too late. Torn and severely stretched ligaments usually require surgery. But hyperextension can often be corrected if it is detected early. People prone to hyperextension can use their muscles to help maintain each joint's natural range of motion. They can support the role of one connective tissue by consciously activating another connective tissue. With enough practice, their muscles will prohibit the joint from moving beyond its normal range of motion.

Muscles

Muscles are soft, pink, vascularized tissues that attach to bones to create movement in your skeleton. They are composed of bundles of muscle fiber that travel in a single direction, and the direction of that fiber determines the direction of muscular action. Each muscle's force and direction is also determined by its origin and insertion, i.e. where it starts and where it ends. The origin and insertion of each muscle is marked by tendons, which are thick bands of connective tissue composed of strong collagen fibers. Tendons are more resilient than ligaments but less resilient than muscles.

Muscle fibers are like a bunch of tiny rubber strands stretched along a bone. These individual strands are bundled into sets of ropes, and the ropes are then wrapped in a sheath of connective tissue. The sheath is gathered into a single bundle by your tendons, which exist at either end of the muscle, and the tendons attach the entire muscle bundle to the bone(s). Muscles narrow considerably as they insert into tendons, and that's where they are most vulnerable to rips and tears. Always avoid pain in those areas, such as the top of your hamstrings, where they attach to your sit bones. Push the stretch into the middle of your muscles, where they are broadest, strongest, and most resilient.

When it comes to muscle fiber, we believe there is more strength in length than in bulk. Lengthening your muscles requires refinement and attenuation of your muscle fibers, and the most effective way to affect muscle fiber is to increase the duration of your poses. Holding poses for longer periods of time will rearrange muscle fiber in a permanent way. Generating internal body heat through dynamic movement—i.e. doing a lot of poses with shorter timings—will also affect your muscles, but the physiological changes created by heat are temporary; they disappear once the muscle has cooled. The physiological changes created by duration are much more significant.

Refining your muscle fiber also involves an evolution in the relationship between your muscles and your mind. Your body is governed by strong behavioral habits. When your mind needs to create movement, it usually stimulates the same set of muscles because those are the only muscles that have been trained to listen. Your mind communicates with these muscles through a set of well-worn neurological pathways because those are the only pathways currently open. You are capable of much more sophisticated mind-body communication, but because daily life demands efficiency, your actions are simplified to follow the path of least resistance. Yoga will change these habits. It will improve your connectivity by creating new pathways in your neuromuscular communication and penetrating parts of your tissue that are currently asleep.

ATROPHY AND SPASTICITY. Muscles can be shorted by trauma and lack of use. Trauma usually results in muscle spasticity and lack of use results in muscle atrophy. In both cases, the muscle fibers become bunched, contracted, and disorganized. In a practical sense, these two very different conditions produce a similar result: muscles that cannot do their job. These dysfunctional muscles can trigger an antalgic reaction that affects the rest of your body as the surrounding muscles and bones alter their function to compensate for the loss.

SPASTICITY AND THE NEUROSYMPATHETIC REFLEX. When your connective tissue is injured, your body activates a defensive reaction called the neurosympathetic reflex. This reflex is designed to stabilize the injured area while your body activates its internal healing process. It begins when muscles near the damaged tissue become agitated in response to the injury. The nervous system senses this agitation, and in an attempt to restore balance it tells the muscles to contract. The muscles begin to contract while they are still agitated, and these opposing actions cause a change in muscle tone called spasticity. A spastic muscle is pulled taught like a bowstring, but it cannot release its tension because the nervous system is telling it to remain contracted. It lives in a hypertonic state that makes it weak, difficult to control, and unable to perform its normal duties.

Spastic muscles will not respond to normal stretching. The constant hypertonic state squeezes all the fluid out of them and leaves them very brittle, so they are more likely to tear than stretch. The most effective way to release a spastic muscle is to reset the connection between the brain and the muscle, similar to the way you reset an electrical circuit in your house. The rapid exchange between the muscle and the nervous system has overloaded the muscle's nerve receptors, in the same way a power surge can overload an electrical circuit. The spastic muscle gets stuck halfway between "on" and "off," just like an overloaded circuit. But you cannot simply push an overloaded circuit back to its "on" position; you have to turn it all the way off to reset the connection between the circuit and the electrical feed. Once the connection is reset, you can turn the circuit back "on" and resume its connection with the proper amount of electrical stimuli.

Spastic muscles require a similar "reset" button, and it is called "approximating" the muscle. Approximating a muscle resets its nerve receptors by bringing the muscle's origin and insertion closer together. It's like folding the muscle in half. It pushes the muscle from halfway on to fully off so it can resume its normal muscle tone. Approximation resets the feedback loop between the muscle and the brain, and once the neurological channels are clear, they can resume normal communication.

Most yogic actions seek to lengthen your muscles by moving their origins and insertions farther apart, but approximation does the exact opposite. This is one of yoga's many lessons: sometimes you have to go backward to make progress. Parts of your body may need to lengthen, but other parts may need to approximate; and it's all part of the journey toward understanding your Self.

SPASTICITY IN THE PSOAS. Many of us live with spastic muscles. Our bodies are unconsciously braced against the trauma of past injuries and chronic imbalances. This constant hypertonic state creates a spinal pathology based on antalgia, the body's ability to compensate for pain through posture and motion. Antalgic reactions are most pronounced when muscle spasticity occurs in deep structural muscles, such as the psoas.

There are two posas muscles in your body. They sit on either side of your lumbar spine, one on the left and one on the right, and in a perfect world they are identical. They originate on the transverse processes of the vertebrae between T12 and L5; the left psoas attaches to the left transverse processes of those six vertebrae, and the right psoas attaches to the right transverse processes. Both posas muscles stretch down along the front of your spine and cross in front of your SI joint (left and right, respectively) and then slide underneath the angular

Functional Anatomy

ligament that defines the bottom of your abdomen (i.e. your leg crease). They continue down across the front of each hip socket and wrap underneath your legs to insert at the lesser trochanters—those little knobs on the inside of your thigh bones, just under the "neck" of the femur.

The psoas muscles bridge the space between your torso and legs and govern the relationship between them. They keep your torso upright above your pelvis, which is a pretty important job. They're also the primary catalyst of full spinal flexion, such as a forward bend like *uttanasana*, and they lift you out of that forward bend as well. They're the only muscles that can lift your legs higher than your hips, and they also work to externally rotate both legs. Contracting the posas on one side will spin that leg outward (external rotation) because the muscle inserts on the underside of your thigh bone.

The psoas can become spastic in response to trauma, disc injuries, and instability in the SI joint. These injuries may be centered on one side of the spine but they always cause a reaction in both psoas muscles: the one closest to the injury becomes hypertonic (overly toned; spastic) and the one on the other side becomes hypotonic (too little tone; atrophied). It is the same neurosympathetic reflex we described earlier, and it creates a spiral in the spine that can eventually resemble scoliosis.

The lunges are a fantastic way to start working with your psoas muscles. Lunges expand the space between the lumbar spine and the femur, thus moving the origin and insertion of each psoas away from each other. They also work with each side individually so you can get a sense of which psoas is more contracted. But alignment is extremely important. The psoas is a very deep muscle that bridges several major joints and it can easily recruit flexibility from these joints. Monitor your body closely to ensure the psoas is not affecting the alignment of your lumbar spine, SI joint, hip socket, and femur.

AGONIST / ANTAGONIST RELATIONSHIPS. Muscles can be organized into pairs governed by a nervous system response called the agonist/antagonist relationship. These muscle pairs are usually separated by a large bone and most of them are in your arms and legs. The agonist/antagonist relationship is quite simple: when you engage the muscle on one side of the bone, your brain tells the muscle on the other side of the bone to release. It is a pre-programmed neurological response that creates movement by balancing muscular action on either side of the bone. The muscle that contracts is the agonist and the muscle that releases is the antagonist, and the relationship changes depending on the nature of the movement. When you straighten your leg, your quadriceps are the agonist and your hamstrings are the antagonist; contracting your quadriceps makes your hamstrings release. But the relationship changes when you bend your knee; the hamstrings become the agonist and the quadriceps become the antagonist.

The most useful agonist/antagonist muscle relationships exist between the quadriceps and hamstrings and the biceps and triceps. These muscle groups create a two-for-one deal: if you focus on engaging the agonist muscle, your nervous system will automatically tell the antagonist muscle to relax. In the straight leg standing poses, learning to fully engage your quadriceps will automatically release your hamstrings. Releasing your hamstrings stacks your femur bone directly over your lower leg and creates a straight line from your foot to your hip. Utilizing this relationship in the arms is more individually specific because the balance between biceps and triceps varies widely from person to person but it is equally effective.

NEUROMUSCULAR COMMUNICATION. There are several types of nervous system feedback loops between your muscles and your brain. The shortest one operates between your sensory nerves and the spinal cord. The messages do not go up to your brain for processing; they are processed right in the spinal cord itself. These short loops create the fastest muscular reaction, the kind that tells you to pull your hand away when you touch something hot. They are essential to your ability to sense and avoid injuries, but they don't create the kind of voluntary movement needed to activate your muscles in yoga.

The largest set of feedback loops involves communication between your brain and your muscles. Different parts of your brain are responsible for different types of movement, and the two main categories are voluntary movement and involuntary movement. Voluntary movement is when you tell your muscles to complete an action, such as lifting your arms in surya namaskar A. Most of your appendicular skeleton is governed by this type of voluntary movement. Involuntary movements are activated by more subconscious stimuli, such as telling the muscles of your heart to beat and telling your psoas muscles to keep you standing upright. You don't have to think about these muscles to make them work because they are governed by a more primitive, autonomic part of your brain.

Functional Anatomy

The other side of this neuromuscular feedback loop allows your muscles to talk to your brain. Messages that come from your muscles are generated by muscle spindles, which are sensory receptors that live in the middle of every muscle. They communicate the state of your muscle fiber to your brain. Reflexes go from the muscle to the brain and back to the muscle, and they also go from the brain to the muscle and back to the brain. It is an intricate set of actions and reactions that are primarily aimed at balance, and in your body, the quest for balance is called homeostasis.

SYMPATHETIC & PARASYMPATHETIC NERVOUS SYSTEM. Your nervous system can be further divided into two sections based on the type of messages they generate. The parasympathetic nervous system is the calming part of your nervous system. Stimulating this system facilitates your "rest and digest" functions: digestion, sleep, and procreation. The sympathetic nervous system is the exciting part of your nervous system. Stimulating this system incites the "fight or flight" reflex associated with increased stress and physical activity.

These two systems are simultaneously active at all times, but they trade dominance in response to external stimuli. For example: when you are busy at work, the sympathetic nervous system may be at 90% and the parasympathetic will be at 10%; you are focused, tense, and have little to no appetite. When you're carefree and content, the pendulum swings back toward the parasympathetic system; you eat, sleep well, and maybe even get frisky with your partner. These two systems work together to maintain balance amidst the challenges and rewards of daily life. Neither system will ever be 100% dominant because you need both of them to survive. The pendulum is constantly swinging between them to create homeostasis.

Homeostasis is your equilibrium. It comes from the Greek homeo, which means constant or equal, and stasis, which means stable. Every one of your internal systems has its own homeostatic set point; the place where it is perfectly balanced. Body temperature is a perfect example. The homeostatic set point for internal body temperature is usually 98.6°F. If your body goes above this temperature, your brain initiates a complex set of interactions—everything from sweating to dilating certain blood vessels—to bring it back to normal. The quest for homeostasis can affect any and every bodily system, but it always works in the same way. It responds to change by initiating a set of actions to bring you back to your equilibrium because being away from your equilibrium is bad for your longevity.

The parasympathetic and sympathetic nervous systems have a homeostatic set point, a place where they are perfectly balanced. If you lived in a cave with no external stimuli, these two nervous system interactions would keep your body and mind balanced at all times. But most of us do not live in caves. We have jobs, families, and obligations, and this external stimulus affects our ability to maintain homeostasis between the two systems.

Your individual homeostatic set point is determined by your life experiences. A stressful life swings your set point permanently in the direction of the sympathetic nervous system, leaving your "fight or flight" system on overdrive. Your equilibrium becomes a state of constant activation. It becomes harder to activate your parasympathetic reflex, the one that lets you rest, digest, and procreate. Most people live in this sympathetic state because our world feeds on the sympathetic nervous system; it tells us we need to be active, productive, consumptive, and watchful at all times. The things that stimulate our parasympathetic reflex, the calm and content side, are few and far between. This constant sympathetic overdrive can create anxiety and depression, which are really two sides of the same hyper-sympathetic imbalance.

Yoga can help you regain balance between these two nervous system reflexes. It will enhance your parasympathetic reflex and turn down your sympathetic reflex (increase your calm and decrease your agitation). The early stages of your relationship with yoga will simply bring you back to your homeostatic set point, wherever that set point may be. If you live in a state of sympathetic overdrive, yoga will bring you back to your starting point: to the place where your body and mind are in balance. That balance point will feel normal, even if it's slightly skewed toward the sympathetic, because it's your set point. That's why you always feel so great when you leave your mat. You have given yourself enough space and time to regain your natural balance. It's the reset button.

Over time, yoga can permanently change the homeostatic set point that exists between the two systems. It will alter the balance between your parasympathetic and sympathetic reflexes. For most of us, yoga initiates a shift toward the parasympathetic system. Your body and mind become more resistant to the stressful external stimuli of life because your homeostatic set point is no longer tipped toward the sympathetic reflex; the "fight or flight" reflex becomes less touchy.

Functional Anatomy

EDDIE:
Yoga is not about the quality of your tissue, it is about training your mind. We are all given a vehicle to work with; some of us have flexible tissue and some of us have stiff tissue, but both types of tissue provide an opportunity to hone your mind. It's all about your mind. The yoga Sutras say very little about the body and *asana*; they instruct us to calm the fluctuations of the self-limiting, self-defeating tendencies of the mind. That's what it's all about. We get to play in these fun and challenging poses, and there are definite health benefits, but in the end it's about your mind.

Functional Anatomy

The parasympathetic nervous system becomes more active, receptive, and easier to reach. All the systems associated with the parasympathetic system—sleep, digestion, and reproduction—regain their natural balance. Your natural homeostatic state will reflect more relaxation and less anxiety, and your entire body will benefit from the shift.

Your homeostatic set point is a strongly entrenched body mechanism, just like your body temperature. It's probably not going to change very quickly. But you are hard-wired toward homeostasis, and using yoga to accommodate homeostasis on a daily basis will plant the seed for a life-altering shift in your homeostatic set point.

GENERAL CONTRAINDICATIONS

Hatha yoga is all about balance. Stiff people are looking for flexibility and flexible people are looking for stiffness. Most people do not fall 100% into either category. Parts of your anatomy may be stiff and other parts may be flexible, and you need to figure out which is which. The most important thing is finding the middle path for your unique anatomy and having the intelligence to adjust the path as you evolve along it.

Stiff People

Being stiff is not a bad thing. It has nothing to do with your inherent value as a human being or your ability to do yoga. It's not a personality flaw and it's not a lifetime sentence, unless you allow it to be. But yoga for stiff people is different than yoga for flexible people so you need to know if you're stiff. It's not a value judgment; it's about personal responsibility, safety, and sustainability.

Stiff bodies are at risk of congestion and atrophy. Your body dehydrates as you age and the limited movement you could muster in your youth will disappear. Your organs will solidify and shrivel. It's not pretty, but age can turn an already stiff person into a slab of concrete. If you are deeply interested in your longevity, you must become more flexible.

FLEXION. Stiff people are most at risk during forward bends. Tight hamstring muscles keep your pelvis stuck in place, and when you start to bend forward, the bend happens in your lower back instead of your hips. Your lumbar discs (the ones in your lower back) are the most vulnerable discs in your spine. Bending from your lower back pushes their natural bulge sideways and backward into the exact place they're most at risk of rupturing. It's especially problematic in seated forward bends because your hips are stuck to the floor; your stiff legs and pelvis cannot rotate so all the movement gets pushed into your lumbar spine. Deepening the bend by pulling your torso toward your feet puts even more dangerous leverage into your lumbar discs, and worst of all, it will never penetrate your hamstrings because the action is coming from your back instead of your legs.

If your legs are stiff it is safest to do moderate forward bends like box on the wall and *parsvottanasana* against a wall or with a chair. Box on the wall protects the natural curve of your lumbar spine while providing leverage to safely pursue your stiff hamstrings. It also uses the action of your arms and legs to decompress your lumbar discs. Your upper body extends toward the wall and your legs reach away from it, and these opposing actions create traction in your lower back. Box on the wall is a fantastic way to relieve painful pressure on your lumbar discs, and it also addresses the root anatomical imbalances that created the pain in the first place.

EXTENSION. Stiff people can also be at risk in backbends, specifically in their neck and shoulders. Many people come to yoga with stiff shoulders and a closed chest. Shoulders belong on your back body, but a beginner's shoulders are more in line with their nipples than with the sides of their ribs. The entire shoulder girdle rides forward and up, like a set of shoulder pads too rigid to fit over your torso. These pads create congestion between the top of your thoracic spine and the base of your cervical spine, and they prevent your neck and shoulders from working together in a backbend.

Extension in your cervical spine should always be supported by extension in your thoracic spine, i.e. by lifting your chest and moving your shoulders toward your back body. These actions create space around the base of your neck and facilitate a smooth transition from your thoracic vertebrae to your cervical vertebrae. But if your shoulders, neck, and chest are stuck in place, backbends get pushed into the space between your Atlas (C1) and occipital condyles (at the base of your skull). This joint is more capable of bending than any other joint in your upper spine, so if your neck and shoulders will not move, the Atlas will move for them. The Atlas is particularly at risk of subluxation (shifting out of place) because it does not have an intervertebral disc to help hold it in place.

The safest backbends in yoga are the simple backbends, including *setu bandha sarvangasana* (bridge) and *supta virasana*. These poses encourage movement between the shoulders and chest without endangering the cervical spine. Poses like *chataranga dandasana* may be too advanced for stiff introductory students, even though it's in a very basic sequence, so please listen to your body and modify accordingly.

Functional Anatomy

ASANA FOR STIFF PEOPLE. The three most important poses for stiff people are box on the wall, *parsvottanasana* (intense side stretch pose) against the wall, and *salamba sarvangasana* (supported shoulderstand) with props. We'll explain why these poses may be helpful to you and you can find step-by-step instructions for each pose in the Practice section.

BOX ON THE WALL. Stiff people are usually shorter on the inside of their limbs than on the outside. This imbalance makes it difficult to evenly distribute weight in your hands and feet because the outsides are always closer to the ground than the insides. In poses that use the hands, the pointer finger knuckle is usually pulled away from the mat and the weight falls to the outer wrist. This can make *surya namaskar A* problematic for people with a stiff upper body. All the beautiful movement of *surya namaskar A* gets transferred to your delicate outer wrist instead opening your chest, shoulders, and spine.

If you are a stiff person, *surya namaskar A* may not the best practice for you. The sequence involves complex movements that can wreak havoc on a stiff body. That doesn't mean you will never do *surya namaskar A*, it simply means you should utilize static poses to develop balance in your arms and legs before pursuing *surya namaskar A*. It is safer to use poses like box on the wall and downward dog to extend the inseam of your arms without endangering your wrists, elbows, and shoulders.

PARSVOTTANASANA. In the standing poses, the imbalance in your legs can make the back of your feet heavier than the front. When you bend forward in a standing pose all your weight falls to the outer ankle and outer heel of your front leg. The outer heel turns white because all the blood is being pushed out of it, and the big toe bone gets pulled away from the mat. The best way to address this imbalance is to start with the simplest standing pose, *parsvottanasana*, and do it against a wall: press the big toe bone of your front leg into the bottom of the wall, with your toes pointing up the wall, and then reach your hands up the wall. *Parsvottanasana* is the simplest standing pose because it allows you to focus on one leg at a time, and it also puts your leg right in front of you; you are looking at it for the duration of the pose. Adding the wall protects your lower back by eliminating the forward bend. It also gives you something to press your big toe bone into, which helps keep weight in the front of your foot instead of the outer heel.

SHOULDERSTAND. Shoulderstand takes your shoulders away from your neck and puts them on your back body, where they belong, but you must use props to make shoulderstand safe and effective for a stiff body. The best prop is a metal folding chair with the backrest removed, plus a couple of thick folded blankets. The back of the chair supports your legs and the front edge of the seat supports your pelvis. This creates a supported extension (backbend) between your chest and your legs and facilitates a lift in your tailbone that opens the front of your pelvis. The blankets go underneath your shoulders to create a safe space for your neck, and they also help put the action of the pose into your shoulders. Straightening your arms to hold the back chair legs provides even more leverage into your shoulders and increases the opening in your chest.

Without props, shoulderstand quickly becomes neckstand: a precarious balancing act on the most delicate part of your spine. Stiffness in your chest and shoulders pushes all the weight of your body into your neck, usually right into the 7th cervical vertebrae (the one that sticks out at the very bottom of your neck). Stiffness in your pelvis prohibits you from leveraging your legs away from your chest, and the pose becomes a forward bend instead of a backbend. If that description sounds like your current shoulderstand, please stop doing it. It is not effective or beneficial, and in reality, it's not shoulderstand. Use props to mold your anatomy toward the true shape of shoulderstand so you may eventually do this magnificent pose without their assistance.

EVOLUTION. These three poses illustrate a fundamental principle of our yoga: if a pose is endangering your anatomy, you must rewind that pose to its most basic anatomical action and find a simple way to learn that action. You can develop balance in your hands by turning *adho mukha svanasana* into box on the wall. You can develop balance in your feet by simplifying all the standing poses into *parsvottanasana* against a wall. Once you have developed balance in your appendicular skeleton, you can safely move forward to more "advanced" *asanas*. Rewinding the pose is not an impediment to your relationship with yoga; it is the key to your relationship with yoga. It will unlock the potential of your body and your life.

Functional Anatomy

Yoga works from the outside to the inside: from your appendicular skeleton to your axial skeleton. Developing balance in your hands and feet will address stiffness in your shoulders and hips, and developing clarity in your shoulders and hips will develop clarity in your spine. Developing clarity in your spine will address congestion in your organs and the larger systems that govern your life: the nervous system and endocrine system. But to get there, you have to start with your hands and feet. Simplifying *asana*s to emphasize their most basic action will develop intelligence in your appendicular skeleton and then translate that intelligence into every part of your being.

Flexible People

Flexibility is neither a blessing nor a curse. It makes some poses really easy and other poses extremely difficult. The hardest thing about being flexible is you have to set your limits because your body will not set them for you. Stiff people can push and push without going too far, but flexible people can push beyond their natural range of motion without "feeling" anything. Unfortunately, your yoga teacher may not be able to help you; many teachers mistake hypermobility for advanced physical capability. A hypermobile individual may be encouraged to push their limits in backbends and forward bends, but, in reality, they should be pulled back to a safer range of motion. This makes the work intensely personal. It requires internal sensitivity and a profound refinement of your proprioception: your internal awareness of your body in space.

HYPEREXTENSION. The strength of a ligament is determined by its collagen fibers. Some people are born with less collagen fiber than others and this lack of stabilizing fibers makes them more prone to ligament laxity. The imbalance comes from your DNA, not from your personality, but your personality can influence the way it is expressed in your body; whether you ignore it, exacerbate it, or address it through the practice of yoga.

Yoga gives you the ability to train your muscles in the face of ligament laxity but it can be a difficult task. Hyperextension doesn't always hurt so you may have to learn to see hyperextension without pain's clear and urgent messages. Once you have identified your hyperextension you can begin the long process of training your muscles to support your joints. You can eventually train your body to detect hyperextension without looking at it, and the micro-adjustments that address your hyperextension will become automatic. They will become a natural part of your quick mental checklist for each pose.

Dealing with hyperextension is more individually specific than dealing with stiffness, and it usually requires intelligent, personalized instruction. Someone with chronic shoulder dislocation can get a huge amount of healing from handstand and downward dog, but only if those poses are properly taught and practiced. If we told everyone with chronic shoulder dislocation to do lots of handstands, we would probably be doing more harm than good. But with proper alignment and supervision, handstand and downward dog can provide a framework for stabilizing a dislocated shoulder. Both of these poses approximate the shoulder joint and develop musculature around the joint capsule to balance the ligament laxity.

The most common joints to suffer from hyperextension in yoga are in the appendicular skeleton: elbows, knees, and ankles. Most of these areas can be protected by the combination of muscle balance and attention to detail we described above. But ligament laxity can also affect joints that are involved with your posture, such as T12 and your SI joints. Hyperextension in these joints is much more difficult to address but we can look at a few ways to avoid destabilizing them in the first place.

FLEXION. Forward bends like *uttanasana* and *paschimottanasana* stretch your legs by bringing your head toward your feet. It seems logical that getting your head closer to your feet will create a deeper forward bend, but that's not the case; deepening the bend comes from the action of your legs, not your torso, head or neck. Unfortunately, we see lots of flexible people opening their chest in forward bends, attempting to lengthen their spine by sliding their ribs down their thighs. This creates an extension (backbend) within the action of a forward bend, and these two opposing actions confront each other at your pelvis.

Opening your chest initiates a lift at the bottom of your spine and forces your tailbone away from your pubic bone. Lifting your tailbone separates your sit bones and opens the bottom of the pelvic girdle—the exact opposite action of *mula bandha*. It puts pressure on the top of your sacrum, and if your SI joint is hypermobile, it can cause your sacrum to shift. This may sound extreme, but we see it in almost every workshop and teacher training and it needs to be addressed. Opening the base of the pelvis in this way is called nutation of the pelvis and it's only supposed to happen in childbirth.

Functional Anatomy

The best way to avoid movement in your sacrum is to utilize the action of *mula* and *uddiyana bandha*. *Mula bandha* pulls your sit bones toward each other and moves your tailbone in the direction of your pubic bone; these actions stabilize the base of your spine. *Uddiyana bandha* supports the natural curve of your sacrum and encourages your lower floating ribs to move toward your pelvis. The *bandha*s combine to honor the energetic direction of the forward bend; strength in your pelvis and legs and softness in your spine. The energy of your torso is passive, and the line from your sacrum to your occiput becomes an even arc instead of a straight line.

EXTENSION. We have mentioned several ways flexible people can be at risk in backbends, but the most common are hinging in T12 and hyperextending the labrum. You can address hinging in T12 by pressing backbends into your thoracic spine, which is the most difficult part of your spine to bend. You can also work on balancing the effort between your arms and legs to create an even, less angular arc in your spine.

Addressing extension in the hip socket employs the same concept: never press the action of a pose into a single joint; the action should always be shared. Lunges and standing poses that extend the pelvis, such as *virabhadrasana A*, should be balanced by extension in your upper body and supported by the musculature of your legs. Without the musculature of your legs, the weight of the pose can sink into your hip socket and put hyperextending pressure on your labrum. The best poses for developing balanced musculature around your pelvis are the simple standing poses, like *parsvottanasana*, and the stabilizing practice of *mula* and *uddiyana bandha*.

PRACTICE SEQUENCES

All of these sequences have been tried and tested but they may not be perfect for your anatomy. As always, your practice should serve you. Stay connected to your breath and your body. Do not pursue poses that feel unsafe and always listen closely to early indications of pain.

We recommend keeping a journal to monitor your evolution. Use it to record your personal practice sequences and any classes you attend. Even though we've been doing yoga for decades, we still write our sequences before we practice or teach. The sequence may change while we're on the mat, but writing it down allows us to analyze what changed and why we changed it. Monitoring those changes is a huge part of developing a deeper understanding of yoga and of your Self.

The practice sequences in this book are separated into sun and moon. Sun sequences contain energetic *ha* poses and moon sequences contain restorative, introspective *tha* poses. Sequences are listed in order of length but it's easy to make them shorter or longer by adjusting the amount of time you spend in each pose. You can also change the intensity of a sequence by substituting specific poses: if you're not ready for a long *adho mukha svanasana*, substitute box on the wall. If you're not ready for *urdhva dhanurasana*, do *setu bandha sarvangasana* instead. You're the boss.

When designing your own sequences, try to follow the shape of a bell curve: smooth ascent, rounded peak, and smooth descent. Begin with a gentle warmup and gradually build intensity until reaching your peak around a specific set of poses. Descend from the peak with a series of increasingly gentle and calming poses, roughly equal in length to the ascent. And always make time for everyone's favorite pose: *savasana*.

Timings are a matter of personal preference. Holding poses for longer periods of time will affect your muscle fiber and direction, while more dynamic movement—i.e. doing a lot of poses with shorter timings—will affect the quality of your connective tissue. You may gravitate toward one or the other but we recommend striking a healthy balance: some days you "play" and other days you "stay." The ultimate goal is finding a sustainable practice, one that becomes part of your daily life. Doing a little bit of yoga on a regular basis is much more effective than doing massive amounts of yoga sporadically.

NICKI:
After you do a certain pose, do you feel better? If yes, then keep doing it. But if you feel worse, stop doing it. Try something else—yoga has a lot to offer. And learning to do that in your practice will teach you to do it in your life. You will slowly learn to do the things that serve you and to stop doing the things that bring you pain.

Practice Sequences

There are certain poses we often hold for specific amounts of time. Some of our general guidelines are below. Shorter times are well suited to an introductory practitioner and longer times reflect a more intermediate practice.

Adho mukha svanasana, uttanasana & box on the wall:
2-5 minutes

Surya namaskar A:
5-10 full rounds

Lunges & standing poses:
1-5 minutes per side (left and right), repeat 2-3x each

Surya namaskar B:
3-7 full rounds

Adho mukha vrksasana:
4x for 1 minute each, with 1 minute rest in *uttanasana*

Backbends:
3x for 1 minute each with 1 minute rest

Salamba sarvangasana:
5-15 minutes, including *halasana*

Seated hip openers:
3-5 minutes

Viparita karani:
10-15 minutes

Now get on your mat and have some fun!

SUN SEQUENCES

1. Marmas	1. Balasana
2. Vajrasana 1-3	2. Adho Mukha Svanasana
3. Simhasana	3. Balasana
4. Surya Namaskar A	4. Uttanasana
5. Lunges 1-5	5. Vajrasana 1-3
6. Surya Namaskar B	6. Uttanasana
7. Standing Back Arch	7. Simhasana
8. Ustrasana	8. Uttanasana
9. Setu Bandha Sarvangasana	9. Trikonasana
10. Urdhva Dhanurasana	10. Parsvakonasana
11. Bharadvajasana	11. Parsvottanasana
12. Salamba Sarvangasana	12. Virabhadrasana B
13. Halasana	13. Supta Pandagusthasana
14. Savasana	14. Viparita Karani
	15. Savasana

Practice Sequences

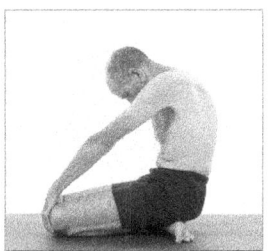

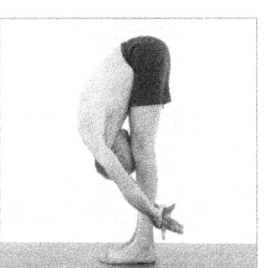

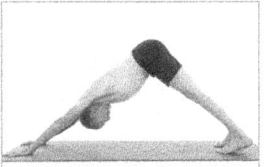

Practice Sequences

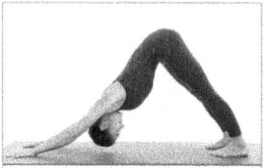

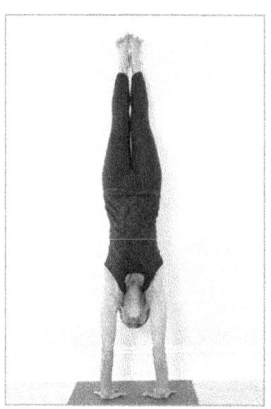

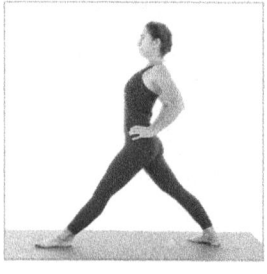

1. Balasana
2. Adho Mukha Svanasana
3. Balasana
4. Adho Mukha Vrksasana
5. Balasana
6. Adho Mukha Svanasana
7. Parsvottanasana
8. Virabhadrasana A
9. Parsvottanasana
10. Trikonasana
11. Salamba Sarvangasana
12. Halasana
13. Gomukhasana
14. Little Hip Opener
15. Savasana

1. Seat
2. Marmas
3. Adho Mukha Svanasana
4. Vajrasana 1-3
5. Uttanasana
6. Adho Mukha Svanasana
7. Surya Namaskar A
8. Lunges 1-5
9. Standing Back Arch
10. Ustrasana
11. Setu Bandha Sarvangasana
12. Urdhva Dhanurasana
13. Lower Back Release
14. Bharadvajasana
15. Savasana

Practice Sequences

1. Balasana
2. Adho Mukha Svanasana
3. Adho Mukha Vrksasana
4. Supta Padangusthasana
5. Adho Mukha Svanasana
6. Trikonasana
7. Virabhadrasana B
8. Trikonasana
9. Virabhadrasana B
10. Trikonasana
11. Parsvakonasana
12. Trikonasana
13. Parsvakonasana
14. Salamba Sarvangasana
15. Halasana
16. Savasana

1. Adho Mukha Svanasana
2. Adho Mukha Vrksasana
3. Trikonasana
4. Parsvakonasana
5. Parsvottanasana
6. Parvritta Parsvakonasana
7. Ardha Chandrasana
8. Adho Mukha Svanasana
9. Standing Back Arch
10. Ustrasana
11. Setu Bandha Sarvangasana
12. Urdhva Dhanurasana
13. Jathara Parivartanasana
14. Supta Pandangusthasana
15. Salamba Sarvangasana
16. Savasana

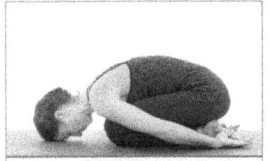

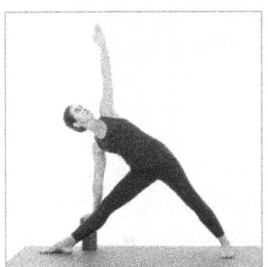

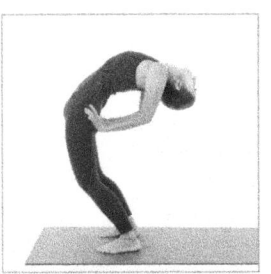

Practice Sequences

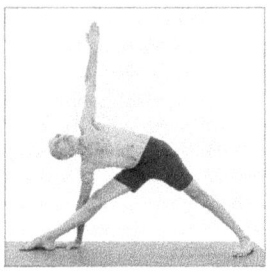

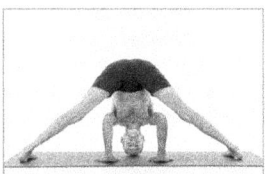

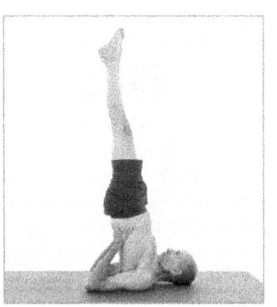

1. Balasana
2. Adho Mukha Svanasana
3. Supta Padangusthasana
4. Virabhadrasana B
5. Parsvakonasana
6. Trikonasana
7. Ardha Chandrasana
8. Parsvottanasana
9. Trikonasana
10. Utkatasana
11. Virasana
12. Baddha Konasana
13. Upavistha Konasana
14. Baddha Konasana
15. Supta Padangusthasana
16. Savasana

1. Seat
2. Marmas
3. Uttanasana
4. Adho Mukha Svanasana
5. Balasana
6. Adho Mukha Svanasana
7. Lunges 1-5
8. Parsvakonasana
9. Trikonasana
10. Virabhadrasana B
11. Parsvottanasana
12. Parvritta Trikonasana
13. Parsvottanasana
14. Prasarita Padottanasana A-D
15. Salamba Sarvangasana
16. Supta Padangusthasana
17. Savasana

1. Balasana
2. Adho Mukha Svanasana
3. Adho Mukha Vrksasana
4. Adho Mukha Svanasana
5. Surya Namaskar A
6. Lunges 1-5
7. Surya Namaskar B
8. Parsvakonasana
9. Parsvottanasana
10. Virabhadrasana B
11. Trikonasana
12. Virabhadrasana A
13. King Arthur
14. Setu Bandha Sarvangasana
15. Urdhva Dhanurasana
16. Salamba Sarvangasana
17. Savasana

1. Marmas
2. Uttanasana
3. Vajrasana 1-3
4. Adho Mukha Svanasana
5. Balasana
6. Uttanasana
7. Surya Namaskar A
8. Lunges 1-5
9. Surya Namaskar B
10. Trikonasana
11. Parsvakonasana
12. Parsvottanasana
13. Virabhadrasana B
14. Setu Bandha Sarvangasana
15. ArdhaJathara Parivartanasana
16. Jathara Parivartanasana
17. Savasana

Practice Sequences

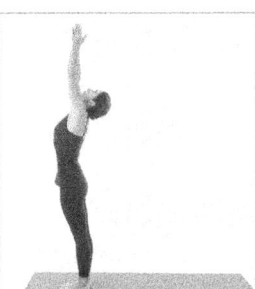

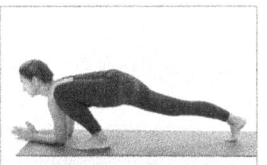

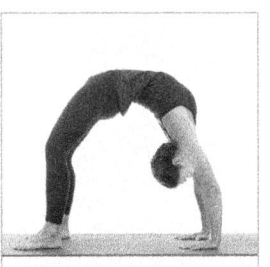

Practice Sequences

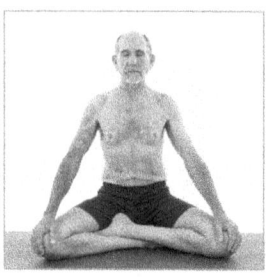

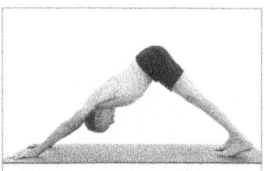

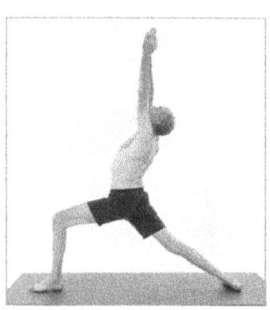

1. Seat
2. Marmas
3. Adho Mukha Svanasana
4. Balasana
5. Simhasana
6. Adho Mukha Svanasana
7. Balasana
8. Surya Namaskar A
9. Lunges 1-5
10. Surya Namaskar B
11. Standing Back Arch
12. Ustrasana
13. Setu Bandha Sarvangasana
14. Urdhva Dhanurasana
15. Ardha Jathara Parivartanasana
16. Jathara Parivartanasana
17. Savasana

1. Seat
2. Marmas
3. Adho Mukha Svanasana
4. Balasana
5. Adho Mukha Svanasana
6. Balasana
7. Simhasana
8. Uttanasana
9. Surya Namaskar A
10. Lunges 1-4
11. Surya Namaskar B
12. Standing Back Arch
13. Ustrasana
14. Setu Bandha Sarvangasana
15. Ardha Jathara Parivartanasana
16. Little Hip Opener
17. Supta Gomukhasana
18. Savasana

Practice Sequences

1. Adho Mukha Svanasana
2. Balasana
3. Prasarita Padottanasana
4. Trikonasana
5. Prasarita Padottanasana
6. Ardha Chandrasana
7. Virabhadrasana A
8. Prasarita Padottanasana
9. Parsvottanasana
10. Prasarita Padottanasana
11. Parvritta Trikonasana
12. Prasarita Padottanasana
13. Parsvakonasana
14. Prasarita Padottanasana
15. Baddha Konasana
16. Upavistha Konasana
17. Gomukhasana
18. Savasana

1. Marmas
2. Vajrasana 1-3
3. Adho Mukha Svanasana
4. Surya Namaskar A
5. Surya Namaskar B
6. Parsvakonasana
7. Trikonasana
8. Virabhadrasana B
9. Parsvottanasana
10. Virabhadrasana A
11. Prasarita Padottanasana A-D
12. Supta Virasana
13. Setu Bandha Sarvangasana
14. Supta Padangusthasana
15. Bharadvajasana
16. Ardha Jathara Parivartanasana
17. Salamba Sarvangasana
18. Savasana

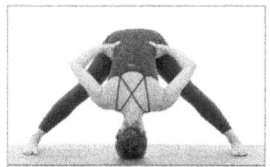
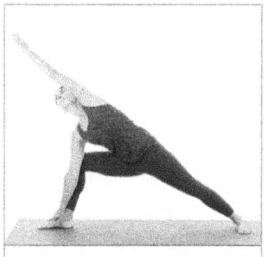
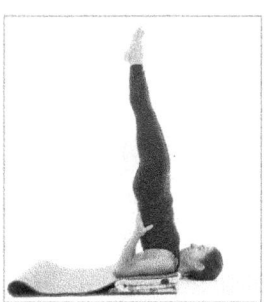

Practice Sequences

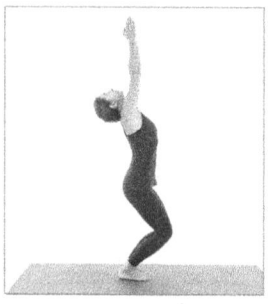

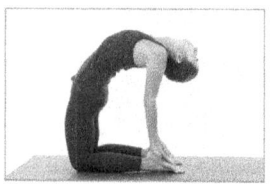

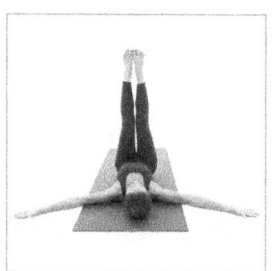

1. Seat
2. Marmas
3. Adho Mukha Svanasana
4. Virabhadrasana B
5. Trikonasana
6. Parsvakonasana
7. Parsvottanasana
8. Parvritta Trikonasana
9. Virabhadrasana A
10. Trikonasana
11. Ardha Chandrasana
12. Utkatasana
13. Supta Virasana
14. Ustrasana
15. Setu Bandha Sarvangasana
16. Urdhva Dhanurasana
17. Little Hip Opener
18. Savasana

1. Seat
2. Marmas
3. Adho Mukha Svanasana
4. Balasana
5. Adho Mukha Svanasana
6. Surya Namaskar A
7. Lunges 1-5
8. Surya Namaskar B
9. Trikonasana
10. Parsvakonasana
11. Adho Mukha Svanasana
12. Adho Mukha Vrksasana
13. Virabhadrasana A
14. Standing Back Arch
15. Ustrasana
16. Urdhva Dhanurasana
17. Jathara Parivartanasana
18. Savasana

Practice Sequences

1. Seat
2. Marmas
3. Adho Mukha Svanasana
4. Balasana
5. Adho Mukha Svanasana
6. Surya Namaskar A
7. Lunges 1-5
8. Adho Mukha Svanasana
9. Adho Mukha Vrksasana
10. Uttanasana
11. Surya Namaskar B
12. Standing Back Arch
13. Setu Bandha Sarvangasana
14. Urdhva Dhanurasana
15. Ardha Jathara Parivartanasana
16. Salamba Sarvangasana
17. Little Hip Opener
18. Savasana

1. Seat
2. Marmas
3. Uttanasana
4. Box on the Wall
5. Balasana
6. Adho Mukha Svanasana
7. Balasana
8. Adho Mukha Svanasana
9. Lunges 1-5
10. Parsvakonasana
11. Trikonasana
12. Virabhadrasana A
13. Parsvottanasana
14. Parvritta Trikonasana
15. Supta Padangusthasana
16. Supta Baddha Konasana
17. Janu Sirsasana
18. Viparita Karani
19. Savasana

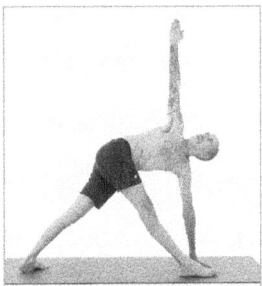

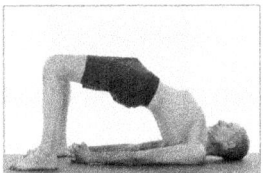

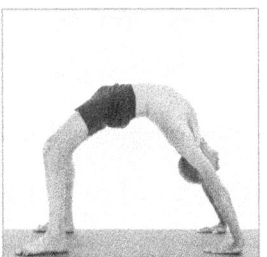

Practice Sequences

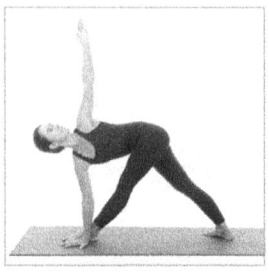

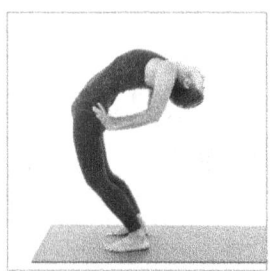

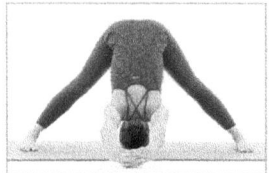

1. Marmas
2. Vajrasana 1-3
3. Adho Mukha Svanasana
4. Surya Namaskar A
5. Lunges 1-4
6. Surya Namaskar B
7. Virabhadrasana B
8. Trikonasana
9. Parsvakonasana
10. Parsvottanasana
11. Virabhadrasana A
12. Parvritta Trikonasana
13. Standing Back Arch
14. Setu Bandha Sarvangasana
15. Urdhva Dhanurasana
16. Ardha Jathara Parivartanasana
17. Jathara Parivartanasana
18. Gomukhasana
19. Savasana

1. Virasana
2. Uttanasana
3. Virasana
4. Uttanasana
5. Adho Mukha Svanasana
6. Balasana
7. Supta Padangusthasana
8. Adho Mukha Svanasana
9. Trikonasana
10. Prasarita Padottanasana A
11. Parsvakonasana
12. Prasarita Padottanasana B
13. Utkatasana
14. Uttanasana
15. Utkatasana
16. Parsvottanasana
17. Prasarita Padottanasana C
18. Little Hip Opener
19. Gomukhasana
20. Savasana

1. Marmas
2. Uttanasana
3. Vajrasana 1-3
4. Adho Mukha Svanasana
5. Balasana
6. Adho Mukha Svanasana
7. Simhasana
8. Uttanasana
9. Urdhva Hastasana
10. Vrksasana
11. Garudasana
12. Surya Namaskar A
13. Lunges 2-5
14. Trikonasana
15. Parsvakonasana
16. Parsvottanasana
17. Virabhadrasana B
18. Prasarita Padottanasana A
19. Supta Padangusthasana
20. Savasana

1. Seat
2. Marmas
3. Adho Mukha Svanasana
4. Balasana
5. Vajrasana 1-3
6. Uttanasana
7. Vrksasana
8. Garudasana
9. Surya Namaskar A
10. Lunges 1-4
11. Parsvottanasana
12. Virabhadrasana A
13. Parsvottanasana
14. Supta Padangusthasana
15. Baddha Konasana
16. Gomukhasana
17. Box/Double Pigeon
18. Supta Baddha Konasana
19. Balasana
20. Savasana

Practice Sequences

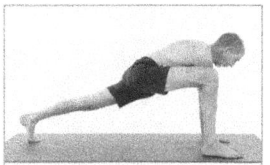

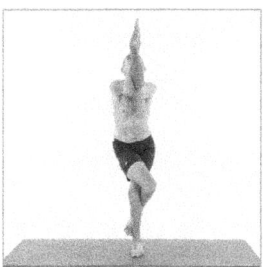

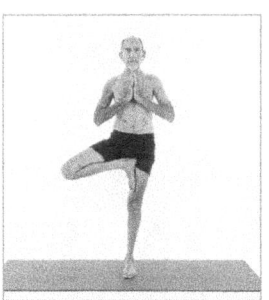

Practice Sequences

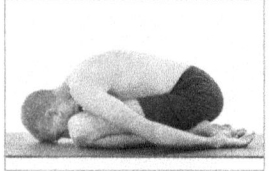

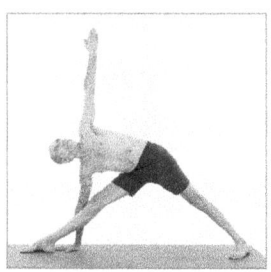

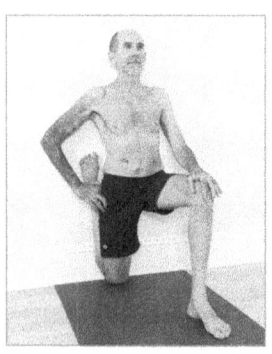

1. Marmas
2. Vajrasana 1-3
3. Uttanasana
4. Simhasana
5. Uttanasana
6. Adho Mukha Svanasana
7. Balasana
8. Adho Mukha Svanasana
9. Trikonasana
10. Parvritta Trikonasana
11. Parsvakonasana
12. Parsvottanasana
13. Virabhadrasana A
14. Virabhadrasana B
15. King Arthur
16. Supta Pandagusthasana
17. Salamba Sarvangasana
18. Halasana
19. Setu Bandha Sarvangasana
20. Savasana

1. Seat
2. Balasana
3. Adho Mukha Svanasana
4. Balasana
5. Adho Mukha Svanasana
6. Parsvottanasana
7. Virabhadrasana A
8. Trikonasana
9. Ardha Chandrasana
10. Trikonasana
11. Parsvottanasana
12. Virabhadrasana A
13. Trikonasana
14. Ardha Chandrasana
15. Trikonasana
16. Baddha Konasana
17. Upavistha Konasana
18. Supta Padangusthasana
19. Jathara Parivartansana
20. Gomukhasana
21. Savasana

1. Seat	1. Marmas
2. Marmas	2. Simhasana
3. Uttanasana	3. Adho Mukha Svanasana
4. Adho Mukha Svanasana	4. Surya Namaskar A
5. Uttanasana	5. Surya Namaskar B
6. Surya Namaskar A	6. Trikonasana
7. Surya Namaskar B	7. Virabhadrasana B
8. Trikonasana	8. Virabhadrasana A
9. Ardha Chandrasana	9. Lunges 1-5
10. Trikonasana	10. Uttanasana
11. Virabhadrasana B	11. Utkatasana
12. Parsvakonasana	12. Uttanasana
13. Trikonasana	13. Trikonasana
14. Parsvottanasana	14. Parsvottanasana
15. Adho Mukha Svanasana	15. Parvritta Trikonasana
16. Lunges 1-5	16. Parsvottanasana
17. Standing Back Arch	17. Supta Virasana
18. Urdhva Dhanurasana	18. Setu Bandha Sarvangasana
19. Jathara Parivartanasana	19. Bharadvajasana
20. Salamba Sarvangasana	20. Salamba Sarvangasana
21. Savasana	21. Savasana

Practice Sequences

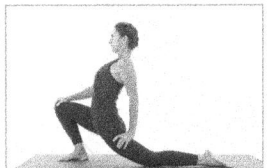

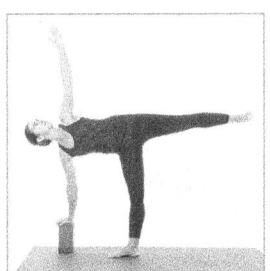

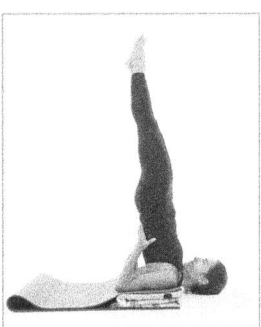

Practice Sequences

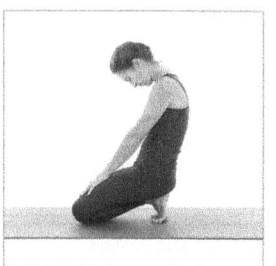

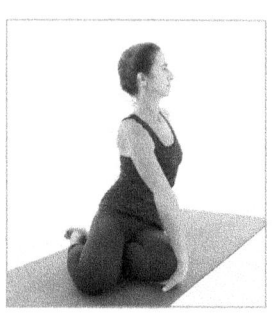

1. Seat	1. Marmas
2. Marmas	2. Uttanasana
3. Adho Mukha Svanasana	3. Vajrasana 1-3
4. Balasana	4. Uttanasana
5. Adho Mukha Svanasana	5. Urdhva Hastasana
6. Balasana	6. Adho Mukha Svanasana
7. Adho Mukha Vrksasana	7. Balasana
8. Vajrasana 1-3	8. Vrksasana
9. Simhasana	9. Garudasana
10. Surya Namaskar A	10. Surya Namaskar A
11. Lunges 1-5	11. Surya Namaskar B
12. Surya Namaskar B	12. Trikonasana
13. Parsvottanasana	13. Parsvottanasana
14. Trikonasana	14. Parvritta Trikonasana
15. Parvritta Trikonasana	15. Parsvottanasana
16. Uttanasana	16. Virabhadrasana A
17. Standing Back Arch	17. Standing Back Arch
18. Setu Bandha Sarvangasana	18. Ustrasana
19. Urdhva Dhanurasana	19. Setu Bandha Sarvangasana
20. Jathara Parivartanasana	20. Bharadvajasana
21. Gomukhasana	21. Jathara Parivartanasana
22. Savasana	22. Salamba Sarvangasana
	23. Savasana

Practice Sequences

1. Marmas
2. Adho Mukha Svanasana
3. Balasana
4. Adho Mukha Svanasana
5. Surya Namaskar A
6. Lunges 1-5
7. Surya Namaskar B
8. Virabhadrasana A
9. Parsvottanasana
10. Trikonasana
11. Parsvakonasana
12. Trikonasana
13. Ardha Chandrasana
14. Virabhadrasana A
15. Parsvottanasana
16. Virabhadrasana A
17. Parvritta Trikonasana
18. Prasarita Padottanasana
19. Baddha Konasana
20. Upavistha Konasana
21. Gomukhasana
22. Bharadvajasana
23. Savasana

1. Vajrasana 1-3
2. Adho Mukha Svanasana
3. Balasana
4. Adho Mukha Vrksasana
5. Surya Namaskar A
6. Surya Namaskar B
7. Lunges 2-4
8. Parsvottanasana
9. Trikonasana
10. Parsvakonasana
11. Ardha Chandrasana
12. Virabhadrasana B
13. Virabhadrasana A
14. King Arthur
15. Standing Back Arch
16. Ustrasana
17. Setu Bandha Sarvangasana
18. Urdhva Dhanurasana
19. Little Hip Opener
20. Ardha Jathara Parivartanasana
21. Jathara Parivartanasana
22. Salamba Sarvangasana
23. Savasana

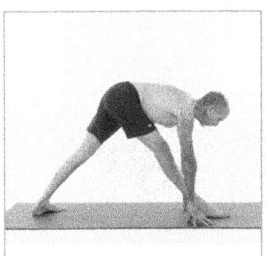

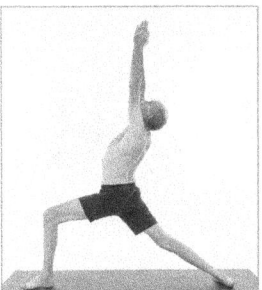

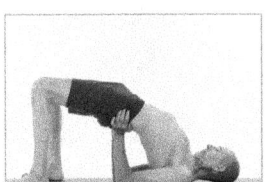

MOON SEQUENCES

Practice Sequences

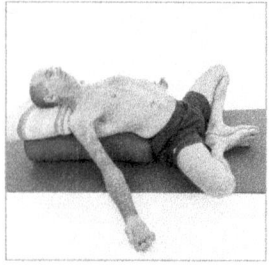

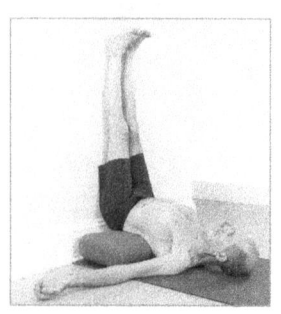

1. Balasana
2. Adho Mukha Svanasana
3. Cross Bolster
4. Janu Sirsasana
5. Supta Baddha Konasana
6. Upavistha Konasana
7. Bharadvajasana
8. Viparita Karani
9. Savasana

1. Box/Double Pigeon
2. Gomukhasana
3. Virasana
4. Upavistha Konasana
5. Baddha Konasana
6. Simhasana
7. Baddha Konasana
8. Viparita Karani
9. Savasana

1. Balasana
2. Supta Padangusthasana A
3. Supta Padangusthasana B
4. Supta Baddha Konasana
5. Balasana w/Bolster
6. Janu Sirsasana
7. Cross Bolster
8. Bharadvajasana
9. Viparita Karani
10. Savasana

1. Balasana
2. Adho Mukha Svanasana
3. Balasana
4. Adho Mukha Svanasana
5. Lunges 2 & 3
6. Vajrasana 1-3
7. Box on the Wall
8. Supta Virasana
9. Supta Padangusthasana
10. Setu Bandha Sarvangasana
11. Viparita Karani

Practice Sequences

1. Marmas
2. Vajrasana 1-3
3. Virasana
4. Supta Virasana
5. Upavistha Konasana
6. Supta Baddha Konasana
7. Janu Sirsasana
8. Gomukhasana
9. Box/Double Pigeon
10. Simhasana
11. Salamba Sarvangasana
12. Viparita Karani

1. Balasana
2. Adho Mukha Svanasana
3. Supta Padangusthasana
4. Box/Double Pigeon
5. Gomukhasana
6. The Beach
7. Gomukhasana
8. Baddha Konasana
9. Upavistha Konasana
10. Baddha Konasana
11. Simhasana
12. Viparita Karani

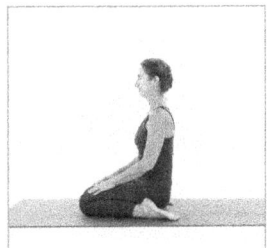

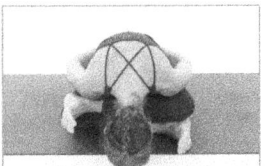

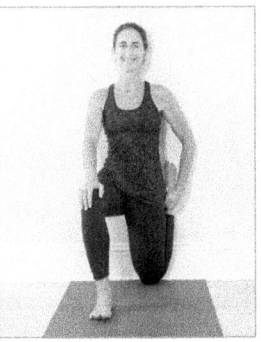

1. Supta Virasana
2. Upavistha Konasana
3. Baddha Konasana
4. Upavistha Konasana
5. Supta Padangusthasana
6. King Arthur
7. Janu Sirsasana
8. Gomukhasana
9. Box/Double Pigeon
10. Simhasana
11. Salamba Sarvangasana
12. Viparita Karani
13. Savasana

Practice Sequences

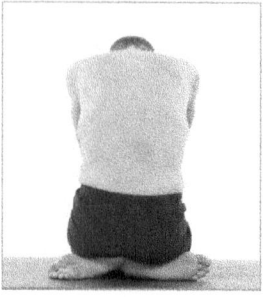

1. Marmas
2. Vajrasana 1-3
3. Simhasana
4. Uttanasana
5. Balasana
6. Upavistha Konasana
7. Baddha Konasana
8. Gomukhasana
9. Box/Double Pigeon
10. Supta Virasana
11. King Arthur
12. Supta Padangusthasana
13. Viparita Karani

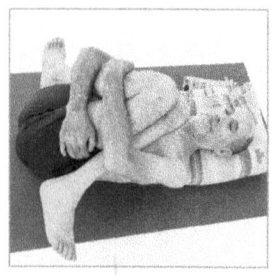

1. Virasana
2. Uttanasana
3. Box on the Wall
4. Balasana w/Bolster
5. Supta Virasana
6. Balasana
7. Supta Baddha Konasana
8. Gomukhasana
9. Upavistha Konasana
10. Bharadvajasana
11. Little Hip Opener
12. Supta Gomukhasana
13. Viparita Karani
14. Savasana

1. Supta Virasana
2. Uttanasana
3. Simhasana
4. Baddha Konasana
5. Upavistha Konasana
6. Box/Double Pigeon
7. Gomukhasana
8. Bharadvajasana
9. Janu Sirsasana
10. Supta Padangusthasana
11. Salamba Sarvangasana
12. Viparita Karani
13. Savasana

Practice Sequences

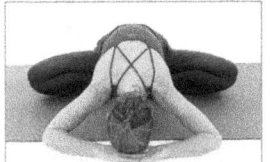

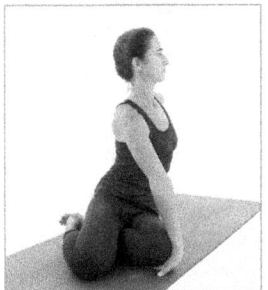

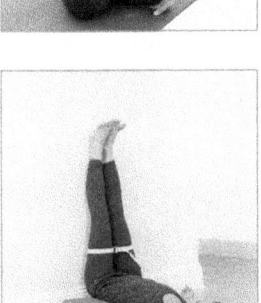

1. Balasana
2. Adho Mukha Svanasana
3. Marmas
4. Vajrasana 1-3
5. Simhasana
6. Uttanasana
7. Gomukhasana
8. Upavistha Konasana
9. Baddha Konasana
10. Box/Double Pigeon
11. Virasana
12. Supta Virasana
13. King Arthur
14. Supta Padangusthasana
15. Savasana

Practice Sequences

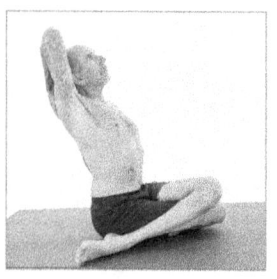

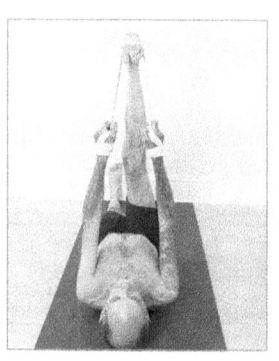

1. Vajrasana 1-3	10. Baddha Konasana
2. Simhasana	11. Bharadvajasana
3. Adho Mukha Svanasana	12. King Arthur
4. Supta Virasana	13. Supta Padangusthasana
5. Upavistha Konasana	14. Setu Bandha Sarvangasana
6. Baddha Konasana	15. Salamba Sarvangasana
7. Box/Double Pigeon	16. Viparita Karani
8. Gomukhasana	17. Savasana
9. Upavistha Konasana	

1. Vajrasanas	11. Supta Virasana
2. Simhasana	12. Janu Sirsasana
3. Adho Mukha Svanasana	13. Gomukhasana
4. Balasana	14. Bharadvajasana
5. Upavistha Konasana	15. Janu Sirsasana
6. Baddha Konasana	16. Supta Padangusthasana B
7. Gomukhasana	17. Setu Bandha Sarvangasana
8. Box/Double Pigeon	18. Salamba Sarvangasana
9. Supta Virasana	19. Viparita Karani
10. Supta Padangusthasana	20. Savasana

LIST OF ASANA

Adho Mukha Svanasana	94
Adho Mukha Vrksasana	199
Ardha Chandrasana	169
Ardha Jathara Parivartanasana	186
Baddha Konasana	215
Balasana	82
Bharadvajasana	183
Box on the Wall	81
Cross Bolsters	242
Double Bolster	239
Fifth Lunge	120
First Lunge	110
Fourth Lunge	117
Garudasana	167
Gomukhasana	224
Janu Sirsasana (Variation)	231
Jathara Parivartanasana	187
King Arthur	173
Little Hip Opener	222
Marmas	61
Parsvottanasana	138
Parvritta Trikonasana	147
Prasarita Padottanasana A-D	151
Salamba Sarvangasana	294
Samastiti	90
Second Lunge	112
Setu Bandha Sarvangasana	191
Setu Bandha Sarvangasana with Two Bolsters	241

Simhasana	75
Standing Back Arch	178
Supta Baddha Konasana	217
Supta Gomukhasana	226
Supta Padangusthasana A	233
Supta Padangusthasana B	235
Supta Virasana	209
Surya Namaskar A	96
Surya Namaskar B	124
Tadasana	92
The Beach Pose	228
The Box	220
The Seat	57
Third Lunge	114
Upavistha Konasana	212
Urdhva Dhanurasana	180
Urdhva Hastasana	93
Ustrasana	176
Uttanasana	77
Utthita Parsvakonasana	159
Utthita Trikonasana	143
Uttkatasana	124
Vajrasanas	70
Viparita Karani	201
Virabhadrasana A	126
Virabhadrasana B	163
Virasana	207
Vrksasana	166

ABOUT THE AUTHORS

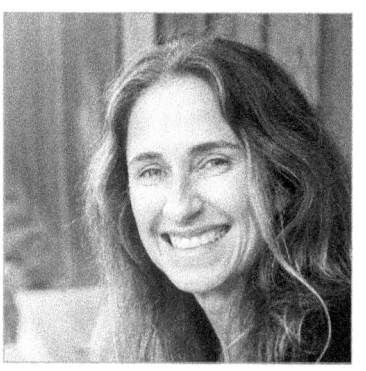

Nicki Doane is the co-founder of Maya Yoga and owner of the Maya Yoga Studio on Maui, Hawaii. She has been practicing since 1988 and is considered one of the world's top teachers. She leads workshops and Teacher Training courses nationally, internationally, and online. She lives off the grid in paradise on Maui's North Shore.
www.nickidoane.com

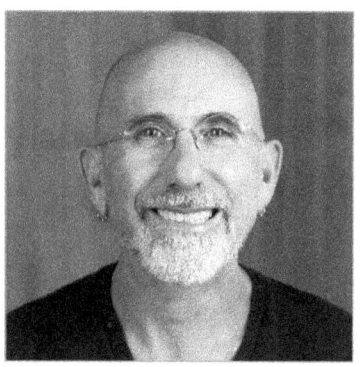

Eddie Modestini is the co-founder of Maya Yoga. He has been practicing yoga since 1983 and has studied extensively with the world's top teachers. He teaches nationally and internationally and is considered a teacher of teachers. He currently teaches *Yoga on the Inside* with his partner Kristin Bosteels.
www.yogaontheinside.com

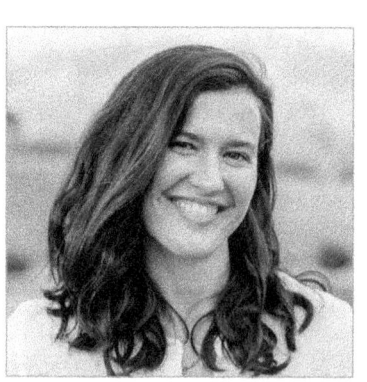

Kaitlin Childers has been studying yoga with Nicki and Eddie since 2010 and began compiling material for this book in 2012. As part of her research she completed four 200-hr. certifications and three 500-hr. certifications. She lives in Healdsburg, CA with her husband and two children and runs a small-production wine label called **Camp Rose Cellars.**

www.ingramcontent.com/pod-product-compliance
Lightning Source LLC
Chambersburg PA
CBHW080354030426
42334CB00024B/2874